The
Encyclopedia of

ADDICTIVE DRUGS

The
Encyclopedia of

ADDICTIVE DRUGS

RICHARD LAWRENCE MILLER

GREENWOOD PRESS
Westport, Connecticut • London

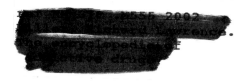

Library of Congress Cataloging-in-Publication Data

Miller, Richard Lawrence.
    The encyclopedia of addictive drugs / Richard Lawrence Miller.
      p. cm.
    Includes bibliographical references and index.
    ISBN 0–313–31807–7 (alk. paper)
    1. Drugs of abuse—Handbooks, manuals, etc.   I. Title.
  RM316.M555   2002
  615′.78—dc21   2002075332

British Library Cataloguing in Publication Data is available.

Library of Congress Catalog Card Number: 2002075332
ISBN: 0–313–31807–7

First published in 2002

Greenwood Press, 88 Post Road West, Westport, CT 06881
An imprint of Greenwood Publishing Group, Inc.
www.greenwood.com

Printed in the United States of America

The paper used in this book complies with the
Permanent Paper Standard issued by the National
Information Standards Organization (Z39.48–1984).

10 9 8 7 6 5 4 3 2

Contents

Introduction

The Encyclopedia of Addictive Drugs will save readers many hours of time that would otherwise be spent tracking down basic facts in science journals and libraries. This book is useful to a wide variety of persons—from a student doing a term paper to reporters preparing a story, from parents reading that story to a narcotics law enforcement officer needing extra information for a public presentation.

In writing this book the approach has been multidisciplinary, meaning that perspectives from several fields of research have been pulled together. The same substance may mean different things to a chemist, a biologist, a physician, or an anthropologist. Thousands of scientific reports were sifted for information and concepts that will be meaningful to readers seeking basic information about specific substances and about drugs in general.

The core of this book is an alphabetical listing of substances. Some are not ordinarily thought of as drugs, but all have been misused in ways indistinguishable from drug abuse. While information in the individual listings and elsewhere may refer to various physical effects, such information does not constitute medical advice. Anyone with a medical difficulty needs to consult a medical practitioner, not this book.

In addition to meaty information about what drugs do, this book includes trivia that might interest, for example, a student preparing a report or a homework assignment. For instance, some individual listings of drugs mention little-known military usage that might intrigue teens interested in the armed forces. Some experiments are mentioned not because they are necessary to know about, but because they might add depth to a term paper or inspire a student to pursue a new angle. Material about effects on pregnancy is inherently important but might also have special interest for female readers.

In addition to alphabetical listings of substances, this book includes a section about drug types in which substances are arranged in general categories, such as stimulants, with further grouping by classes of stimulants (amphetamine, anorectic, cocaine, pyridine alkaloid). Such an arranging of drugs puts them in a broader context of information. A chemist knows that a certain element has particular characteristics because of its place in the periodic table, and a biologist knows that a certain organism will have particular characteristics because of its species classification. A reader of this book can automatically glean information about an individual substance because of the way it is classified. For example, everything said in this book about stimulants applies to the class of stimulants known as amphetamines; everything said about amphetamines applies to the particular drug **methamphetamine**. (Substances printed in **bold** have main entries in this book's alphabetical section.) A reader familiar with basics about stimulants and who only needs a few specifics about methamphetamine can quickly find those details. A reader who needs to understand more about the general nature of stimulants can find that background information as well. Persons desiring to go deeper than the summaries of scientific information in alphabetical entries can consult reliable sources listed at the end of each entry. Many of those sources list still more references.

This book concludes with a guide to finding general information about drugs. Here readers are directed not only to ostensibly neutral sources of information but also to sources taking explicit and differing stances on various aspects of drug use.

The index lists street names and other alternate names (used in various communities at various times), giving page numbers where information can be found about those drugs.

Descriptions of individual drugs in the alphabetical section of this book present the scientific consensus about those substances, based mainly upon reports from refereed science journals. A refereed journal is one that does not merely accept an author's word but instead has the articles critiqued and approved by assorted experts prior to publication. Articles in such journals are fundamental sources of scientific information. Although findings reported in this book come from scientific investigations around the world, not everyone agrees with what scientists discover about drugs. Sometimes scientists themselves disagree with one another. The history of science is filled with detection of errors, and future research will no doubt provide new understandings of these drugs. This book, however, presents scientific consensus concerning these drugs as the twenty-first century begins.

DRUG ABUSE

Drug abuse is an emotionally charged topic involving more than facts about pharmaceuticals. Personal and moral values are involved, as are fears that sometimes transform into anger. The author of this book has studied drug abuse questions since the 1980s; visited with prosecutors, judges, and health care givers, along with drug abusers and their families; drafted drug control legislation introduced by Republican and Democratic legislators; testified before legislative committees; and given public presentations. In all settings, facts have rapidly disappeared in discussion of the topic.

For most of the twentieth century, addiction was considered a physical effect of some drugs. If a drug failed to produce physical symptoms associated with addiction, the substance was classified as nonaddictive. In the 1980s, however, some researchers began arguing that addiction could exist without associated physical symptoms, that mental craving alone was enough to power addiction.[1] An important boost to acceptance of that concept came in 1987 when the American Psychiatric Association declared that "**cocaine** dependence" did not require physical dependence for diagnosis.[2] The APA stated, "Continuing use of **cocaine** appears to be driven by persistent craving and urges for the substance rather than attempts to avoid or alleviate withdrawal symptoms."[3] That approach yielded a broader understanding: that people could be addicted to things other than drugs, a new and controversial concept but one that was becoming more accepted as the twenty-first century began.

Regardless of whether addiction can be more of a mental process than a physical one, the likelihood of a user developing a harmful relationship with drugs is greater with some substances than with others. The harm may be physical. The harm may be disruption of a user's life. Experience shows, for example, that **cocaine** is far more risky to use than **caffeine**.

Some drugs can be used so much that they and a person's body develop what may be called a physical resonance. That is not a standard drug abuse term, but it communicates the concept more vividly than other terminology. *Resonance* means that an individual's body has adapted to the drug in such a way that stopping use of the drug makes a person feel ill. Symptoms depend on the drug and can range from a runny nose to convulsions. Not all drugs can produce such a state, but those that can are traditionally called addictive. Indeed, appearance or nonappearance of an "abstinence" or "withdrawal" syndrome of illness upon sudden end to drug dosage used to be considered a definitive test of whether a drug is addictive and whether a user is an addict. Some specialists might use the term *neuroadaptation* for the mechanism that creates resonance, but here more conservative language that asserts less about roles of the brain and nervous system will be used.

Resonance is typically, and somewhat misleadingly, called "dependence" by many persons. An addict who temporarily feels sick upon stopping a drug but who later feels better is not really "dependent" on it, in the ordinary dictionary sense of that word's meaning. Granted, physical dependence upon a drug is possible, in the dictionary sense, regardless of whether the underlying mechanism is neuroadaptation. An example is a diabetic who needs insulin. Cutting off insulin supply would make the diabetic sicker and sicker, so the person truly is dependent on the drug. Its presence is necessary for good health. Normally, however, that is not what is meant by saying a drug abuser is dependent on a substance; rather, one means the abuser will feel temporarily ill if dosage suddenly stops. Nonetheless, some drug addictions can involve the dictionary meaning of dependence. For example, persons *extremely* addicted to alcohol or barbiturates can die if cut off from their supply. Death typically comes from cascading problems culminating in convulsions. That dismal outcome is uncommon but possible. In addition, *dependence* is sometimes used in contexts making it synonymous with *addiction*, perhaps referring to persons undergoing treatment to break dependence on some drug they crave and are unable to stop taking. Because *dependence* has multiple meanings, the term is not ideal. However, this book uses the term because of its familiarity to specialists, despite its potential for causing confusion among general readers.

The concepts of addiction and dependence differ. Someone who takes a lot of barbiturates may experience both states. Someone who uses a lot of **marijuana** may experience neither. Knowing the differences between those two concepts can help a person spot confusion in rhetoric about drug abuse.

A person who has dependence on a drug may experience an abstinence or withdrawal syndrome if the supply runs out. The syndrome may begin several hours or several days after drug use stops, depending on how long a drug and its by-products last in the human body. Different drugs have different withdrawal symptoms, and they are specified in this book's alphabetical listings. Often a withdrawal symptom is the opposite of what a drug does. For example, if a drug constipates a person, withdrawal from that drug may include diarrhea. If a drug makes a person sleepy, withdrawal may include insomnia. Sometimes the withdrawal syndrome can be avoided if dosage is gradually reduced rather than stopped suddenly. At times the syndrome is avoided by substituting another drug that has "cross-tolerance" with the first one. Cross-tolerance means that one drug can substitute for another in some ways, typically in ways that prevent a withdrawal syndrome from emerging. A classic example allows **methadone** to be substituted for **heroin**. This book's alphabetical section notes cross-tolerance among assorted drugs. Cross-tolerance is a concept that differs from tolerance described below.

Tolerance means that as time passes, a person must use more and more of a drug to get the same effect. Such an outcome is a traditional sign of addiction. Tolerance can develop to some effects of a drug and not to others. For example, an amphetamine addict may become tolerant to euphoric properties of the drug, but not to its poisonous qualities. A **cocaine** addict may build tolerance to appetite-loss properties of the drug but not to other actions. The opposite may also happen, in which a person becomes sensitized to a drug and needs less and less. Evidence for such a development has been seen in humans with **DOM** and benzodiazepines and in animals with **cocaine** and **DMT**. Such a development, however, would not be considered evidence of addiction. Tolerance can have a strong mental component; the same phenomenon can be seen in reduced pleasure gained from continual indulgence in wild music events or a particular food or shopping. Recreational and medical users can take the same drug, often with medical users never developing tolerance—perhaps because of the purpose for which they take the drug and not because of its chemistry, although that possible explanation is not yet confirmed. Some experts argue that tolerance is indeed a physical effect, caused by organic brain changes induced by a drug. Ultimately those experts are correct: All mental feelings and processes result from changes in the brain's electrochemical activity. Some of these changes can even be measured and correlated with broad psychological characteristics. For example, changes in brain waves and emotions can be seen after some drugs are administered. Our understanding of such things remains crude, however. We don't know how brain chemicals and electricity induce a person to love someone or hate an idea. Ultimately some still unknown physical process may explain why people who take a drug for pleasure develop a tolerance to its effects, while people who take the same substance for medical purposes never experience a change in what the drug does.

From a purely physical standpoint, someone who has recreationally abused a drug for years may indeed be able to tolerate a stronger dose than someone who takes the same drug for the first time. The abuser's body may develop physical adaptations permitting high doses. For instance, body chemistry can change in ways that counteract a drug, requiring more and more of the substance to overcome the change. Nonetheless, for many practical purposes we can say the cause of tolerance is psychological. This was implied in medical research comparing the amount of **meperidine** required to relieve pain in appendectomy patients.[4] The study was conducted in Beirut and examined records of patients who underwent surgery before, during, and after a brutal civil war that destroyed much of that city. For pain relief, prewar patients needed more of the drug than wartime or postwar patients did. Researchers concluded that part of the reason was a psychological change in how pain was evaluated during those years of brutality. The study did not directly investigate tolerance, but it did demonstrate that a change in attitude can change the amount of drug effect perceived by users.

Change in attitude illustrates the influence of set and setting on drug effects. *Set* describes someone's basic personality and expectations about what a drug does. *Setting* is the environment in which drug use occurs. Rat experimentation[5] demonstrated that the setting in which a drug is administered can alter the amount of tolerance, with those conditions demonstrating a psychological component in physical tolerance. Countless human examples demonstrate that set and setting can determine how much effect a given drug dose produces, whether it is pleasant or unpleasant, even whether a dose is tolerable or fatal.

Dosage affects a drug's impact. Overdose of most drugs can produce serious unwanted effects, including death. In addition to the amount of drug, the method of dosage (injection, oral, smoking, or other routes) can make a huge difference in effects. The same amount of drug can have a much different impact depending on route of administration. A "safe" dose by one route can be fatal by another. An effect at one dosage level may be the opposite of what happens at a different dosage level. Sometimes a drug can cause a condition that it is supposed to prevent. Such paradoxical actions illustrate hazards involved in reckless drug use.

Taking more than one drug of a given type can be expected to increase effects typical of that type. For example, a person who ingests the depressant **alcohol** simultaneously with an opiate depressant will normally experience deeper depressant effects than if just one of the drugs was used. Taking a normal dose of several drugs from one type can be the practical equivalent of overdosing on any one of them. Taking drugs of different types can also be hazardous. For example, the stimulant **cocaine** and the depressant **heroin** do not cancel each other's effects if taken together; instead, the body may be assaulted from different directions simultaneously and break down under the attack.

HOW ARE ABUSE RISKS MEASURED?

Historical experience shows addiction to be more likely with some drugs than with others, just as some road intersections are more hazardous than others even though anyone might drive through them safely at a given time. Whether the subject be drugs or intersections, persons concerned about dangers attempt to discover if similarities exist. Do certain characteristics of intersections (speed limits, stop signs, obscured vision) indicate whether danger is more likely? Characteristics of drugs, particularly their chemical formulas, are examined to determine similarities that might indicate whether particular drugs have more addictive or abuse potential than others. For example, the shape of a drug's molecule may determine how a user's body reacts, so drugs with molecules of a similar shape might be expected to have similar effects. Also, new substances derived from an old drug may be assumed to have similarities to the old drug.

Schedules

In the United States the result has been a blend of science and law called "scheduling," set up in 1970 by the federal Comprehensive Drug Abuse Prevention and Control Act, which replaced all previous federal narcotics laws. (The legal definition of "narcotics" includes stimulants such as cocaine and hallucinogens such as **LSD**.) Scheduling is an ongoing process affected by the same influences that shape other laws. Sometimes Congress or a state legislature puts a drug in a particular schedule. Sometimes a federal or state official does so. Like all law, scheduling has an element of arbitrariness, enhanced as federal statutes interact with state laws and local ordinances. Nonetheless, even though results can be puzzling, basic principles in scheduling are clear.

In the United States drugs are either scheduled or unscheduled. Unscheduled drugs may be benign or highly dangerous, available over the counter or by prescription only, perhaps even available to children through a plant growing wild in the woods. A hospital emergency room may deal with someone who uses an unscheduled drug, but the U.S. Drug Enforcement Administration probably will not. Almost all drugs are unscheduled, whether they be pharmaceutical creations from a laboratory or natural products harvested from the soil.

Scheduled drugs are theoretically ranked by their potential for abuse. Not all abuse is addictive, but the rankings imply that some drugs are more of an addiction hazard than others. At the time this book was written, five schedules existed. Generally drugs in a lower-numbered schedule are considered more prone to abuse than those in higher-numbered schedules. Heroin is a Schedule I drug. A cough medicine available without prescription might be in Schedule V. Schedule I is also used for abused drugs having no medical use approved by regulatory agencies in the United States. Thus Schedule I includes marijuana even though decades of research have shown it to be more benign than most drugs listed in other schedules. Schedule I also includes some drugs (**dextromoramide, dipipanone, phenoperidine**, and others) used routinely by doctors in other countries but that lack approval from U.S. authorities. So although Schedule I is often viewed as a list of the most dangerous drugs, relatively harmless ones are listed if they are unapproved for medical use in the United States, while drugs that can easily kill even when administered in a hospital setting are listed in schedules indicating less danger of abuse. Still, the general rule is that drugs are scheduled according to their abuse potential, with drugs in lower-numbered schedules having more abuse potential than drugs in higher-numbered schedules. Some illicit drug makers try to avoid scheduling regulations altogether by tweaking the chemical composition of a substance just enough that it is no longer the molecule defined in a schedule. Such "designer drugs" remain legal until schedules are updated again.

Schedule I is for drugs ruled as being most prone to abuse, lacking generally accepted use in the American health care system, and being so dangerous that health practitioners cannot safely administer these drugs to patients. Except for specially authorized scientific studies, possession of a Schedule I substance is illegal under any circumstance. No physician can authorize a patient to use a Schedule I item. Schedule II is for drugs ruled as being most prone to abuse but in use in the American health care system and carrying the potential to cause major physical or mental dependence upon continued usage. Schedule III is for drugs ruled as being less prone to abuse; these are generally accepted by the American health care system but pose risks of "moderate or low" physical dependence or "high" psychological dependence. Schedule IV is for drugs ruled as being still less prone to abuse; these are generally accepted by the American health care system and are less likely to result in physical or psychological dependence than Schedule III substances. Schedule V is for drugs least prone to abuse; they are generally accepted by the American health care system and are less likely to result in physical or psychological dependence than Schedule IV compounds.

This book's alphabetical listings give each drug's federal schedule status. States also have schedules. At times, state and federal schedules may not "match" for a particular drug. For example, under international treaty the U.S. government put **flunitrazepam** in Schedule IV, but federal authorities believed it should be Schedule I. So states have been encouraged to put the substance in Schedule I. Sometimes federal authorities change a drug's schedule, and states may lag behind in conforming. For practical purposes, federal and state schedules have equal legal standing. A drug user who runs afoul of a state schedule can be punished as severely as a person who runs afoul of a federal schedule. A further complication is that although a drug that is unlisted in any schedule is presumed to be unscheduled, official pages of schedules do not necessarily specify all scheduled substances. Sometimes the official pages have not caught up with official decisions; sometimes a chemical is covered if it is derived from a scheduled substance, without a separate listing for the chemical being required. The list of sources at the end of this book tells how to find the official pages of schedules.

For many years, stimulants, depressants, and hallucinogens basically comprised the entire contents of schedules. In the 1990s another type of drug was added, anabolic steroids. Various types of steroids exist. The anabolics can be used to build muscle mass and have long been popular among athletes seeking an edge in competitions. Anabolic steroids can have other effects as well, effects particularly harmful to young persons whose bodies are still developing. Attainment of adult height can be thwarted, and sexual organs can be damaged. Rising concern about injury to younger athletes caused the strict regulations of scheduling to be applied to these drugs, although other types of control (requiring prescriptions and suppressing nonmedical sales) had long been in place.

Scheduling is an element of law enforcement. Penalties for illegal use or possession of a drug depend partly upon its schedule. A related purpose of scheduling involves control of scheduled substances through tracking prescriptions written by health care practitioners and by tracking inventory records of pharmacies.

Pregnancy Categories

Legal drugs are placed in a Pregnancy Category, a system used to classify the risk of birth defects if the substance is used by a pregnant woman. Different countries have different systems of categories. The alphabetical entries in this book use the U.S. Food and Drug Administration system that was in place as the twenty-first century began.

Pregnancy Category A. Studies using pregnant women do not show birth defects caused by the drug in the first trimester, and evidence has not emerged showing risk later in pregnancy.

Pregnancy Category B. Studies using pregnant women have not been conducted, but experiments with pregnant animals fail to demonstrate birth defects. Alternatively, animal experiments have produced birth defects, but studies using pregnant women have not.

Pregnancy Category C. Animal experiments have produced birth defects, but no studies have used pregnant women to examine the potential for human birth defects. Alternatively, no animal or human studies have been conducted to determine the drug's potential for causing birth defects.

Pregnancy Category D. Studies or reports of clinical experience indicate that the drug causes human birth defects, but using the drug during pregnancy may be so important to the woman's health that fetal risk is justified (for example, no acceptable alternative therapy is available to deal with the woman's illness).

Pregnancy Category X. Animal or human studies or clinical reports indicate the drug causes birth defects, and the drug's potential benefits for a pregnant woman's health do not justify risk to fetal development (for example, acceptable therapies are available that do not involve the drug).

Often a birth defect is thought of as something apparent upon birth, but scientists have found that some problems from fetal drug exposure such as cancer do not become evident until adulthood. And even though problems might not be observed among infants of women who used a certain drug during pregnancy, that fact does not necessarily mean the drug has no impact on fetal development. Drugs discussed in this book typically affect a user's brain, suggesting that they may be particularly prone to harming fetal brain and nervous system development. Due to the course of fetal development, those effects may occur in a later stage of pregnancy than types of harm involving bones or other organs. In addition to matters affecting fetal development, pregnancy can alter a drug's effect on the woman, for example, causing a dose to last longer than in a nonpregnant woman. That, in turn, could cause a pregnant woman to receive a cumulative overdose if she uses an amount suitable for a nonpregnant woman.

STATISTICS

Numbers are a common element in articles and speeches about drugs. Numbers can seem to provide precise information. Occasionally, however, the precision is illusory. For example, a study[6] of drug deaths in major U.S. cities during the early 1970s found that 60% of deaths in New York involved methadone, but it was involved in under 1% of deaths in Los Angeles and 0% in Chicago. Depending on which city's experience someone was inclined to cite, methadone could be made to appear as a major or as an insignificant problem. Statistics may lump substances together, perhaps saying that a particular percentage of persons who died had marijuana or cocaine in their blood. Those are two very different drugs. What percentage was marijuana and what percentage was cocaine? What percentages were at a level of intoxication? Would intoxication have had anything to do with the cause of death? If so, was the death due to a poisonous effect of the drug, or was it due to a poor decision while intoxicated? Many statistics offer no answers to such questions. Even when statistics are both reliable and meaningful, often they are rapidly outdated.

For all those reasons, *The Encyclopedia of Addictive Drugs* offers few statistics. Numbers found in this book are solid and should still have meaning years from now. The list of general sources at the end of this book includes Internet Web sites that can provide the latest statistics. They may be accurate, but (as indicated above) their meaning may be uncertain.

NOTES

1. For an overview see J. Orford, "Addiction as Excessive Appetite," *Addiction* 96 (2001): 15–31. For example, cocaine was long considered non-addictive because usage did not produce physical symptoms of addiction. In the 1980s this traditional understanding was challenged by research reports such as F.H. Gawin and H.D. Kleber, "Abstinence Symptomatology and Psychiatric Diagnosis in Cocaine Abusers: Clinical Observations," *Archives of General Psychiatry* 43 (1986): 107–13; H.D. Kleber and F.H. Gawin, "In Reply," *Archives of General Psychiatry* 44 (1987): 298; H.D. Kleber, "Epidemic Cocaine Abuse: America's Present, Britain's Future?" *British Journal of Addiction* 83 (1988): 1364. Those challenges met skepticism or even outright rejection from A.E. Skodol, "Diagnostic Issues in Cocaine Abuse," in H.I. Spitz and J.S. Rosecan, eds., *Cocaine Abuse: New Directions in Treatment and Research* (New York: Brunner/Mazel, 1987), 120; D.W. Teller and P. Devenyi, "Bromocriptine in Cocaine Withdrawal—Does It Work?" *International Journal of the Addictions* 23 (1988): 1197–1205; A.S.V. Burgen and J.F. Mitchell, *Gaddum's Pharmacology*, 9th ed. (Oxford: Oxford University Press, 1985), 76; J.E.F. Reynolds. *Martindale: The Extra Pharmacopoeia*, 28th ed. (London: The Pharmaceutical Press, 1982), 914; J.M. Arena, ed., *Poisoning: Toxicology, Symptoms, Treat-*

ments, 5th ed. (Springfield, IL: Charles C. Thomas, 1986), 557; *Drug Facts and Comparisons*, 1990 ed. (St. Louis: Facts and Comparisons, 1989), 2078; A. Goth, *Medical Pharmacology: Principles and Conduct*, 11th ed. (St. Louis: C.V. Mosby Company, 1984), 350; B.K. Colasanti, "Contemporary Drug Abuse," in C.R. Craig and R.E. Stitzel, eds., *Modern Pharmacology*, 2d ed. (Boston: Little, Brown and Company, 1986), 620; F.J. Goldstein and G.V. Rossi, "Pharmacological Aspects of Drug Abuse," in A.R. Gennaro, ed., *Remington's Pharmaceutical Sciences*, 17th ed. (Easton, PA: Mack Publishing, 1985), 1351; G.K. McEvoy, ed., *American Hospital Formulary Drug Service Information* (Bethesda, MD: American Society of Hospital Pharmacists, 1989), 1508; Sidney Kaye, *Handbook of Emergency Toxicology: A Guide for the Identification, Diagnosis, and Treatment of Poisoning*, 5th ed. (Springfield, IL: Charles C. Thomas, 1988), 272; R.E. Gosselin, R.P. Smith, and H.C. Hodge, *Clinical Toxicology of Commercial Products*, 5th ed. (Baltimore: Williams & Wilkins, 1984), III–117.

2. *Diagnostic and Statistical Manual of Mental Disorders*, 3rd ed., rev. (Washington, DC: American Psychiatric Association, 1987), 166–68.

3. Ibid., 179.

4. H.K. Armenian, M.A. Chamieh, and A. Baraka, "Influence of Wartime Stress and Psychosocial Factors in Lebanon on Analgesic Requirements for Postoperative Pain," *Social Science and Medicine* 15E (February 1981): 63–66.

5. J. Vila, "Protection from Pentobarbital Lethality Mediated by Pavlovian Conditioning," *Pharmacology, Biochemistry, and Behavior* 32 (1989): 365–66; R.E. Hinson and S. Siegel, "Pavlovian Inhibitory Conditioning and Tolerance to Pentobarbital-Induced Hypothermia in Rats," *Journal of Experimental Psychology: Animal Behavior Processes* 12 (1986): 363–70.

6. E.C. Dinovo et al., "Analysis of Results of Toxicological Examinations Performed by Coroners' or Medical Examiners' Laboratories in 2000 Drug-Involved Deaths in Nine Major U.S. Cities," *Clinical Chemistry* 22 (1976): 847–50.

Drug Types

This section of the book groups drugs in common ways that help readers make basic distinctions among them. For example, a drug grouped here among stimulants has basic differences from one grouped with depressants. Likewise, all drugs in the same classification share common attributes. Many details about drugs in the following classes are in the alphabetical listings of specific substances, in addition to the general overview below.

STIMULANTS

As the name implies, these drugs stimulate the user. A trucker might use stimulants to drive a cargo cross country without rest. A soldier might use them to perform strenuous action that would otherwise be impossible. Stimulants frequently achieve such ends by drawing upon a person's reserves of stamina and energy. Occasional use in that way can help accomplish tasks, and if a person is able to rest and recuperate afterward, perhaps no harm is done. Abusing powerful stimulants, however, is like burning a candle at both ends to produce more light. The quick burst of energy may be followed by collapse.

Not all stimulants are powerful. Some are so mild that they are readily available in certain foods such as **caffeine** in coffee, tea, and soda. A person taking a few ounces of such a beverage will likely need no recuperation at all from the stimulative action. Nonetheless, multiple doses of caffeine can produce a strong effect, and some natural products can be massaged to increase the dose. Caffeine is far less powerful than **cocaine**, but a person using a lot of caffeine can become as jittery and hyperactive as a person using a little cocaine. A mild drug can be abused.

Using potent pharmaceutical stimulants is a way to improve feelings of well-being because increased energy can improve self-confidence regardless of any other effects on body chemistry. Such a mental state can make current problems seem less troublesome. They may not go away, but worries about them can decline. That effect of stimulants can be seductive. Moreover, if that is the reason someone uses stimulants, stopping the drug can be doubly difficult. Not only are feelings of self-confidence and energy replaced by self-doubt and exhaustion, but problems that never went away will probably seem all the worse. And indeed they may really be worse if the stimulant user has taken no effective action to deal with them.

For information about specific stimulants not otherwise classified below, see the entries on: **caffeine**, **modafinil**, **pemoline**, and **yohimbe**.

Amphetamine Class

Amphetamine stimulants are pharmaceutical products created in laboratories, not harvested or refined from natural products. When amphetamines debuted under the brand name Benzedrine during the Great Depression of the 1930s, they were an ingredient used for inhalers that people would sniff to relieve stopped-up noses. Another effect was a burst of energy and alertness, sometimes accompanied by a brightening of mood into euphoria, and people began using the nonprescription inhalers for recreational purposes. Such drugs were called Cartwheel, Euphodine, and Halloo-wach. Amphetamines became accepted therapeutically as a treatment for depression and worked best if a person simply had difficulty coping with stress during part of a day, as a dose wears off quickly and can leave a person feeling lower if nothing has changed in the situation causing the stress. For example, a dose might deal effectively with occasional aggravation in the workplace but not work so well for a person who stayed at home all the time with continual depression. In the 1930s oral tablets of Benzedrine ("Bennies") became available. Both inhalers and tablets tended to promote insomnia, and that effect was soon used medically to fight narcolepsy, an affliction in which a person suddenly falls asleep numerous times throughout the day. The drug was also used to treat Parkinson's disease, epilepsy, and alcoholism and to help persons suffering from attention deficit hyperactivity disorder (ADHD). ADHD begins in childhood and involves difficulty in paying proper attention to surroundings while also acting restless. Usually the condition goes away as children grow older, but it can continue into adult life. Treating the condition with a stimulant may sound counterproductive, but experience shows that low doses of amphetamine class stimulants can ease ADHD. Practitioners had to learn caution in prescribing to children, however, as occasionally this treatment could intensify rather than diminish the undesired conduct.

World War II brought wide use of amphetamines as military forces on all sides issued "pep pills" to give personnel an edge in combat. The most prominent combat pills were Benzedrine (amphetamine sulfate), Dexedrine (**dextroamphetamine**), and Methedrine (**methamphetamine**). Combining such drugs with hard physical labor can be risky, with a user crumpling from overexerting the heart and overheating the whole body, an additional combat hazard for users. In contrast to some other military forces, the United States did not routinely issue the pills except to bomber crews. Nonetheless, the drug was freely available to U.S. personnel who wanted it and was a standard item in survival packs. To improve alertness, national leaders such as British Prime Minister Winston Churchill and, later on, President John F. Kennedy freely used amphetamines as well.[1] Kennedy's New Frontier rhetoric was characterized by his frequent call for "vigor," a prime effect of amphetamines, and a state of being that was important to him.

In athletic events, long-standing records fell after amphetamines became available; speculation exists about whether diet and training were solely responsible for a sudden burst of feats that no human had ever been able to perform. We know for sure that racehorses were doped with amphetamines in that era.

The wartime habit of using amphetamines to increase worker productivity made a peacetime transition in Japan and Sweden, where amphetamine abuse became a major concern in the 1950s. In the United States concern also grew with publicity about dangerous ingestion of these tablets by exhausted long-haul truckers. Even though federal officials had cracked down on "upper" sales at truck stops and gas stations, in 1965 the Interstate Commerce Commission (ICC) described amphetamines as a serious threat to motorists sharing the road with trucks, a claim disputed by the American Trucking Association.[2]

Reports that a drug is used for recreation traditionally raise suspicions about it in America, and an undercurrent of such reports about amphetamines picked up strength in the 1950s. Members of New York's fashionable "beautiful people" who used the drug were called the Benzedrine Set, and in Hollywood the tablets were called "Dolls." Connoisseurs began dosing themselves simultaneously with barbiturate depressants for what was called "a bolt and a jolt." At the social scale's other end, investigators confirmed a brisk business at various prisons where guards were illicitly selling inhalers to prisoners. Outside the jails, crimes against property and persons were attributed to inhalers.

Although restrictions governed sales of inhalers, they were officially nonprescription and priced under a dollar. One inhaler would yield the equivalent of 25 Benzedrine tablets. The original manufacturer of amphetamine sulfate, along with competitors who produced the drug, tried to mix substances into inhalers that would thwart misuse. Abusers found ways to overcome those deterrents, however.

Hearing about alleged results of amphetamine abuse may have been exotic entertainment for most Americans, but they became alarmed by stories of pleasure usage by youths. Inhaler parties by teenagers became so notorious around Kansas City, Missouri, that a U.S. senator introduced federal legislation to curb inhaler sales (Kansas City merchants were retailing hundreds more a week than would be expected in a medicinal context).[3] Pharmaceutical companies began withdrawing brands from the market, and in 1959 the U.S. Food and Drug Administration (FDA) announced that the product would henceforth be available by prescription only.

In the 1960s amphetamines received publicity as an element of the hippie pharmacopeia, with that association promoting disdain for a type of drug that had originally been welcomed by ordinary people. Illicit usage of injectable amphetamines became known as "speeding," a reference to hyperactivity resulting from such needle work. Federal authorities placed new restrictions on these stimulants during the 1960s. Varieties available from drugstores declined, as did physicians' ability to prescribe them. The 31 million prescriptions made in 1967 comprise a number never equaled since.

Amphetamines stimulate the central nervous system (the brain and associated anatomy). At one time evidence of damage to nerve cells was not clear enough to satisfy some credible researchers that such a hazard exists, despite any theoretical reasons for concern, but in the 1990s evidence was becoming persuasive. Among other things, researchers have found that persons who continually abuse amphetamines and persons with a certain type of organic brain injury ("focal damage to orbitofrontal PFC [prefrontal cortex]") have similar problems in making decisions.[4] Severity correlates to length of amphetamine abuse. Nonprescription sales have long been banned in Sweden due to kidney system damage, and amphetamines are suspects in liver damage involving hepatitis. Amphetamines also excite the heart, increasing pulse rate and blood pressure. Normally cardiac effects are unharmful but can be risky at high doses. To a lesser extent, amphetamines help to open air pathways in the lungs while stimulating breathing. A less welcome action can be promotion of muscle and vocal tics, causing users to jerk or cry out uncontrollably. This problem, however, applies more to persons already troubled by tic afflictions than to persons having no such disability. Amphetamines can also cause rashes or hives. Libido can also change, perhaps involving a stronger sex drive, perhaps involving impotence.

Various foods and drugs can interact with amphetamines. Vitamin C and fruit juices lessen amphetamine effects, while common stomach antacid preparations increase them. Amphetamines can boost actions of widely prescribed psychological medicines called tricyclic antidepressants, an interaction also affecting heart action. Amphetamines can counteract medicines intended to control high blood pressure and can also release extra noradrenaline hormone that is stored in the bodies of people taking monoamine oxidase inhibitors (MAOIs, found in some antidepressants and some Parkinson's disease medication). That release can raise blood pressure enough to create headaches while simultaneously raising body temperature enough to kill a person. The danger of MAOI interaction is far less with oral amphetamine dosage than with intravenous injection, and some medical practitioners have simultaneously prescribed oral forms of amphetamine and MAOI drugs, believing that probable benefits outweigh possible risks. Lithium carbonate, a medicine used to control manic behavior, can reduce central nervous stimulation caused by amphetamines.

Psychological effects vary. In addition to results that many persons would find attractive (noted above), users can also become grouchy, jittery, unable to sleep, and suspicious of other persons. Someone highly intoxicated on amphetamines can act mixed up and pugnacious, be frightened, and have hallucinations. This type of drug promotes impulsive actions—not a good consequence if a user is angry and afraid. Overindulgence can leave a person tired, peevish, confused, and depressed when the drug session ends. A serious abuser can develop symptoms duplicating schizophrenia.

Over time some abusers feel a need to increase dosages in order to get the same effects that lower doses once provided. That suggests an abuser has developed "tolerance" to the drug, a classic component of addiction. In contrast to abusers of other drugs, amphetamine abusers commonly fight tolerance not by gradually increasing their dose but by alternating between periods of little use and binges of massive use, a practice promoting inconsistent behavior that can bewilder acquaintances. Despite all of this, into the 1980s amphetamines were described as not addictive.

Although amphetamines have a long history and widespread usage, their potential for causing cancer is unknown; necessary animal experiments had not been conducted as the twentieth century closed. Abnormal fetal development has occurred in mice receiving over 40 times the maximum safe human dose, but normal development of offspring has occurred despite administration of 12.5 times the maximum human dose to rats and 7 times the maximum to rabbits.[5] One human study noted a tendency for more cleft palates than usual if mothers used amphetamines during the first two months of pregnancy.[6] Amphetamines easily pass from a pregnant woman into the fetal blood supply. Standard medical advice cautions pregnant women against using the drug without first discussing the issue with a physician. Some studies claim to find that children born of women who abused amphetamines during pregnancy will have long-term problems with personality and intelligence—but these same women abused other drugs as well; some were displeased about their pregnancies; and about 80% of children in one study had been taken away from the mothers and put into foster homes.[7] Problems faced by such youngsters may well originate outside amphetamines. Tracking amphetamines' physical effect on offspring is easier. Babies from women who abused amphetamines during pregnancy can exhibit anxiety and physical discomfort suggesting dependence and withdrawal. We know that excessive use by a pregnant woman can promote premature birth and reduce a newborn's weight. Genetic predisposition appears to influence how much this type of drug will affect fetal development.

Amphetamines enter human milk and can reach levels three to seven times higher than shown in maternal blood, so nursing mothers can be dosing their infants. Because this kind of drug can act as an appetite suppressant, causing a person to take in inadequate nutrition, that effect is still another concern if infants receive amphetamines through a mother's milk.

For information about specific amphetamine class stimulants, see alphabetical listings for: **dextroamphetamine**, **ephedrine**, **khat**, **ma huang**, **methamphetamine**, **methcathinone**, and **methylphenidate**.

Anorectic Class

Many persons in the United States consider themselves overweight. That self-perception may be more prevalent than obesity itself, but even so, by medical standards a good 33% to 50% of Americans are overweight.[8] That condition can aggravate or even cause serious physical afflictions such as diabetes, high blood pressure, and heart disease. Persons seeking slimness and who are dissatisfied with results from changes in diet and exercise may seek pharmacological help.

The first diet drug to receive scientific endorsement was thyroid hormone. Its use for this purpose began in the 1890s on the theory that it would boost a person's metabolism and thereby promote faster use of calories. The same theory made dinitrophenol a standard diet drug before World War II. Although it boosted metabolic rate, it also boosted rates of cataracts and of harm to the peripheral nervous system (which involves the functioning of various organs and muscles). For those reasons the drug was abandoned. In the 1930s amphetamines became available and quickly became a popular diet aid despite their potential for abuse.

Many stimulants suppress appetite, and some are used as medicines to help people lose weight. Those medicines are called "anorectics." Their stimulant effects may be lower than drugs in other classes but can still have potential for abuse and addiction. For that reason, many anorectics are scheduled substances.

Such drugs are casually described as appetite suppressants, but not all promote weight loss in that way. For instance, some may affect the way food is absorbed in the body; some increase a person's rate of metabolism so the person burns more calories; some make a person more physically energetic. Question has even been raised about whether a stimulant's anorectic action simply comes from elevating the mood of depressed people and thereby reducing their need to gain comfort from eating. Mechanisms by which anorectics work are poorly understood.

Indeed, whether they work at all is uncertain. Compared to placebos, most studies show additional weight loss among persons taking anorectics to be measurable but barely noticeable; some studies show anorectics to be no more effective than placebos. In experiments where anorectics work well, skeptics wonder if results come from factors other than the drug, such as rapport between physician and patient, belief that the substance would work, or even from basics such as controls on food intake during the experiment. Scientists directing one study of anorectics concluded that sensations of appetite suppression were so subtle that a user could miss them unless the person was trying to be aware of them.[9] The effectiveness of an anorectic declines as weeks go by, through development of tolerance. A telling exception to development of tolerance is methylcellulose, an unscheduled substance used to increase bulk of consumed food and thereby increase the physical feeling of fullness. The substance has no psychological effect, and no tolerance develops. Methylcellulose is also among the least effective dieting aids.

Abusers of stimulant anorectics exhibit symptoms similar to those found among abusers of amphetamines, from skin rash to psychosis. Some persons using anorectics properly under medical supervision experience muscle pain and cramps, weariness, peevishness, depression, difficulty in thinking. That group of symptoms is the same as those undergone by persons trying to cope with lack of food regardless of drug use, a coincidence raising question about whether some undesired effects attributed to anorectics are simply undesired effects of being hungry.

A harsh fact about anorectics is that weight lost while using them tends to return if a person stops taking the drugs (and generally they are intended for short-term use only). Behavioral therapy teaches people how to change their eating and exercise habits. A comparison study[10] not only found behavioral therapy superior to anorectic therapy in preventing regain of lost pounds but also found behavioral therapy to be more effective alone than when using anorectics along with it—a troubling result for advocates of anorectics. Skeptics ask whether drugs that produce only mild temporary improvement in a chronic condition are worth anything.

For information about specific anorectic class stimulants, see alphabetical listings for: **benzphetamine, diethylpropion, fenfluramine, mazindol, phendimetrazine, phenmetrazine, phentermine,** and **sibutramine.**

Cocaine Class

As decades change, so do attitudes toward cocaine. In the latter 1800s it was widely used by ordinary middle-class Americans and had a reputation no worse than **alcohol** or tobacco. In the years before World War I, news media stories tied the drug to African Americans and crime, and public opinion transformed the substance from a commonplace item into a substance used mainly by social deviants. Cocaine received little attention from the 1960s illicit drug culture, which seemingly considered cocaine an archaic item no longer of interest. In the 1970s cocaine was portrayed as a drug used by wealthy "beautiful people," and in the 1980s it was portrayed as a poor ghetto dweller's drug. In the 1800s cocaine was considered highly addictive, but from the 1950s into the 1980s it was described as nonaddictive. By the 1990s cocaine was called the most addictive drug known, and demand for the product resulted in accessibility likened to fast-food hamburgers. Although tolerance develops with abuse of most stimulants and was reported with cocaine in the 1800s, in the 1970s and 1980s a scientific consensus held that tolerance did not develop among cocaine abusers. On the contrary, abuse was believed to sensitize people taking the drug, allowing them to achieve the same effects with smaller and smaller doses. Yet by the 1990s cocaine addicts were believed to have a compulsive desire to take more and more of the drug. They were seen to engage in the same kind of binge habit exhibited by amphetamine abusers.

Although a chemical formula stays unaltered as decades pass, ways of using a substance can change. Long ago cocaine was used to make mildly stimulating drinks. Velo-Coca and Vin Mariani were popular cocaine beverages of the nineteenth century, the latter endorsed by notables such as Thomas Edison, Jules Verne, and Pope Leo XIII. The soft drink Coca-Cola originally contained cocaine, but the drug was dropped from the soda early in the twentieth century. These old beverages, however, had about the same relation to cocaine as beer has to white lightning moonshine. A pint of beer and a pint of white lightning may both contain alcohol, but their impact on a user will likely differ. Compared to full-strength pharmaceutical cocaine, old cocaine beverages were relatively weak concoctions.

Some notables are famed for their use of the full-strength product, the most famous example being that of the pioneering psychiatrist Sigmund Freud. When he no longer found the drug useful, he tapered off and eventually quit with no particular difficulty. His example has been duplicated by many other users. He and they were persons enjoying lives of fulfillment in which cocaine was simply one part. In contrast, persons who are dissatisfied with their lives, for whom cocaine brings relief of unhappiness, may face a harder struggle in giving up the drug if it begins degrading the quality of their lives. The more needs a drug satisfies for a person, the stronger its appeal. Some needs may be biological; a study of identical twins finds their cocaine usage patterns to be remarkably similar.[11] Some needs may derive from a person's life situation.

Cocaine abuse is normally part of a multiproblem lifestyle. A study of homeless cocaine abusers found that achieving abstinence was easier for them if they obtained shelter and employment.[12] Compared to the whole population, cocaine addicts are much likelier to be addicted to gambling as well.[13] Alcoholism and suicidal thoughts increase the likelihood that a person who uses cocaine will become addicted.[14] One study of persons being treated for cocaine abuse found over one half to be jobless and over one third to have jail records.[15] A survey of crack smokers found that over one third had been physically attacked over a one-year period.[16] Five years of records at one hospital showed the following primary reasons for admission of cocaine-using patients: assaults, stabbings, and bullet wounds.[17] Such persons obviously face serious challenges other than cocaine; any inability to cope with the drug is but a single element in a general inability to cope with life.

For information about specific cocaine class stimulants, see alphabetical listings for: **coca** and **cocaine**.

Pyridine Alkaloids Class

Tobacco and **areca nut** are the most widely used substances containing drugs from this class. Although most Americans think of tobacco's **nicotine** as a recreational drug, it has had agricultural functions as a pesticide and for ridding farm animals of worms. Nicotine is readily absorbed through the skin and causes "green tobacco sickness" among farmworkers who handle leaves, a poisoning sometimes severe enough to require hospitalization. The tobacco plant has been known to kill livestock that eat it. Humans have also been poisoned when attempting to use tobacco as food, such as by boiling greens.

Tobacco apparently originated in the Americas, where native peoples did not seem to regard it as a recreational substance. Their uses were spiritual and medical. Even in the twentieth century some native peoples used tobacco to treat conditions ranging from chills to infections and snake bites. When Europeans discovered tobacco in the New World, they removed it from the cultural context in which its primary uses had been medical and spiritual. Used without those restrictions, hazards became obvious soon enough. Lacking the shared social values that had long limited tobacco's use in the New World, Europeans attempted to control the substance by law. Property of cultivators and traffickers became subject to forfeiture in Hungary and Russia and even Japan. In the 1600s smoking was condemned by the pope and by King James of England, and smokers were condemned to death in Turkey, Iran, Russia, and some German states. Legal harshness, however, was unable to substitute for the social values that had limited consumption in lands where tobacco originated.

We often measure drug addiction by the amount of drug used, assuming that the more a person uses, the stronger the drug's hold. Researchers have found this assumption to be incorrect for nicotine. Measured by strength of dependence symptoms, a person who smokes more than a half pack of tobacco cigarettes each day may be no more addicted than a person who smokes just half a pack,[18] meaning the lighter smoker may have just as much trouble quitting as the heavier smoker.

Among cigarette users, the amount of smoking depends in part on the tobacco's nicotine content, but other factors are also involved. During the 1990s in the United States female smokers tended to have a higher degree of tobacco addiction than male smokers did (measured not in number of cigarettes smoked but in strength of addiction symptoms such as tolerance, withdrawal, and difficulty in reducing consumption).[19] Whites had stronger levels of addiction than did members of other races.[20] Adolescents tended to smoke fewer cigarettes than middle-aged persons, but despite adolescents' lower usage, their addiction symptoms were just as strong as those found in heavier-smoking middle-aged persons.[21] Older smokers were the least addicted even though they were the heaviest users.[22] Researchers are unsure whether such differences are caused by biology or culture or a combination.

In the United States tobacco smoking is associated with being an adult, and adolescents may take up the practice partly as a symbol of their passage into adulthood. Role models are also important; a prominent person who smokes may inspire admirers to do so. Celebrity endorsements of cigarettes were once routine in advertising, but the admired person can also be a personal acquaintance. A survey in Spain revealed that the role model of teachers who smoke seems to be a major factor in starting the habit among students there.[23]

The popularity of smoking among American teenagers declined in the 1970s and 1980s but increased in the 1990s. A cancer statistics authority reported that by 1997 over 33% of American high schoolers were using cigarettes.[24] A study of Taiwanese high school students published in 1999 found a much lower usage rate, more like 10%.[25] In 1999 a survey of over 14,000 young adult American college students found about 33% using some sort of tobacco product, mostly cigarettes.[26] The latest statistics can be found through the "Sources for More Information" at the end of this book.

For information about specific pyridine alkaloids class stimulants, see alphabetical listings for: **areca nut** and **nicotine**.

DEPRESSANTS

Depressants generally have the opposite effect of stimulants. Many depressants are used as sedatives or tranquilizers, terms often used as if they mean the same thing even though some experts would dispute such interchangeable usage of the terms sedative and tranquilizer. Depressant drugs slow a person down, and one result can be reduction of tension, which in turn can improve a mentally depressed mood. Depressant withdrawal symptoms typically include uneasiness and sleeping difficulty. If dependence is strong enough, withdrawal may also involve tremors, loss of strength, delirium, and seizures. Gradual reduction in dosage may help avoid withdrawal symptoms, but much depends on the particular drug and the strength of dependence.

For information about specific depressants not listed among the following classes, see alphabetical listings for: **alcohol, chloral hydrate, ethchlorvynol, GHB, glutethimide, ketamine, mandrake, meprobamate, methaqualone, PCP, pentazocine, zaleplon,** and **zolpidem.**

Barbiturate Class

Barbiturates were introduced into medical practice during the early 1900s, for combating insomnia, anxiety, and seizures. Despite occasional flurries of concern, not until the 1960s did much alarm grow about barbiturates in the United States. Members of a U.S. Senate subcommittee began portraying the drug class as a menace in the 1970s, and afterward stricter controls were put on use.

Barbiturates and alcohol have similar effects. If someone intoxicated by alcohol takes barbiturates, the drunkenness will deepen as if more alcohol had been swallowed. Pharmaceutical effects of alcohol alone can kill a person who overdoses, and adding barbiturates can transform a session of social drinking into a fatal one. More than one person has died by taking barbiturate sleeping pills with alcohol instead of water.

The similarity of alcohol and barbiturates is also shown by the appearance of a serious withdrawal syndrome called delirium tremens in alcohol and barbiturate abusers who are cut off from their drug. Lesser withdrawal symptoms for both drugs may include perspiring and vomiting. Barbiturate withdrawal may involve dizziness, tremors, fidgety behavior, edgy feelings, and insomnia. Even with strict medical supervision, withdrawal can be fatal. Tolerance can develop. More details can be found in alphabetical entries for specific barbiturates.

A person using barbiturates should take the same precautions as a person using alcohol, for example, using care about running dangerous machinery such as automobiles.

Barbiturates can cause reflex sympathetic dystrophy of the arm, a disease in which a hand loses bone density and becomes painful and difficult to move. This class of drugs may also cause a syndrome that produces pain in the shoulder and hand, interfering with their movement. Extended dosage with barbiturates may cause rickets, a disease in which bones soften. One of the most dangerous effects of barbiturate overdose is temporary stoppage of electrical activity in the brain, which could lead to premature declaration of a patient's death, particularly if the patient is being treated for some injury without caregivers knowing about the person's barbiturate usage.

This class of substances may interfere with blood thinner medicine, with birth control pills, and with other female hormone medications. Barbiturates may extend the time that an MAOI dose lasts.

In animal experiments barbiturates have encouraged the development of cancer.

When used by pregnant women, barbiturates can cause birth defects ranging from internal organ deformities to malformations of the face. If a pregnant woman uses barbiturates regularly, her offspring may be born resonant with them. This class of drugs passes into the milk of nursing mothers and may depress consciousness, pulse rate, and respiration of nursing infants.

For information about specific barbiturate class depressants, see alphabetical listings for: **butalbital, mephobarbital, pentobarbital,** and **phenobarbital.**

Benzodiazepine Class

Benzodiazepines became widely available for medical purposes in the 1960s and replaced barbiturates in treatments of many conditions. Benzodiazepines proved themselves less prone to abuse than barbiturates, in addition to being safer—accidental overdose is unlikely because the amount needed for a medical effect is so much smaller than a poisonous amount. In addition to reducing anxiety, benzodiazepines may improve quality of sleep—from fighting insomnia to eliminating sleepwalking. This class of drugs is also used to calm people and to treat convulsions. Some users experience mild euphoria.

As might be expected with drugs that promote sleep, benzodiazepines can worsen reaction time, vigilance, and thinking abilities and therefore should be used cautiously if a person is operating dangerous machinery such as an automobile. Problems may also develop for persons who are already unsteady on their feet, such as elderly persons prone to falling. The substances can also cause memory trouble, typically difficulty in recalling recent experiences. Headache, peevishness, confusion, and tremors may occur. In unusual cases rageful outbursts may occur. These are "paradoxical reactions," meaning they are the opposite of what would be expected from the drug. Expressions of rage possibly emerge because the drug reduces anxiety in a person who is angry about something, and less anxiety can lead to less inhibition against doing something.

Over a 12-year span a practitioner observed patients taking benzodiazepines to treat serious sleep problems such as night terrors and sleepwalking. The practitioner found that 2% of this population (not 2% of all patients but just those using benzodiazepines against these sleep disorders) occasionally abused them,[27] and this population base included persons with a previous history of drug abuse; thus we can expect benzodiazepine abuse to be even lower in a general population. Among persons treated for drug abuse, benzodiazepines are among the least-abused substances. Experiments giving free access to benzodiazepines to persons undergoing treatment for drug abuse revealed little interest in those compounds.[28] This class of depressants can be highly popular among special populations, however. One study noted that 30% of alcoholics were using benzodiazepines.[29] When benzodiazepines were given to rats in experiments, the animals' consumption of alcohol increased,[30] suggesting that human benzodiazepine usage might increase alcohol's appeal. Although benzodiazepines are administered to treat alcohol withdrawal, combining the two substances recreationally is a dangerous mix that can prove fatal.

Different benzodiazepines have differing attractiveness to abusers. Measured by amount of misuse, claims made by misusers about drug effects, mental and physical effects verified in scientific experiments, and impressions reported by medical caregivers, **diazepam** is considered to have one of the greatest potentials for abuse. **Alprazolam** and **lorazepam** have similar, but lower, risk. **Halazepam** and **oxazepam** seem to be among the least risky for abuse.

Tolerance to some benzodiazepine effects can develop (many details are in this book's alphabetical section). Dependence can also emerge, with a withdrawal syndrome similar to those of alcohol and barbiturates. Often the syndrome may be avoided by gradual reduction of dosage.

Small studies have found that women who use benzodiazepines during pregnancy produce infants who are smaller than normal.[31] Children in one of these studies[32] rapidly caught up in some growth perimeters, but at the age of 18 months head size still remained smaller than normal. Facial deformities were common. The children had persistent trouble with muscle control. Similar findings in another small study[33] included mental retardation, but still another study[34] noted that such children also had heavy fetal exposure to alcohol, exposure that is known to produce mental retardation. Thus the actual role of benzodiazepines was unclear.

Some of these reports did not track outcomes past infancy. Research tracking children up to four years of age found that early problems attributed to benzodiazepines cleared up in most of them.[35] When teachers were asked to evaluate schoolchildren who had fetal exposure, the instructors found no difference between them and classmates.[36]

Researchers who investigated the outcome of thousands of pregnancies found no evidence that benzodiazepines cause cleft palate.[37] A large study involving hundreds of pregnancies found birth defects to be no more likely among women who used benzodiazepines than among women who did not use them; and even when malformations occurred, no particular kind of birth defect tended to appear in benzodiazepine offspring.[38] Drugs that cause fetal harm generally cause particular types of damage; lack of a particular type with benzodiazepines suggests that the drug was not the cause of observed malformations. Some investigators believe they have detected a particular birth defect pattern, but such findings have been questioned.[39] As the twenty-first century began, a research team reported evidence that benzodiazepines may damage fetal brain development.[40] Science has not yet rendered a verdict on the safety of benzodiazepines during pregnancy. Infants with fetal exposure can be born dependent on this type of drug. It passes into breast milk, but the amount from lower-dosage levels probably has no effect on nursing infants.

For information about specific benzodiazepine class depressants, see alphabetical listings for: **alprazolam, chlordiazepoxide, clonazepam, clorazepate, diazepam, estazolam, flunitrazepam, flurazepam, halazepam, lorazepam, midazolam, oxazepam, prazepam, quazepam, temazepam,** and **triazolam.**

Opiate Class

Along with alcohol, opiates are the oldest known depressants. At one time the term *narcotic* referred specifically and only to opiates, but when drug control laws were strengthened in the early twentieth century the language of those laws expanded the dictionary definition of *narcotic* and made it a synonym for all controlled drugs.

Although opiates have various medical uses, the main therapeutic application is pain control. Other common uses are for fighting coughs and reducing diarrhea. Some other therapeutic uses of specific opiates are given in this book's alphabetical listings of drugs.

The chance of medical opiate usage turning a person into an addict is slim. Very few persons receiving medical opiates find them attractive, and almost all patients who enjoy opiates already have a drug abuse problem. Researchers examined records of 11,882 patients who received narcotics and found 4 with a subsequent addiction problem who lacked a prior drug addiction history.[41] The chance of developing dependence is higher, but a patient can be weaned off opiates in ways that avoid withdrawal symptoms.

Illicit users of opiates generally seek to achieve a mental state of indifference in which problems and frustrations no longer feel bothersome. A person high on opiates is oblivious to the world and unlikely to bother anyone. Some users experience euphoria.

Classic unwanted actions from opiates are constipation, urinary difficulty, low blood pressure, and breathing trouble. MAOI drugs, described earlier, may interact dangerously with opiates. In contrast to such problems, a desirable drug interaction is that opiates may boost pain relief from aspirin.

Originally the phrase "being hooked on a drug" referred to being so resonant with (that is, dependent on) an opiate that a withdrawal syndrome occurred if dosage stopped. Symptoms of opiate withdrawal are similar to those of influenza: sweats, goose bumps, muscle aches, cramps, runny nose, diarrhea, and sleep difficulties. Although conscienceless and irresponsible addicts may be particularly short-tempered and dangerous if undergoing withdrawal, for other persons the experience is miserable, but not horrible, and usually lasts only a few days. Traditionally those few days are the extent of withdrawal, but some authorities believe a subsequent stage of withdrawal occurs in which a person experiences aches, insomnia, and grouchiness for several months. Such symptoms, however, may simply be signs that the psychological buffer provided by opiate use is no longer available.

Drug addiction "maintenance" programs are designed to supply enough drug to hold off withdrawal but not enough to produce recreational sensations. Unless participants supplement the legal dosage with illicit supplies, such persons will not experience opiate effects enjoyed by addicts. Someone on a maintenance dose can adequately perform job duties and safely operate a motor vehicle. Performance may not be as sharp as in a drug-free state, but performance is in the normal range.

Opiates have a wide range of effects on fetal behavior. If a pregnant woman uses opiates regularly the fetus soon adapts to the presence of the drug and seems to develop normally, although an infant can be born resonant with (that is, dependent on) the drug and undergo withdrawal. Intermittent use of opiates is more damaging to a fetus than regular use, with the changing drug environment causing extra stress as a fetus copes with one condition and then another. Opiates cause fetal metabolism to increase, diverting energy away from body development. Infants born to opiate users are commonly smaller than normal, and early slowness of brain development has been observed. Evidence exists that fetal exposure causes long-lasting problems in children, involving impulsiveness and inattention, but some researchers feel that home environment (often involving a single-parent opiate abuser with additional problems) is a better explanation for those difficulties.

For information about specific opiate class depressants, see alphabetical listings for: **buprenorphine, codeine, dihydrocodeine, etorphine, heroin, hydrocodone, hydromorphone, morphine, nalbuphine, opium, oxycodone, pholcodine,** and **thebaine.**

Opioid Class

Opioids are often called opiates, which is satisfactory for practical purposes because the two classes of drugs basically produce the same effects in the same way. A technical difference exists between the two classes, however. If the history of a product were traced backward through its manufacturing processes, opiates generally would begin with the **opium** plant, but opioids would generally begin in a laboratory. Despite this technical distinction, the terms *opiates* and *opioids* are often used synonymously. Some of these substances are called "semisynthetic" and are referred to as "opiate/opioid." Some opiates, such as morphine, can even be manufactured wholly in a laboratory without starting from the natural product opium; thus the same chemical can be either an opiate or an opioid.

For information about specific opioid class depressants, see alphabetical listings for: **butorphanol, dextromethorphan, dextromoramide, dextrorphan, diphenoxylate, dipipanone, fentanyl, ketobemidone, LAAM, levorphanol, meperidine, methadone, oxymorphone, phenoperidine, piritramide, propoxyphene, remifentanil,** and **trimeperidine.**

STEROIDS

The steroids governed by schedules of controlled substances are anabolic steroids. Anabolic substances build up parts of living organisms, as opposed to catabolic substances, which decompose those parts. Anabolic steroids are abused mainly by persons desiring to increase muscle mass, such as competitive athletes and body builders. Steroids can improve muscle strength in females and in castrated males, but scientific evidence is weaker for intact males. Still, steroids do seem to promote muscle mass, endurance, and overall athletic performance while dosage continues. Some scientists suspect that any performance enhancement experienced from anabolic steroids comes not from muscle power but from psychological effects, with the drugs increasing a user's aggressiveness. Anabolic steroids can produce mania, anger, impulsiveness, euphoria, and feelings of invincibility—a combination that may lead some users into harmful social interactions. The combination can produce other types of unwise behavior as well, such as extravagant expenditures of money and taking reckless physical risks. Reports exist of paranoia and hallucinations developing while using steroids and disappearing when steroid usage is stopped.

Sports governing authorities banned the use of anabolic steroids by competitors. Some athletes ignore the ban in hopes of avoiding detection. Various other drugs are prohibited as well, but in 1988 most of the failed drug tests ordered by the International Olympic Committee revealed anabolic steroids, the most common one being **nandrolone**.[42] Below that elite level, athletic use of steroids seems uncommon. In the 1990s a study involving 58,625 college students found only 175 steroid takers to study.[43] That small group also had a much higher consumption of other drugs, legal and illegal, than the average student—suggesting that the steroid abusers were predisposed to use drugs for coping with all sorts of life situations, not just sports. Similar association of steroids with other illicit drug usage is found at the high school level.[44] High school steroid statistics are often based on the concept of "lifetime use." Lifetime use means a person has taken a steroid at least once, which is not the same as regularly taking them. The number of regular users will be much smaller than the number of "lifetime" users.

Anabolic steroids are related to **testosterone**. Most, if not all, are androgens, substances promoting male characteristics. A female who uses those drugs may develop facial hair and a deeper voice, along with unwanted changes in sexual organs. In a young person who is still growing, androgens can prematurely halt further growth and thereby cause a smaller adult stature. Among persons of either gender and any age, androgens may alter blood composition and increase the body's retention of various minerals. That retention is not necessarily good. For example, sodium retention promotes bloating and can be inadvisable for persons with heart trouble. Liver damage and reduction of male fertility may occur due to anabolic steroids. Extended use of the substance may worsen cholesterol levels, thereby narrowing blood vessels, and such narrowing promotes heart attack and stroke years later. Steroid abusers tend to take far higher doses than are considered medically safe, thus further increasing the risks. Oral and slow-release under-the-skin implant formats of anabolic steroids can be processed in ways that will physically permit them to be injected. Such a practice is highly dangerous, as noninjectable formats of drugs have components that are not designed for direct introduction into the bloodstream.

Anabolic steroid dependence is reported with withdrawal symptoms that can include weariness and depression. Use by a pregnant woman can permanently masculinize a female fetus.

For information about specific anabolic steroids, see alphabetical listings for: **boldenone, ethylestrenol, fluoxymesterone, methandriol, methandrostenolone, methyltestosterone, nandrolone, oxandrolone, oxymetholone, stanozolol, testolactone, testosterone,** and **trenbolone**.

HALLUCINOGENS

Although various drugs cause hallucinations, some drugs are so notable for such an effect that they are classified as hallucinogens. Controversy exists about what a hallucination is. Is it a bluish tint to colors in a normal scene? Is it wavy motions in a solid and stationary object? Is it shapes in fireplace flames transforming into animal heads? Is it something that goes away if someone's eyes open? Is it a creature that appears out of nowhere and provides mystical insights? Is it sensations of floating? Is it a different flow of time? Is it cross-wiring of senses, where colors are heard and smells are seen? Specialists may quibble, but this book classifies all such experiences as hallucinations.

Many people dislike hallucinatory experiences, especially people who like to be in control of themselves and of situations around them. Such people often find hallucinations not only unpleasant but downright frightening. Other people find the sensations intriguing and pleasurable.

Scientific interest in hallucinogens began to emerge in the 1800s, blossoming in the 1950s and 1960s. In those latter times hallucinogens were popularly identified with beatniks and hippies, and social disapproval of those lifestyles promoted legal restrictions on hallucinogens that terminated almost all scientific research regarding these substances. Thus much of the scientific data is old.

For information about specific hallucinogens, see alphabetical listings for: **AET, amanita, belladonna, bufotenine, DET, DMT, DOB, DOM, dronabinol, ergot, ibogaine, jimson weed, LSD, marijuana, MDA, MDEA, MDMA, mescaline, morning glory, nutmeg, peyote, psilocybin, 2C-B,** and **yage.**

INHALANTS

Although some authorities consider inhalants to be depressants, and inhalants have hallucinogenic qualities, for several reasons this book lists inhalants as a substance type in their own right. First, despite easy availability, inhalants are among the most dangerous of abused substances. There is no range of inhalants, some of which are benign and some of which are risky, as there is with stimulants or depressants. All inhalants are dangerous despite wide variations in their chemistry, and this sets them apart from other types of drugs. Second, inhalants are generally used by inhaling them in their gaseous state (which is not the same as smoking and also differs from eating a solid or drinking a liquid). That dosage format sets them apart from other drugs. Third, inhalants are used mainly by younger persons (typically teenage males), a usage pattern that also sets inhalants apart from other drugs.

With some inhalants the amount needed to produce a recreational effect is close to a fatal dose, and deadly outcomes demonstrate that the difference was too close for some deceased users to handle. In addition, strenuous exercise seems related to inhalant death, troublesome for users at dance clubs. The products are often flammable, sometimes producing serious physical injury unrelated to pharmacology. Some users act as if they do not realize they need a continual supply of oxygen, and they administer inhalants in ways that cause suffocation. In addition to all these acute dangers, long-term use of many inhalants can produce nerve damage, impairing the ability to use arms and legs and hands and feet, damage verified scientifically. Another type of long-term damage appears to be assorted types of psychoses. This consequence is harder to verify because inhalant users often take other potent drugs, so proving which mind-altering drug affected the mind can be very difficult. Unquestionably, however, inhalant users can develop states of mind interfering with—or even preventing—their ability to function in society. Admittedly, some users avoid serious outcomes, just as some car drivers run red lights without harm. Escape, however, does not mean that danger should be disregarded.

Generally, adult drug users shun most inhalants except as a choice of desperation if nothing else is available. Inhalant users tend to be teenagers or younger, perhaps because other drugs of abuse (even alcohol and tobacco) are harder for some young persons to obtain. Sniffing is often a social event with acquaintances rather than a solitary pastime. As the 1960s began, the average age among 130 glue sniffers in Denver was 13.[45] In this group 124 were male; most were lower-class Hispanics in trouble with school or law enforcement authorities; many had emotional problems. Another study found glue sniffers to have personalities matching those of alcoholics.[46] **Gasoline** sniffers are often emotionally deprived teens from troubled families, typically living lower-class lives in rural areas, often members of native populations whose cultures have been devastated (American Indians in the United States, aborigines in Australia, Island peoples in the Pacific). Case studies of **butane** sniffers tell of lonely persons with difficulties at school or at home. A psychological test of 59 inhalant abusers[47] found them to be impulsive persons with little respect for authority. Most research finds inhalant users to be unhappy persons marginalized by society. Yet not all researchers find that inhalant users are social misfits from dysfunctional families; some appear to be ordinary persons, though still youthful.

That difference in findings—most researchers saying inhalant abusers are social misfits, with some researchers contending inhalant abusers are normal—deserves an attempt at explanation. Many inhalant researchers work where inhalant abuse has been publicized as a major community problem, and those places tend to have populations of socially marginalized people. Researchers commonly study persons receiving medical attention for inhalant abuse, and sometimes the medical attention is received involuntarily by court order. Such persons may be no more typical of inhalant users than hospitalized alcoholics receiving court-ordered treatment are typical of most alcohol users. And the definition of "user" may influence understanding. A user who sniffs several times a day is not the same kind of user who sniffed with some friends once or twice over a period of several years. Although most research finds inhalant abusers to be troubled outcasts, it is possible that such typical findings are due to the demographics of the population being studied.

For information about specific inhalants, see alphabetical listings for: **butane**, **ether**, **freon**, **gasoline**, **mothballs**, **nitrite**, **nitrous oxide**, **TCE**, and **toluene**.

NOTES

1. W.P. Czerwinski, "Amphetamine-Related Disorders," *Journal of the Louisiana State Medical Society* 150 (1998): 491; R. Reeves, "President's Health the Great Coverup of JFK Years," *Kansas City Star*, Oct. 11, 1992, K4; R. Reeves, *President Kennedy: Profile of Power* (New York: Simon & Schuster, 1993), 178, 243, 648n. 146; T.C. Reeves, *A Question*

of Character: A Life of John F. Kennedy (New York: The Free Press, 1991), 295–96; C.D. Heymann, *A Woman Named Jackie* (New York: Lyle Stuart, 1989), 296–319.

2. R. King, *The Drug Hang-up* (New York: W.W. Norton, 1972), 271, 283–85.

3. C.O. Jackson, "The Amphetamine Inhaler: A Case Study of Medical Abuse," *Journal of the History of Medicine and Allied Sciences* 26 (1971): 187–96. The author is also indebted to Jackson's article for other colorful examples of amphetamine's history.

4. R.D. Rogers et al., "Dissociable Deficits in the Decision-making Cognition of Chronic Amphetamine Abusers, Opiate Abusers, Patients with Focal Damage to Prefrontal Cortex, and Tryptophan-Depleted Normal Volunteers: Evidence for Monoaminergic Mechanisms," *Neuropsychopharmacology* 20 (1999): 322–39.

5. "Adderall," "Dextrostat," and "Dexedrine," in *Physicians' Desk Reference*, 56th ed. (Montvale, NJ: Medical Economics Company, 2002), 1513, 3231, 3237.

6. L. Milkovich and B.J. van den Berg, "Effects of Antenatal Exposure to Anorectic Drugs," *American Journal of Obstetrics and Gynecology* 129 (1977): 637. See also M.A. Plessinger, "Prenatal Exposure to Amphetamines: Risks and Adverse Outcomes in Pregnancy," *Obstetrics and Gynecology Clinics of North America* 25 (1998): 119–38.

7. L. Cernerud et al., "Amphetamine Addiction during Pregnancy: 14-Year Follow-up of Growth and School Performance," *Acta Paediatrica* 85 (1996): 204–8; L. Billing et al., "The Influence of Environmental Factors on Behavioural Problems in 8-Year-Old Children Exposed to Amphetamine during Fetal Life," *Child Abuse and Neglect* 18 (1994): 3–9. See also M. Eriksson et al., "Cross-sectional Growth of Children Whose Mothers Abused Amphetamines during Pregnancy," *Acta Paediatrica* 83 (1994): 612–17.

8. C.M. Apovian, "The Use of Pharmacologic Agents in the Treatment of the Obese Patient," *Journal of the American Osteopathic Association*, pt.2, 99 (1999, Suppl.): S2–S7; W.S. Poston II et al., "Challenges in Obesity Management," *Southern Medical Journal* 91 (1998): 710–20.

9. S.B. Penick and J.R. Hinkle, "The Effect of Expectation on Response to Phenmetrazine," *Psychosomatic Medicine* 26 (1964): 369–73.

10. J. Mellar and L.E. Hollister, "Phenmetrazine: An Obsolete Problem Drug," *Clinical Pharmacology and Therapeutics* 32 (1982): 672.

11. K.S. Kendler et al., "Illicit Psychoactive Substance Use, Heavy Use, Abuse, and Dependence in a U.S. Population–Based Sample of Male Twins," *Archives of General Psychiatry* 57 (2000): 261–69.

12. J.B. Milby et al., "Initiating Abstinence in Cocaine Abusing Dually Diagnosed Homeless Persons," *Drug and Alcohol Dependence* 60 (2000): 55–67.

13. G.W. Hall et al., "Pathological Gambling among Cocaine-Dependent Outpatients," *American Journal of Psychiatry* 157 (2000): 1127–33.

14. C.S. Lopes and E.S. Coutinho, "Transtornos mentais como fatores de risco para o desenvolvimento de abuso/dependência de cocaína: Estudo caso-controle" (Mental disorders as risk factors for the development of cocaine abuse/dependence: Case-control study), *Revista de Saude Publica* 33 (1999): 477–86 (abstract in English).

15. Hall et al., "Pathological Gambling among Cocaine-Dependent Outpatients."

16. H.A. Siegal et al., "Crack-Cocaine Users as Victims of Physical Attack," *Journal of the National Medical Association* 92 (2000): 76–82.

17. C.R. Schermer and D.H. Wisner, "Methamphetamine Use in Trauma Patients: A Population-Based Study," *Journal of the American College of Surgeons* 189 (1999): 442–49.

18. D.B. Kandel and K. Chen, "Extent of Smoking and Nicotine Dependence in the United States: 1991–1993," *Nicotine and Tobacco Research* 2 (2000): 263–74.

19. Ibid.

20. Ibid.

21. Ibid.

22. Ibid.

23. M.A. Hernández-Mezquita et al., "Opinión de los directores escolares sobre la influencia de factores del medio escolar en la actitud de niños y jovenes ante el tabaco" (Influence of school environment on student's attitudes about tobacco consumption in the opinion of the headmasters), *Anales Españoles de Pediatría* 52 (2000): 132–37 (abstract in English).

24. G.A. Giovino, "Epidemiology of Tobacco Use among U.S. Adolescents," *Nicotine and Tobacco Research* 1 (1999, Suppl. 1): S31–S40.

25. M.Y. Chong, K.W. Chan, and A.T. Cheng, "Substance Use Disorders among Adolescents in Taiwan: Prevalence, Sociodemographic Correlates and Psychiatric Comorbidity," *Psychological Medicine* 29 (1999): 1387–96.

26. N.A. Rigotti, J.E. Lee, and H. Wechsler, "U.S. College Students' Use of Tobacco Products: Results of a National Survey," *Journal of the American Medical Association* 284 (2000): 699–705.

27. C.H. Schenck and M.W. Mahowald, "Long-Term, Nightly Benzodiazepine Treatment of Injurious Parasomnias and Other Disorders of Disrupted Nocturnal Sleep in 170 Adults," *American Journal of Medicine* 100 (1996): 333–37.

28. D.A. Ciraulo, "Abuse Potential of Benzodiazepines," *Bulletin of the New York Academy of Medicine* 61 (1985): 728–41.

29. L. Walters and P. Nel, "Die Afhanklikheidspotensiaal van die Bensodiasepiene: Toepassing van die Resultate van die Behandeling van die Alkoholonttrekkingsindroom" (The addiction potential of benzodiazepines. Application of the results of treatment of alcohol withdrawal syndrome), *South African Medical Journal* 59 (1981): 115–16 (abstract in English). See also L. Walters and P. Nel, "Pharmacological Requirements of Patients during Alcohol Withdrawal," *South African Medical Journal* 59 (1981): 114.

30. A.H. Soderpalm and S. Hansen, "Benzodiazepines Enhance the Consumption and Palatability of Alcohol in the Rat," *Psychopharmacology* 137 (1998): 215–22.

31. In addition to other studies cited in this paragraph, see L. Laegreid, G. Hagberg, and A. Lundberg, "The Effect of Benzodiazepines on the Fetus and the Newborn," *Neuropediatrics* 23 (1992): 18–23.

32. L. Laegreid, G. Hagberg, and A. Lundberg, "Neurodevelopment in Late Infancy after Prenatal Exposure to Benzodiazepines—A Prospective Study," *Neuropediatrics* 23 (1992): 60–67.

33. L. Laegreid, "Clinical Observations in Children after Prenatal Benzodiazepine Exposure," *Developmental Pharmacology and Therapeutics* 15 (1990): 186–88. See also G. Viggedal, "Mental Development in Late Infancy after Prenatal Exposure to Benzodiazepines—A Prospective Study," *Journal of Child Psychology and Psychiatry, and Allied Disciplines* 34 (1993): 295–305.

34. U. Bergman et al., "Effects of Exposure to Benzodiazepine during Fetal Life," *Lancet* 340 (1992): 694–96. See also J.A. Kuller et al., "Pharmacologic Treatment of Psychiatric Disease in Pregnancy and Lactation: Fetal and Neonatal Effects," *Obstetrics and Gynecology* 87 (1996): 789–94; S.D. Silberstein, "Headaches and Women: Treatment of the Pregnant and Lactating Migraineur," *Headache* 33 (1993): 536.

35. P.R. McElhatton, "The Effects of Benzodiazepine Use during Pregnancy and Lactation," *Reproductive Toxicology* 8 (1994): 461–75.

36. L. Stika et al., "Effects of Drug Administration in Pregnancy on Children's School Behaviour," *Pharmaceutisch Weekblad: Scientific Edition* 12 (1990): 252–55 (abstract in English).

37. A. Czeizel, "Lack of Evidence of Teratogenicity of Benzodiazepine Drugs in Hungary," *Reproductive Toxicology* 1 (1987–1988): 183–88. See also Kuller et al., "Pharmacologic Treatment of Psychiatric Disease in Pregnancy and Lactation: Fetal and Neonatal Effects."

38. A. Ornoy et al., "Is Benzodiazepine Use during Pregnancy Really Teratogenic?"

Reproductive Toxicology 12 (1998): 511–15. See also P.R. McElhatton et al., "The Outcome of Pregnancy in 689 Women Exposed to Therapeutic Doses of Antidepressants: A Collaborative Study of the European Network of Teratology Information Services (ENTIS)," *Reproductive Toxicology* 10 (1996): 285–94.

39. L. Laegreid et al., "Congenital Malformations and Maternal Consumption of Benzodiazepines: A Case-Control Study," *Developmental Medicine and Child Neurology* 32 (1990): 432–41; P.R. McElhatton, "The Effects of Benzodiazepine Use during Pregnancy and Lactation," *Reproductive Toxicology* 8 (1994): 461–75; U. Bergman, "Pharmacoepidemiological Perspectives on the Suspected Teratogenic Effects of Benzodiazepines," *Bratislavske Lekarske Listy* 92 (1991): 560–63 (abstract in English).

40. J.W. Olney et al., "Environmental Agents That Have the Potential to Trigger Massive Apoptotic Neurodegeneration in the Developing Brain," *Environmental Health Perspectives* 108 (2000, Suppl. 3): 383–88.

41. J. Porter and H. Jick, "Addiction Rare in Patients Treated with Narcotics," *New England Journal of Medicine* 302 (1980): 123.

42. "Nandrolone decanoate," in *Therapeutic Drugs*, ed. C. Dollery, 2d ed. (New York: Churchill Livingstone, 1999), N29.

43. P.W. Meilman et al., "Beyond Performance Enhancement: Polypharmacy among Collegiate Users of Steroids," *Journal of American College Health* 44 (1995): 98–104.

44. R.H. du Rant, L.G. Escobedo, and G.W. Heath, "Anabolic-Steroid Use, Strength Training, and Multiple Drug Use among Adolescents in the United States," *Pediatrics* 96 (1995, pt. 1): 23–28.

45. H.H. Glaser and O.N. Massengale, "Glue-Sniffing in Children: Deliberate Inhalation of Vaporized Plastic Cements," *Journal of the American Medical Association* 181 (1962): 300–304.

46. P.W. Lewis and D.W. Patterson, "Acute and Chronic Effects of the Voluntary Inhalation of Certain Commercial Volatile Solvents by Juveniles," *Journal of Drug Issues* 4 (1974): 167.

47. R.J. Goldsmith, "Death by Freon," *Journal of Clinical Psychiatry* 50 (1989): 36–37.

Alphabetical Listings of Drugs

All substances listed here have been declared a public concern by government officials, medical caregivers, or news media. If a listing mentions another drug's name in **bold type**, that drug has an entry of its own in this section of the book.

Some drugs have similar effects. For example, most anabolic steroids promote development of male characteristics when used by females. If an individual anabolic steroid is known to have that effect, that information is given in the individual listing. Such a style might make some entries seem repetitive if someone is looking up one anabolic steroid after another, but this approach improves the odds of important information being communicated. A cross-reference style that expects readers to flip back and forth among pages to "see this" or "see that" in order to avoid repetition might work for scientists, but for readers of this book, ease of usage is more important.

Although many drugs of abuse are described in this section, many others exist that are not included here. The choice of which to include and which to leave out was based on several factors. The first was whether a drug is listed in the U.S. government schedule of controlled substances. Another factor was whether a drug is abused even though it is not a controlled substance. Still another factor was whether enough data exist in the scientific literature to provide solid information. With some drugs described here, scientific information is scanty concerning particular aspects of a given drug, such as potential for causing cancer; that lack is specifically noted where relevant in drug descriptions.

Drugs are alphabetized by common name. Listings are arranged in the following manner:

Pronunciation: The proper way to pronounce a substance's name is given here. Sometimes alternative pronunciations are included.

Chemical Abstracts Service Registry Number: This number (CAS RN) is unique to every chemical, just like a fingerprint or a U.S. Social Security number is unique to each person. Drugs, like people, may go by different names, but different-sounding drugs having the same CAS RN are identical—that is, chemically and structurally the same. The CAS RN can be used to search various databases for more information about a drug and can also be used to confirm that a scientific report is indeed about the drug in question.

Formal Names: Entries in this section are a partial list of brand names and generic names. Some are for combination products including the drug. These names are used by scientists and health care providers.

Informal Names: These are casual and slang terms for the drug. The lists are not necessarily complete, but they do include typical informal names. Some nicknames are used for more than one drug.

Type: The type of drug and its class are given so a reader can refer to pages elsewhere in this book having background information about that substance.

Federal Schedule Listing: The status line gives the drug's legal standing (see page 6 for explanations of "schedules") and the U.S. Drug Enforcement Administration Controlled Substances Code Number if the drug is a controlled substance.

USA Availability: The availability line tells what must normally be done to obtain the substance legally in the United States. Normally Schedule V substances are prescription, but can be nonprescription in some state jurisdictions. A nonprescription item may still have other regulations limiting its availability, such as requiring a purchaser to be an adult or to register the purchase, as with over-the-counter (OTC) codeine-containing cough medicines. A substance may be legally available but may become illegal if used in prohibited ways.

Pregnancy Category: Not all drugs have an official pregnancy category designation. For example, such a rating does not exist for substances lacking official approval for therapeutic use. See page 8 for an explanation of categories.

Occasionally information in one of the above listings could not be verified despite diligent search. In such cases the topic is omitted.

The detailed descriptions of each drug are arranged to cover:

- uses
- drawbacks
- abuse factors
- (some but not all) drug interactions
- cancer (risks)
- pregnancy (effects)
- (in some cases) additional information

Reliable sources of additional scientific information are suggested at the end of each individual substance entry. At the back of this book is a list of general information sources, some of which may have additional data about the substance covered in the alphabetical entry. Many drugs have been studied for decades, and some references reflect the venerable history of such studies.

Drug descriptions occasionally mention the following concepts:

One drug may be stronger than another, but such a comparison depends not only on the effect being measured but on the animal species being tested. Frogs, chickens, and rats may react very differently than humans would to an equivalent dose of various drugs. For example, **bufotenine** and **LSD** effects are thousands of times stronger in humans than in monkeys; a dose that leaves a small monkey unfazed might devastate a human. Animal experiments are useful to know about, but the results do not necessarily extrapolate to humans. When this book compares strengths of drugs, the comparison simply gives a rough idea of strengths and has no bearing on determining what size dose of one drug would be equivalent to another size dose of a different substance.

When one drug is said to "boost" the effect of another, this means the increase is more than would be expected from simply adding the effect of one drug to the other $(1 + 1 = 2)$ but instead involves synergistic chemical and biological processes yielding a total that is more than the combination of parts $(1 + 1 = 3)$.

"Flashback" is an ability (voluntary or involuntary) to reexperience a drug state without taking the substance. Some details about flashback are given in this book's description of **LSD**, although the phenomenon is not limited to that drug (see also, for example, this book's listings about **methamphetamine** and **psilocybin**).

"Polydrug" abuse is a typical element of setting. For example, **heroin** addicts normally abuse other drugs as well. Someone who takes **MDMA** at a dance club may well take **cocaine** at the same time, just as some persons simultaneously smoke tobacco and drink **alcohol**. Even if all the compounds inside an illicit user can be verified, determining which is responsible for which effect can be challenging. This book's alphabetical section presents both the conclusions and doubts that scientists express about polydrug use, along with some classic interactions that occur when more than one drug is taken at the same time. Individuals who get into a medical emergency after drug use should bring samples of substances to health care providers; an item may not be what a user thinks it is, and effective treatment must be based on chemical reality rather than consumer belief.

Animal experiments may show that a drug can cause cancer or birth defects. The practical meaning of such results is sometimes clouded because the same drug may affect different species in different ways. Also animal tests sometimes involve many times the recommended human dose, perhaps levels high enough to poison the animals. These kinds of tests are not meaningless but may involve levels of risk unlikely to be experienced by humans. And yet large doses having no effect on animals do not guarantee a drug's safety for pregnant women. In some countries a compound called thalidomide was approved for human use after animal tests revealed no potential for causing birth defects, but in humans the substance produced severe congenital malformations such as missing or highly deformed limbs.

Experiments testing a drug occasionally produce conflicting results—some may say a drug does something; some may indicate the drug will not do it. These kinds of uncertainties are unsatisfying, but that is the way scientific research operates. Perhaps conflicting results come from differences in dosage size, or the manner in which a dose is given, or diet, or living conditions, or any number of other causes. Perhaps the conflict is due to researcher errors—a classic error being failure to run adequate controls (for example, failing to give the drug and a placebo in the same manner to a large number of the same kind of experimental subjects). The size of a drug experiment can also be a problem. Many involve a handful of volunteers. Conclusions from small studies (that is, studies involving a small number of test subjects) are not as significant as conclusions from studies measuring thousands of persons. Sometimes drug effect information is based on medical case reports, in which something has happened to one person but has not been experimentally tested to determine how typical the effect is. Malnourishment and physical afflictions can affect drug actions. Another tricky angle occurs when reports say a drug is "associated" with an effect, meaning the drug is administered and an effect follows. "Before and after" time sequence is not the same as "cause and effect" (chanting may be associated with the subsequent end of a solar eclipse, but it does not cause the termination). In scientific drug reports what scientists say about drugs can be less certain than what public policymakers say.

This section of the book strives to present the consensus of mainstream scientific thought. However, sometimes the only available information comes from observations lacking experimental confirmation, at the present time; the reader should keep in mind that by definition such observations are not yet part of a consensus even if they are reported in scientific journals.

AET

Pronunciation: ā-ee-tee

Chemical Abstracts Service Registry Number: 2235-90-7

Formal Names: Alpha-Ethyltryptamine, Etryptamine, Monase

Informal Names: Alpha-ET, Alpha-Ethyl, ET, Love Pearls, Love Pills, Trips

Type: Hallucinogen. *See* page 25

Federal Schedule Listing: Schedule I (DEA no. 7249)

USA Availability: Illegal to possess

Pregnancy Category: None

Uses. This substance has been used for decades. It has similarities to **DMT** in chemistry and actions and was made a Schedule I substance partly because some AET effects are reminiscent of **MDMA**. As a Schedule I substance AET has no approved medical use in the United States but has been used elsewhere (in Europe, for example) as an antidepressant.

Intoxication symptoms can resemble those of amphetamine, and urine tests for amphetamine can also pick up AET. When AET was given to rats, in some ways they responded as if they had received either amphetamine or MDMA.

A researcher who used AET reported enjoyable sensations of energy and contentment. As dosage increased, so did euphoria and enjoyment of sensual activity such as eating, music, and sex. In several accounts of effects hallucinations were not reported.

Drawbacks. AET has been associated with agranulocytosis, a blood disease involving development of sores in various places throughout the body.

Abuse factors. Tolerance is reported. Some opiate abusers trying to break their addiction have used AET to ease opiate withdrawal symptoms.

Drug interactions. AET is a monoamine oxidase inhibitor (MAOI), a type of drug that can interact dangerously with some of the other drugs described in this book.

Cancer. Not enough scientific information to report.

Pregnancy. Not enough scientific information to report.

Additional scientific information may be found in:

Daldrup, T., et al. "Etryptamine, a New Designer Drug with a Fatal Effect." *Zeitschrift für Rechtsmedizin* 97 (1986): 61–68 (article in German, but summary available in English).

Huang, X.M., M.P. Johnson, and D.E. Nichols. "Reduction in Brain Serotonin Markers by Alpha-Ethyltryptamine (Monase)." *European Journal of Pharmacology* 200 (1991): 187–90.

Krebs, K.M., and M.A. Geyer. "Behavioral Characterization of Alpha-Ethyltryptamine, a Tryptamine Derivative with MDMA-Like Properties in Rats." *Psychopharmacology* (Berlin) 113 (1993): 284–87.

Morano, R.A., et al. "Fatal Intoxication Involving Etryptamine." *Journal of Forensic Sciences* 38 (1993): 721–25.

Alcohol

Pronunciation: AL-kuh-hall

Chemical Abstracts Service Registry Number: 64-17-5

Formal Names: Ethanol, Ethyl Alcohol, Hydroxy Ethane

Informal Names: Liquor

Type: Depressant. *See* p. 19

Federal Schedule Listing: Unlisted

USA Availability: Freely available to adults; various jurisdictions limit access to minors; some pharmaceutical preparations are prescription

Uses. Various kinds of alcohol exist; many are poisonous, such as wood alcohol, and are not intended for drinking. Those types are not substances of abuse and are not discussed in this book.

In former times physicians prescribed alcohol as a treatment for assorted afflictions. That usage is largely outmoded, but alcohol is still a common ingredient in cough remedies, is applied to skin as a disinfectant, and is a component of some injectable solutions. Alcohol is used as a partial antidote for methanol poisoning associated with inhalant abuse, and it is used to combat glycol poisoning. In some medical procedures alcohol is administered to create a form of anesthesia called a nerve block. Around 1970 at one hospital a combination of alcohol and **chloral hydrate** was routinely given to make pregnant women unconscious during labor, although alcohol is also a treatment for stopping premature labor. The substance can be a sleep aid (a "nightcap" drink), but researchers have found that it interferes with dreaming, which is an important component of sleep. Tolerance can develop to sleep-inducing actions, and dream content can become disturbing for awhile after usage stops. Some persons drink alcohol to cope with stress. Evidence exists that moderate consumption of wine may help people live longer by reducing risk of heart disease and cancer.

Drawbacks. As with many other drugs, moderate recreational use can be pleasurable while causing little harm. In contrast, excessive use can not only have psychological effects harmful to family and social functioning but also injure the stomach, liver, kidneys, heart, and brain. Rat experiments have demonstrated damage to the pancreas, damage that is boosted by cigarette smoke. A study found that men with spinal osteoporosis, a disease increasing the likelihood of broken bones, drink more alcohol than persons without the disease; this finding does not mean that alcohol causes the affliction, but it does indicate the need for further research. Alcohol does not make peaceful individuals rageful, but it can lower inhibitions while leaving a person able to act out urges. Thus violent and criminal acts are commonly associated with alcohol intoxication. Impairment of mental and physical activity can occur during acute intoxication, making operation of dangerous machinery (such as automobiles) hazardous. During intoxication sensory perceptions are blunted, reducing awareness of tastes, smells, sounds, and pain.

Lesser known problems are associated with alcohol. Male users experience a decline in **testosterone** levels, and females may experience menstrual difficulties. The nerve inflammation disease beriberi has been linked with alcoholism, and research has raised the possibility that alcoholism can worsen Alzheimer's disease. Some studies report that drinkers have a slightly higher chance of developing cataracts, but a very large study involving 77,466 women found little, if any, relationship between the substance and cataracts. Experiments show that a drink of alcohol encourages more cigarette consumption and that persons who use both alcohol and **nicotine** tend to drink more when cigarettes are unavailable. Although alcohol can make a person feel hotter, that effect is superficial; the substance actually lowers body temperature, making alcohol counterproductive if a chilled person is trying to warm up; the substance should not be given to persons injured by exposure to cold temperatures. Alcoholics commonly have memory trouble, and small studies find that heavy-drinking nonalcoholics have impaired thinking skills even while sober.

Abuse factors. In addition to being a potent intoxicant, alcohol is one of the most addictive substances. Tolerance ("holding your liquor") and dependence may occur. Withdrawal can be dangerous, with death occurring (typically from difficulties leading to convulsions) despite intense medical supervision. The withdrawal syndrome is called delirium tremens. Its symptoms are similar to those of barbiturate withdrawal: weariness, nervousness, perspiration, tremors, vomiting, cramps, high blood pressure, accelerated heartbeat, convulsions, and hallucinations. Symptoms may be worse in elderly persons.

Women tend to be more affected by alcohol than men are because, among other reasons, the drug has more bioavailability in females (more of a given dose is used in females, so they need less quantity than men do in order to reach the same level of effect).

Drug interactions. Alcohol lengthens the duration of effects from **chlordiazepoxide**, **diazepam**, and **lorazepam**. **Cocaine** worsens liver damage caused by alcohol. When rats receiving **morphine** or **methadone** drink alcohol, the alcohol blood level takes longer to increase but then lasts longer, a result suggesting that a human opiate user might have to drink more in order to get an alcohol effect and would then stay intoxicated longer than someone who does not use opiates. Rat studies indicate that steady opiate consumption may intensify alcohol dependence. In rats, alcohol, chlordiazepoxide, and **pentobarbital** all have cross-tolerance with one another, meaning that one will substitute for the other to some extent. So many drugs interact dangerously with alcohol that a person should always check information labels on drug containers before using the substances simultaneously with alcohol.

Cancer. Most laboratory tests give no indication that alcohol has a potential for causing cancer. Nonetheless, mice experimentation indicates that long-term use of alcohol can cause liver cancer. Human reports indicate an increased risk for prostate cancer. Women who take more than two drinks a day have an increased risk of breast cancer. A study of 8,006 Japanese men in Hawaii found an association between alcohol and cancer of the lungs and rectum, but "association" is not the same as cause and effect. Evidence indicates that saliva might transform alcohol in ways that promote oral cancer.

Pregnancy. A study of 430 couples in Denmark found fertility to decline among women as their alcohol consumption increased, but no effect was observed on male fertility. In contrast, a study of farm couples in Canada found no difference in fertility between women who did or did not drink alcohol. Still another study, in the Netherlands, found male alcohol consumers to have higher fertility as consumption increased, with no difference in fertility rate between women who drank different amounts. Such findings of sometimes yes, sometimes no, are a classic sign of an "invalid variable," which in this case would mean that no difference in fertility can be attributed to alcohol (although more studies would be needed to reach a firm conclusion, and some authorities say the trend of research indicates that alcohol does reduce female fertility).

A study found that premature infants were more likely among pregnant teenagers who drank alcohol than among those who did not. That effect was not seen among older pregnant women who drank. Other research has noted lower birthweights among children delivered by pregnant alcohol consumers.

A human experiment documented fetal response to two glasses of wine drunk by women whose pregnancies were close to time of delivery: In that experiment fetal respiration and sleep were disturbed—which did not surprise researchers because heavy consumers of alcohol frequently give birth to infants having sleep difficulties. Such newborns may also have tremors and poor reflexes and cry more than normal. Children can be born dependent on the drug.

Alcohol is a well-known cause of birth defects. In mice the substance is known to cause a facial deformity called holoprosencephaly, and a human case report suggests that heavy dosage can do the same in humans. Less dramatic facial characteristics are common after substantial prenatal exposure to alcohol. Other human birth defects attributed to alcohol include kidney, heart, and brain trouble. More subtle damage has been measured as a slight decline in IQ among schoolchildren of mothers who took two or more drinks a day during pregnancy. Male exposure to some drugs can produce birth defects, and researchers have found problems in behavior and thinking skills among children of alcoholic fathers as well as among offspring of pregnant alcoholics. Fetal alcohol syndrome (FAS) is a collection of afflictions observed in children typically born to women who had six or more drinks a day while pregnant. The syndrome may include low birthweight, defective vision, delayed development, specific facial characteristics, trouble with muscles and joints, heart abnormality, and mental retardation. Problems can be long-lasting and even permanent. Prenatal exposure to alcohol can delay motor skill development in children, cause difficulties in maintaining balance, and limit growth in height. Such children may be more impulsive and aggressive. A study of adolescents compared two groups, one born with FAS and another whose mothers drank little or no alcohol during pregnancy. The FAS group showed impairment in some types of memory, attention, thinking, and learning—findings supported by other research as well. Some researchers believe that fetal exposure to alcohol has more to do with teenage drinking than family environment does. Comparing adults with heavy prenatal alcohol exposure to those without such exposure, a small study measured significant psychiatric differences, particularly with the alcohol subjects being more depressed and fearful.

Fetal damage from maternal alcohol use is unquestionable, but the amount of use necessary to cause damage is less certain and can be affected by a woman's general physical condition and lifestyle (including nutrition and other drug usage). Occasional binge drinking and routine heavy drinking are certainly hazardous to fetal development, but for many years pregnant women have used alcohol in moderation without apparent effect on offspring. Nonetheless, in general, women are now advised to avoid any alcohol consumption during pregnancy.

Experimenters note that alcohol consumption reduces mothers' milk production but does not affect energy provided by the milk. Alcohol levels in milk are similar to a mother's blood levels. A nursing infant may be sickened by milk from a mother who abuses alcohol—an infant has not yet developed the proper body chemistry to break down alcohol, so a dose lasts longer in an infant than in an older child or adult.

Additional information. Beverage alcohol is a powerful intoxicant. Alcohol is also probably the most familiar drug, used so freely that many persons regard it solely as a beverage rather than as a drug. Indeed, for many years excessive drunkenness was considered a moral failing rather than a disease, and not until the 1950s was alcoholism officially recognized as an affliction appropriate for medical treatment.

By the 1800s drunkenness had become a major public concern in the United States. Temperance societies, organizations whose members pledged to avoid beverage alcohol and to discourage consumption by other persons, became politically powerful. Before the Civil War such groups had been able to get laws passed outlawing the sale of beverage alcohol in various communities and sometimes throughout entire states. Shortly after World War I this agitation culminated in the Eighteenth Amendment to the Constitution of the United States, giving the federal government power to ban manufacture and sale of beverage alcohol. Although purchase and consumption remained legal, the majority of Americans became so displeased with Prohibition that the Twenty-first Amendment to the Constitution was passed in the 1930s repealing the earlier one.

Additional scientific information may be found in:

Chasan-Taber, L. et al. "A Prospective Study of Alcohol Consumption and Cataract Extraction among U.S. Women." *Annals of Epidemiology* 10 (2000): 347–53.
Curtis, K.M, D.A. Savitz, and T.E. Arbuckle. "Effects of Cigarette Smoking, Caffeine

Consumption, and Alcohol Intake on Fecundability." *American Journal of Epidemiology* 146 (1997): 32–41.

Florack, E.I., G.A. Zielhuis, and R. Rolland. "Cigarette Smoking, Alcohol Consumption, and Caffeine Intake and Fecundability." *Preventive Medicine* 23 (1994): 175–80.

Gronbaek, M., et al. "Type of Alcohol Consumed and Mortality from All Causes, Coronary Heart Disease, and Cancer." *Annals of Internal Medicine* 133 (2000): 411–19.

Jensen, T.K. "Does Moderate Alcohol Consumption Affect Fertility? Follow up Study among Couples Planning First Pregnancy." *BMJ* 317 (1998): 505–10.

Kraus, L., et al. "Prevalence of Alcohol Use and the Association between Onset of Use and Alcohol-Related Problems in a General Population Sample in Germany." *Addiction* 95 (2000): 1389–1401.

Moore, M.H., and D.R. Gerstein, eds. *Alcohol and Public Policy: Beyond the Shadow of Prohibition.* Washington, DC: National Academy Press, 1981.

Phillips, B.J., and P. Jenkinson. "Is Ethanol Genotoxic? A Review of the Published Data." *Mutagenesis* 16 (2001): 91–101.

Pihl, R.O., M. Smith, and B. Farrell. "Individual Characteristics of Aggressive Beer and Distilled Beverage Drinkers." *International Journal of the Addictions* 19 (1984): 689–96.

Pollack, E.S. "Prospective Study of Alcohol Consumption and Cancer." *New England Journal of Medicine* 310 (1984): 617–21.

Weinberg, N.Z. "Cognitive and Behavioral Deficits Associated with Parental Alcohol Use." *Journal of the American Academy of Child and Adolescent Psychiatry* 36 (1997): 1177–86.

Alprazolam

Pronunciation: al-PRAY-zoh-lam (also pronounced al-PRAZ-oh-lam)
Chemical Abstracts Service Registry Number: 28981-97-7
Formal Names: Alplax, Frontal, Solanax, Tafil, Trankimazin, Xanax, Xanor, Zotran
Type: Depressant (benzodiazepine class). *See* page 21
Federal Schedule Listing: Schedule IV (DEA no. 2882)
USA Availability: Prescription
Pregnancy Category: D

Uses. This calming and sleep-inducing substance is probably the most frequently prescribed drug in the benzodiazepine class. Alprazolam is used mainly to help persons suffering from panic attacks and other anxiety disorders, but it is not recommended for posttraumatic stress disorder. The compound can dramatically lessen premenstrual syndrome (PMS) and is routinely given to women of child-bearing age. Improvement of PMS is not invariable, however, and two careful experiments yielded results showing little benefit. Theoretical reasons and results from a rat experiment suggest that alprazolam may help maintain bone mass. That action may be especially important to athletes and elderly women, who commonly suffer loss of bone mass—an affliction making breakage easier. The drug has been tested as an asthma treatment with encouraging results, though reasons for success are unclear. Some researchers believe the drug has potential in diabetes control. In an experiment measuring alprazolam's pain-relieving properties, the drug reduced the severity but not the frequency of chronic tension headaches. The compound has antidepressant and anticonvulsant properties, has been used to treat ringing in the ears and to alleviate tremors and catatonia, and has been found useful in easing **alcohol** withdrawal symptoms in alcoholics. A rat study suggests that alprazolam may also have a place in treating **cocaine** addiction. Measurements find the drug worsens snoring but improves quality of sleep (at least for the snorers).

Drawbacks. Motorists have suffered accidents attributed to drowsiness from alprazolam. Experiments show that the drug reduces startle response in humans, which may mean drivers are less alert or respond less vigorously to situations. Case reports tell of alprazolam (alone and in combination with other medicine) causing the skin to become extra sensitive to sunlight. The compound may produce jaundice.

Although the drug normally encourages eating, about 20% of persons in one study experienced weight loss, along with unwanted effects such as difficulty in controlling muscles (including urinary incontinence), peevishness, bellicosity, and lowering of inhibitions. Researchers generally believe the drug interferes with sexual function in men and women. A case report tells of the drug causing mania with euphoria, high self-confidence, increased energy, and trouble with getting proper sleep—all rather untypical effects. Despite such possibilities, one team reviewing scientific literature found reports of unwanted actions to be uncommon for alprazolam, and another team concluded that alprazolam generally has fewer such reports than other benzodiazepine class drugs. Analysts who examined medical records of 10,895 alprazolam patients found little mention of unwanted effects. In evaluating the infrequent accounts of mania, aggression, hallucinations, or other unexpected psychological reactions to alprazolam, we should remember that many such cases involve persons already exhibiting psychiatric disturbances for which they are receiving the drug. Such reactions may be far less likely in a psychiatrically normal person.

Abuse factors. An experiment showed no tendency for abuse of alprazolam among users even though it is a controlled substance. A 1993 review of human and animal studies of the drug concluded that scientific experimental evidence failed to support a popular belief that abuse of alprazolam was more likely than abuse of other benzodiazepine class drugs. Another 1993 report disagreed but described alprazolam abuse as minuscule and limited to persons already misusing other drugs, particularly opiates and alcohol. Brainwave and other measurements imply that alprazolam has more appeal to alcoholic men than it does to nonalcoholics. Experiments show that persons with a family history of alcoholism tend to experience more pleasure (even euphoria) when taking alprazolam than do persons lacking such a history. Tests find the drug to have stronger effects (positive *and* negative) on women whose fathers were alcoholics, compared to women whose immediate family background does not include alcoholism. When experiments gave drug abusers a choice between **diazepam** or alprazolam, the abusers tried both but found alprazolam more pleasant.

Craving and tolerance do not seem to develop, but alprazolam can produce bodily dependence, which is a traditional sign of addictive potential. Sudden stoppage can cause seizures or delirium, so practitioners customarily wean their patients with tapering dosages. Withdrawal symptoms may include perspiration, tremors, cramps, vomiting, diarrhea, cloudy eyesight, prickling sensations on the skin, and general befuddlement. Convulsions and seizures are reported. One experiment noted that withdrawal signs cleared up in a week.

Drug interactions. Kava is an intoxicating drink prepared from the kava plant, suspected of interacting so seriously with alprazolam that a coma may result. Persons taking antifungus drugs such as itraconazole or ketoconazole are supposed to avoid alprazolam, as those two drugs increase the power and prolong the effect of an alprazolam dose. The heartburn medicine cimetidine (Tagamet), the antidepressant fluoxetine (Prozac), and the pain-relieving opioid **propoxyphene** each lengthen the time an alprazolam dose lasts, and ritonavir (used against the human immunodeficiency virus in AIDS [acquired immunodeficiency syndrome]) can drastically boost the potency of alprazolam. In contrast, alprazolam's effects are reduced by the epilepsy drugs phenytoin and carbamazepine, by the tuberculosis medicine rifampin, and by the asthma medication theophylline. A case of glaucoma resulting in blindness is attributed to a multidrug regimen of antidepressants and antianxiety medicines including alprazolam. Some tests find that the substance worsens reaction time and memory. Taking alprazolam with diazepam can cause persons to forget what happened while they were under the drugs' influence. In one experiment alprazolam by itself seemed to interfere with memory even weeks after taking it, but deeper analysis of the results caused investigators to question any long-lasting effect. Persons functioning adequately while drinking alcohol decline in performance when a dose of alprazolam is added, and the combination may increase hostile attitudes and actions. Findings in a mice experiment showed alprazolam boosting pain relief provided by **morphine**, but a human experiment found no such increase (although alprazolam reduced the typical nausea effect of morphine—a benefit that has also been demonstrated in cancer chemotherapy patients). Alprazolam has crosstolerance with **chlordiazepoxide**.

Cancer. A two-year rat experiment found no evidence that alprazolam causes cancer. Measurements of persons receiving alprazolam for panic disorder indicated the substance does not reduce levels of tumor necrosis factoralpha, a protein that helps the body fight off cancer.

Pregnancy. Alprazolam experimentation with mice yielded no birth defects. Examination of pregnancies in which women used the drug during the first trimester found no more birth defects than would be expected if the drug were not taken at all, but researchers cautioned that the sample sizes (411 in one study and about 200 in another) were too small to reach firm conclusions about the drug's effect on fetal development. A study of 88 infants born to women who used alprazolam during pregnancy found 10 born with "major" deformities. Mice having prenatal exposure to the drug show reduced social interaction, and males are more aggressive than normal. Such mice also exhibit subtle trouble with hind legs.

Clinicians have observed alprazolam to increase the hormone that prepares female breasts for milk production. When combined with the pain reliever tramadol and the antidepressant citalopram, alprazolam has been known to cause excessive milk flow. Alprazolam passes into milk, and nursing is not recommended for mothers taking the drug. In one case an infant even exhibited drug withdrawal symptoms when a nursing mother who was receiving alprazolam ceased nursing.

Additional scientific information may be found in:

Edwards, J.G. "Prescription-Event Monitoring of 10,895 Patients Treated with Alprazolam." *British Journal of Psychiatry* 158 (1991): 387–92.

Jonas, J.M., and M.S. Cohon. "A Comparison of the Safety and Efficacy of Alprazolam versus Other Agents in the Treatment of Anxiety, Panic, and Depression: A Review of the Literature." *Journal of Clinical Psychiatry* 54 (1993, Suppl.): 25–45.

Nishith, P., et al. "Brief Hypnosis Substitutes for Alprazolam Use in College Students:

Transient Experiences and Quantitative EEG Responses." *American Journal of Clinical Hypnosis* 41 (1999): 262–68.

Romach, M.K. et al. "Characteristics of Long-Term Alprazolam Users in the Community." *Journal of Clinical Psychopharmacology* 12 (1992): 316–21.

Rothschild, A.J. "Comparison of the Frequency of Behavorial Disinhibition on Alprazolam, Clonazepam, or No Benzodiazepine in Hospitalized Psychiatric Patients." *Journal of Clinical Psychopharmacology* 20 (2000): 7–11.

Rush, C.R., et al. "Abuse Liability of Alprazolam Relative to Other Commonly Used Benzodiazepines: A Review." *Neuroscience and Biobehavorial Reviews* 17 (1993): 277–85.

Sellers, E.M., et al. "Alprazolam and Benzodiazepine Dependence." *Journal of Clinical Psychiatry* 54 (1993, Suppl.): 64–75.

Spiegel, D.A. "Efficacy Studies of Alprazolam in Panic Disorder." *Psychopharmacology Bulletin* 34 (1998): 191–95.

Amanita

Pronunciation: am-uh-NEYE-tuh
Chemical Abstracts Service Registry Number: None
Formal Names: *Amanita muscaria*
Informal Names: Aga, Fly Agaric
Type: Hallucinogen. *See* page 25
Federal Schedule Listing: Unlisted
USA Availability: Nonprescription natural product
Pregnancy Category: None

Uses. These mushrooms are found in much of the Northern Hemisphere and are known to grow elsewhere. Due to the possibility that an effective dose is close to a poisonous dose, and because of variations in potency, these mushrooms are easily poisonous and have even been mixed with milk as bait to kill flies. Persons seeking amanita sometimes accidentally ingest *Amanita phalloides*, also called Death Cap and Death Cup, which can be deadly poisonous to the kidneys and liver. Confusion with other dangerous mushrooms has also harmed people seeking *Amanita muscaria*.

The *Amanita muscaria* mushroom has been used to treat **alcohol** overdose and to relieve nervousness, fever, and pain of sore throat, nerves, and joints. The natural product contains muscimol, a chemical that initially acts as a stimulant but that can later produce temporary loss of muscular control as the drug action proceeds. Muscarine chloride can be prepared from amanita. In various animal species muscarine chloride can cause spasms and constrictions and lower blood pressure. The relevance of those studies to humans is unclear; for example, a dose that would poison a human leaves a monkey unfazed. **Bufotenine** has been reported in amanita, but the report is disputed. The ibotenic acid in amanita can produce hallucinations; a case report mentions visual hallucinations lasting for days after ingesting the mushroom. The mushroom is said to produce euphoria and to cause changes in sensory perceptions. Some persons consume the fungus for spiritual purpose, a practice that some authorities date back to ancient Buddhist times, with the Buddhists perhaps learning the custom from still older examples among forest peoples in northern Europe and Asia. Usage by Siberian shamans has been documented in modern times. Drug-induced insight into personal psychological issues is reported.

Drawbacks. One user describes the experience as lacking in feelings of happiness, or love, or sexual impulses—a lack that sets amanita apart from many drugs that are used recreationally. A scientist who engaged in self-experimentation had similar results of emptiness. Of 6 subjects who received the mushroom in an experiment, all were nauseated, 2 vomited, 1 had hallucinations, and several had sensory distortions. None cared to repeat the experience. The supervising researcher wondered if variations in supplies of the natural product explained why the experiment's results differed so greatly from hallucinations and pleasures reported by other persons. Personality, expectations, and surrounding environment can shape the experience. A researcher interviewed 18 persons who ate *Amanita muscaria* or *Amanita pantherina*; half had eaten the mushrooms deliberately, and half thought they were consuming something else. Every person who accidentally ate the substance found its actions unpleasant. In contrast, the mushroom's effects were enjoyed by every individual who deliberately ate it.

Because active chemicals from the natural product are excreted into urine, people can dose themselves again by drinking their own urine, a dosage method that may horrify Americans but that a few other cultures have accepted calmly.

Unwanted amanita effects can include twitching, cramps, abdominal discomfort, sweating, nausea, vomiting, diarrhea, dizziness, confusion, rapid heartbeat, difficulty in moving around, high body temperature, and convulsions. Users can become manic and then sleepy, with those conditions alternating back and forth until a person collapses. Scientific journals contain many articles about brain damage caused by ibotenic acid, although conditions of experiments do not necessarily duplicate what happens when mushrooms are eaten. A person who received a dose of ibotenic acid in an experiment developed a headache for two weeks. Under laboratory conditions amanita extracts cause red blood cells to clump together.

Abuse factors. Not enough scientific information to report.

Drug interactions. Not enough scientific information to report.

Cancer. Not enough scientific information to report.

Pregnancy. The muscimol in amanita causes birth defects in rats.

Additional scientific information may be found in:

Davis, D.P., and S.R. Williams. "Amanita Muscaria." *Journal of Emergency Medicine* 17 (1999): 739.

Fabing, H.D. "On Going Berserk: A Neurochemical Inquiry." *Scientific Monthly* 83 (1956): 232–37.

Horne, C.H.W., and J.A.W. McCluskie. "The Food of the Gods." *Scottish Medical Journal* 8 (1963): 489–91.

McDonald, A. "The Present Status of Soma: The Effects of California *Amanita muscaria* on Normal Human Volunteers." In *Mushroom Poisoning: Diagnosis and Treatment*, ed. B.H. Rumack and E. Salzman. West Palm Beach, FL: CRC Press, 1978. 215–23.

Ott, J. "Psycho-Mycological Studies of Amanita: From Ancient Sacrament to Modern Phobia." *Journal of Psychedelic Drugs* 8 (January–March 1976): 27–35.

Areca Nut

Pronunciation: AR-i-kuh nut (also pronounced uh-REE-kuh nut)

Chemical Abstracts Service Registry Number: None

Formal Names: *Areca catechu*

Informal Names: Betel Nut, Katha, Pinang, Pugua

Type: Stimulant (pyridine alkaloids class). *See* page 18

Federal Schedule Listing: Unlisted

USA Availability: Nonprescription natural product, but restrictions apply to interstate commerce

Pregnancy Category: None

Uses. Accounts of areca nuts date back to at least 504 B.C. They are about the size of a cherry and come from palm trees in the Indian Ocean region, grown in countries such as India, China, and the Philippines. Trees reach up to 90 feet in height, and nuts are about an inch in diameter. The product is used not only as a drug but also as a dye and in the leather tanning industry. Drug use of areca nut is common in South Africa, India, Taiwan, and other areas of South Asia and the Pacific basin. The product has been unfamiliar in the United States, but is available and is used in some immigrant communities.

Areca nut is a popular recreational stimulant relieving tension and producing euphoria, regularly used by perhaps 200 million to 600 million persons, making it one of the most popular substances in the world. Users commonly put the nuts in a quid (a chewable cut) as with **coca** or tobacco. Effects may be unpleasant for new chewers: nausea, dizziness, burning sensation in the mouth, a closing sensation in the throat. With perseverance, those unwanted effects are replaced by desired ones. As with **alcohol**, in lands ranging from India to New Guinea areca nut has a place in religious and other ceremonies (engagements to marry, offerings to spirits), but the product's main use is secular. In some places, areca nut is a social lubricant, much as beer is used in the United States. Paraphernalia involved with consuming areca nut may be either utilitarian or highly decorated functional artwork. The product adds a smell to the breath that many people find appealing. As with tobacco quids, users typically spit out areca nut juice, staining walls or other targets. Because such a practice may potentially promote the spread of disease, in some places large cans are lined with plastic bags and used as spittoons.

Comments from one user make the substance sound like fast-acting **caf-**

feine; another user talked of a mild background stimulation accompanied by pleasant enhancements of perception; still another user described a brightening of colors, with motions around him becoming jerky, as in old-time silent movies or modern Internet videos, and said he felt relaxed. (Those descriptions are anecdotal, not from scientific journals.) Areca nut users generally explain the experience as reducing hunger, tiredness, anxiety, and peevishness while increasing contentment and alertness—effects reminiscent of coca chewing. Some people simply use the quids as a cheaper substitute for chewing gum. Areca nut usage is seen more often in older persons than in younger and may therefore be declining. Younger persons do indulge, however. One survey found up to 16% of high school students in Taiwan regularly using the substance. Areca nut and **nicotine** both influence some of the same parts of the central nervous system in similar ways.

Chewers widely believe areca nut aids digestion. Chewing the substance can slow or accelerate pulse rate, raise or lower blood pressure, promote salivation and tremors, and increase body temperature and sweating. Outdoor workers use areca nut to combat cold weather. Areca nut is used to rid humans of worms. The substance is also a treatment for worms and constipation in animals. Traditional healing applications include treatment of edema, hepatitis, gum disease, inadequate urine output, and gastrointestinal complaints including both constipation and diarrhea. Investigators find that areca nut reduces schizophrenia symptoms in schizophrenic chewers. Nonetheless, the natural product has little place in modern medicine.

Some authorities describe areca nut's actions as similar to amphetamine. Although areca nut is a stimulant, its ability to improve workplace performance is unproven. One laboratory study demonstrated that the substance is unlikely to worsen job performance; another laboratory study showed improvement in some reaction time; still another showed longer reaction time. Tests of workers who operated heavy earth-moving equipment while using areca nut found evidence that the men were more alert, but otherwise they exhibited no effect that would influence job performance; measurements included short-term memory, reaction time, and eye-hand coordination.

A chemical refined from areca nut (Areca II-5-C) shows excellent potential as a medicine to reduce blood pressure, even though the natural product tends to raise blood pressure. Experiments with areca nut's pyridine alkaloid arecoline indicate that the chemical can improve memory in mice, and arecoline produces the same benefit in persons suffering from Alzheimer's disease (although improvement may be marginal). Still other chemicals isolated from areca nut seem to have potential for inhibiting formation of plaque on teeth, although in practice areca nut chewers have more plaque than nonchewers. Chewers, however, also seem to have less tooth decay than nonchewers, and areca nut toothpaste has been marketed. Areca nut chewing is linked to a lower prevalence of a bowel disease called ulcerative colitis, but the possible protective effect has not been differentiated yet from tobacco smoking of chewers (nicotine is known to improve ulcerative colitis). One alcohol extract of areca nut has been successfully tested as a treatment for skin wrinkles, making people look younger. Another alcohol extract shows promise in treating inflammations, allergies, and cancer. Burning areca leaves at a campsite helps repel some types of mosquito, effectively enough that researchers say the practice can reduce spread of disease carried by mosquitoes.

Drawbacks. Overindulgence can produce hallucinations and delusions, but those effects are uncommon. Based on chemical properties, theoretical reason exists for expecting areca nut to promote diabetes; animal experiments exploring that hypothesis have been suggestive but not conclusive. Chewing areca nut produces large amounts of blood-red saliva, which over the years can turn teeth brown or black. The physical action of continual chewing day after day appears to promote breakage of tooth roots, while ever-present draining of saliva across corners of the mouth can crack that skin. Areca nut harms the antimicrobial ability of white blood cells, thereby promoting gum disease, but saliva of chewers apparently inhibits bacterial growth. Areca nut inhibits the body's access to vitamin B_1 and reduces metabolism of carbohydrates, a situation that may produce an exhausting disease called beriberi.

The arecoline drug in areca nut can cause asthma. Some researchers speculate that areca nut chewing helps explain why Asians are the predominant ethnic group hospitalized for asthma in Great Britain. Areca nut is known to reduce the healing qualities of asthma medications. Heartbeat abnormalities serious enough to hospitalize people have followed their chewing of areca nut, but a cause-effect relationship has not been established even though arecoline is known to cause cardiac crisis in dogs.

Because of chemical transformations caused by heat, using roasted nut instead of unroasted may reduce short-term adverse effects.

Pan masala is a product including areca nut and other substances. Pan masala interferes with liver activity in rats.

Abuse factors. Some researchers have concluded that areca nut is as addictive as tobacco cigarettes. Unquestionably some users feel a strong continual need for the product; one person spoke of arising in the middle of the night to dose herself. Mild withdrawal symptoms are common but can become strong enough that persons seek medical aid. Withdrawal symptoms can include fatigue, nervousness, depression, trouble with memory and concentration, and paranoia. Compared to nonchewers, generally areca nut chewers are more likely to smoke cigarettes and drink alcohol—although researchers studying schizophrenics find that, compared to nonchewers, schizophrenic areca nut chewers are less likely to use recreational substances causing more damage to themselves than areca nut does.

Drug interactions. Areca nut is believed to interact with psychiatric medicines that can produce tremors and spasms reminiscent of Parkinson's disease, worsening such adverse effects of the medicines. People using a preparation of areca nut and pumpkin seed have experienced dizziness and stomach upset. Animal experiments have identified a chemical in areca nut as an antidepressant operating as a monoamine oxidase inhibitor (MAOI), and various drugs described in this book react badly if used simultaneously with an MAOI.

Cancer. The nut is rich in tannins, chemicals that inhibit utilization of dietary protein and that promote cancer. An experiment injecting an areca nut extract into rats for almost a year and a half gave tumors to every rat. Various other animal experiments also indicate a danger of cancer from using areca nut, but scientists are uncertain that the substance causes cancer in humans unless used in combination with tobacco.

In a mice experiment a small percentage of animals receiving pan masala developed assorted cancers, but animals receiving no pan masala developed no cancers. Humans who habitually chew the nut can get noncancerous and precancerous abnormalities in the mouth. Fatal oral tumors may develop, but reports are not always clear about persons' use of other substances that may promote cancer. Oral submucous fibrosis (OSF) is a serious mouth disease directly attributed to chewing plain areca nut or pan masala. Some victims also chew or smoke tobacco. In evaluating precancerous and cancerous growths in the mouth, however, some researchers analyzing medical cases have found areca nut to be a far more likely cause of such afflictions than tobacco. (That type of research examines outcomes of drug usage, not mechanisms by which usage promotes cancer.) Animal experiments suggest that consuming alcohol may heighten the risk of mouth cancer from pan masala, a suggestion supported by clinical experience. Tests on pan masala users find them to suffer from increased DNA damage in tissues exposed to pan masala, a tendency duplicated in laboratory tests of pan masala and areca nut. Such chromosome damage is suspected of causing mouth, throat, and esophageal cancers ascribed to areca nut. A study examining the combined effects of pan masala, tobacco smoking, and alcohol drinking found that persons who do all three are 123 times more likely to get mouth cancer than persons who do none. Experiments suggest that vitamins A and E might help reduce the health risks of pan masala.

Pregnancy. In male mice pan masala damages chromosomes and sperm, and ingestion of pan masala by male rats has caused their gonads to shrink in weight. Examination of human uterine cells indicates mutation from chewing areca nut preparations. Examination of human white blood cells shows increased chromosome damage in pregnant women who chew areca nut preparations and still more damage if nonpregnant chewers use birth control pills. Chicken experiments produce birth defects when an alcohol extract of areca nut is injected into embryos, but results from chicken embryo testing are not accepted as evidence of human risk. One human study found that pregnant chewers were almost three times more likely to have adverse pregnancy outcomes than nonchewers. Another study found that infants of pregnant chewers had lower birth weight but were also less likely to have jaundice.

Additional information. Betel pepper leaves are chewed, but this plant (*Piper betle*, also called *Piper betel*) is not *Areca catechu*. Betel pepper leaves, areca nut, and mineral lime (not the fruit) are combined into a product called betel. Studies indicate that leaves of betel pepper reduce areca nut's ability to cause chromosome damage. Chewing betel is thought to convert arecoline into arecaidine, which some researchers consider more benign in its effects than arecoline.

Additional scientific information may be found in:

Burton-Bradley, B.G. "Arecaidinism: Betel Chewing in Transcultural Perspective." *Canadian Journal of Psychiatry* 24 (1979): 481–88.

Burton-Bradley, B.G. "Papua and New Guinea Transcultural Psychiatry: Some Implications of Betel Chewing." *Medical Journal of Australia* 16 (1966): 744–46.

Chittivelu, S., and K.S. Chittivelu. "Betel Nut Chewing and Cardiac Arrhythmia." *Veterinary and Human Toxicology* 40 (1998): 368.

Nelson, B.S., and B. Heischober. "Betel Nut: A Common Drug Used by Naturalized Citizens from India, Far East Asia, and the South Pacific Islands." *Annals of Emergency Medicine* 34 (1999): 238–43.

Norton, S.A. "Betel: Consumption and Consequences." *Journal of the American Academy of Dermatology* 38 (1998): 81–88.

Pickwell, S.M., S. Schimelpfening, and L.A. Palinkas. " 'Betelmania.' Betel Quid Chewing by Cambodian Women in the United States and Its Potential Health Effects." *Western Journal of Medicine* 160 (1994): 326–30.

Reichart, P.A., and H.P. Phillipsen. "Betel Chewer's Mucosa—A Review." *Journal of Oral Pathology and Medicine* 27 (1998): 239–42.

Wyatt, T.A. "Betel Nut Chewing and Selected Psychophysiological Variables." *Psychological Reports* 79 (1996): 451–63.

Belladonna

Pronunciation: bell-uh-DON-uh

Chemical Abstracts Service Registry Number: 8007-93-0

Formal Names: *Atropa belladonna*

Informal Names: Black Cherry, Deadly Nightshade, Death's Herb, Devil's Cherries, Devil's Herb, Divale, Dwale, Dwayberry, Great Morel, Love Apple, Murderer's Berry, Naughty Man's Cherries, Poison Black Cherry, Sleeping Nightshade, Sorcerers Berries, Sorcerer's Cherry, Witch's Berry

Type: Hallucinogen. *See* page 25

Federal Schedule Listing: Unlisted as natural product

USA Availability: Nonprescription natural product; some pharmaceutical preparations are prescription

Pregnancy Category: None

Uses. Belladonna bushes thrive in the United States, Europe, North Africa, and Southeast Asia. Some persons seeking a hallucinogenic effect eat the berries. Leaves and roots are used medically. The wood has an even higher drug content but does not seem to be exploited medically. The plant grows wild and has also been cultivated on a commercial scale for the pharmaceutical industry. Drugs found in the plant include atropine, hyoscyamine, and scopolamine, all of which are also found in **jimson weed** and European **mandrake**.

Belladonna substances can ease premenstrual syndrome. They can reduce spasms in smooth muscles of the digestive tract, but they cause tremors or stiffness in other muscles. Heart rate is accelerated. Migraine headaches can lessen. An experiment showed that belladonna can reduce breathing abnormalities in infants. Some medical traditions have used belladonna for reducing sweat and other secretions and against tonsilitis, meningitis, scarlet fever, whooping cough, and epilepsy. At one time medical practitioners gave belladonna to fight Parkinson's disease and drug addiction, but those treatments have been superseded by others. Belladonna preparations have modern usage against vesico-ureteral reflux, a condition in which urine flows back toward the kidney from the bladder. Caregivers have administered belladonna to treat various pains, ranging from kidney stones to sore throat. Belladonna powders and cigarettes have been used against asthma. The natural product is considered effective against afflictions of the gallbladder and liver. Belladonna is used with uncertain results for depression, middle ear inflammation, and some heart complaints and for attempts to promote weight loss. Depending on dosage, the substance can act as a depressant or as a stimulant.

At one time the plant had cosmetic uses from which it supposedly gained its Italian name meaning "beautiful lady." The precise cosmetic usage is uncertain: One authority mentions a rouge; another authority says the substance whitened the skin; still another says that belladonna was simply a medicinal application to remove pimples and other skin blemishes. Many accounts today say that the cosmetic function was to make women more alluring by dilating the eyes' pupils, but those stories do not explain how flirting women would have handled the pain and near-blindness caused by artificial dilation. Modern medicine uses the belladonna component atropine to dilate pupils.

Erotic dreams may occur from ingestion, and reputedly belladonna is considered an aphrodisiac in Morocco. Users have reported hallucinating interactions with landscapes and other persons, experiences so compelling that their hallucinatory nature was unapparent until the belladonna dose wore off.

Drawbacks. Dosage with the natural product belladonna is so risky that persons are routinely advised to use it only under guidance of a trained expert. For example, depending on circumstances a fatal dose can vary by a factor of 10, meaning that a given ingestion might be survivable, but on another occasion one tenth that amount could just as easily be fatal. Three berries have been enough to kill youngsters. People have been poisoned by meat from animals that ate belladonna. Just handling the plant can pass its drugs into cuts and scrapes and even through unbroken skin. During World War II troops stationed in East Africa suffered "wholesale poisoning" from belladonna, presumably due to recreational usage. Yet despite powerful effects on humans, some nonhuman species (including birds, rabbits, pigs, and sheep) can consume the plant without injury—an example of why caution is needed in reaching conclusions from drug experiments on animals.

Experiments show that the scopolamine component of belladonna reduces attention and vigilance while interfering somewhat with memory. Some volunteers testing the drug report dizziness and blurred vision. Nonetheless, aerospace researchers have concluded that scopolamine is a satisfactory motion sickness medicine for active-duty crews.

Belladonna can interfere with urination and bowel movements—drug actions that are sometimes desirable, as in persons who have lost the ability to restrain such body functions. Unwanted belladonna effects include delayed passage of food from the stomach, overheating (aggravated by diminished perspiration), dry mouth, skin rash, glaucoma, hyperactivity, jabbering (or sometimes an opposite inability to speak), mania, anxiety, delirium, and convulsions. Psychedelic drug advocate Timothy Leary is reputed to have claimed he was unaware of anyone ever having a good experience with using belladonna as a hallucinogen, and firsthand accounts do seem mostly negative. Stories say that in olden times belladonna was a component of witch's brews; if so, such persons certainly partook of it for purposes rather different from those of modern recreational drug users. A medical journal author who observed several recreational belladonna sessions judged the substance to be powerful, but none of the users needed medical aid. Modern negative accounts often derive from hospitalized individuals, and they are not necessarily a representative sample of typical users. For example, compilers of one series of case reports noted that six of the seven patients were psychologically abnormal before using belladonna. Another pair of case reports noted that both patients had histories of depression and drug abuse.

Abuse factors. Not enough scientific information to report about likelihood of addiction, tolerance, dependence, or withdrawal.

Drug interactions. Not enough scientific information to report about the natural product.

Cancer. Not enough scientific information to report.

Pregnancy. Belladonna is suspected of causing birth defects if used during pregnancy. Belladonna drugs have been given to pregnant women, however, to control excessive salivation and vomiting, without apparent injury to offspring.

Additional information. "Belladonna" is a nickname for **PCP**, but the substances have no other connection.

Additional scientific information may be found in:

Forbes, T.R. "Why Is it Called 'Beautiful Lady'? A Note on Belladonna." *Bulletin of the New York Academy of Medicine* 53 (1977): 403–6.

Gowdy, J.M. "Stramonium Intoxication: Review of Symptomatology in 212 Cases." *Journal of the American Medical Association* 221 (1972): 585–87.

Nuotto, E. "Psychomotor, Physiological and Cognitive Effects of Scopolamine and Ephedrine in Healthy Man." *European Journal of Clinical Pharmacology* 24 (1983): 603–9.

Schneider, F., et al. "Plasma and Urine Concentrations of Atropine after the Ingestion of Cooked Deadly Nightshade Berries." *Journal of Toxicology: Clinical Toxicology* 34 (1996): 113–17.

Southgate, H.J., M. Egerton, and E.A. Dauncey. "Lessons to Be Learned: A Case Study Approach. Unseasonal Severe Poisoning of Two Adults by Deadly Nightshade (*Atropa belladonna*)." *Journal of the Royal Society of Health* 120 (2000): 127–30.

Benzphetamine

Pronunciation: benz-FET-ah-meen

Chemical Abstracts Service Registry Number: 156-08-1

Formal Names: Didrex, Inapetyl

Type: Stimulant (anorectic class). *See* page 15

Federal Schedule Listing: III (DEA no. 1228)

USA Availability: Prescription

Pregnancy Category: X

Uses. This amphetamine was created in a laboratory in 1953 and is used as an appetite suppressant. Its qualities are similar to **dextroamphetamine**, although users perceive benzphetamine as the weaker of the two in various aspects and—with one notable exception—do not particularly find benzphetamine to be a substitute for dextroamphetamine. The exception is that some persons wanting to boost alertness use benzphetamine in order to avoid the jumpiness caused by dextroamphetamine.

Experiments with rhesus monkeys show dextroamphetamine to be about 14 times stronger than benzphetamine when used as an appetite depressant; in dogs the difference is 5 times. Difference in potency also varies depending on the effect being measured (locomotion, blood pressure). In terms of end result, studies have been inconclusive when comparing benzphetamine, **phenmetrazine**, and dextroamphetamine. One experiment found benzphetamine superior to dextroamphetamine in weight reduction. In that same study benzphetamine maintained appetite reduction longer than other drugs did, but benzphetamine users in another comparison test detected no change in their feelings of hunger. The drug has little effect on levels of blood pressure or blood sugar, which some scientists see as positive factors for hypertensive or diabetic patients.

Benzphetamine is known to cause euphoria, yet that response apparently is uncommon. Volunteers taking the substance in an experiment acted more friendly but not euphoric, although they did feel more energetic. In another study the psychological state of users remained the same as with persons taking a placebo. In contrast to results from animal experiments, electroencephalograms (brain wave readings) taken from humans fail to show brain stimulation by benzphetamine.

Drawbacks. Users occasionally report wooziness, eyesight difficulty, and mild insomnia. The compound's ability to mask fatigue can also cause persons to overextend themselves—a hazard when operating dangerous machinery such as motor vehicles. In an experiment, complaint of dry mouth was routine, and insomnia less so, but the drug did not make people particularly active or ill-tempered. Once ingested, benzphetamine will convert into amphetamine and **methamphetamine** and may cause a person to fail a drug test for those substances, although skilled interpretation of test results can sometimes suggest benzphetamine as the source.

People with diabetes, thyroid trouble, epilepsy, or anxiety should use benzphetamine with caution. Persons with glaucoma, cardiac ailment, high blood pressure, or narrowed arteries are supposed to avoid benzphetamine altogether.

Abuse factors. Experiments with rhesus monkeys have been interpreted as meaning benzphetamine may be more effective in producing desire for the drug than in producing appetite loss. Human tests find the drug about as appealing as phenmetrazine. In an experiment with 75 human subjects, 5 reported experiences likened to those induced by **mescaline**. Drug abusers may find benzphetamine attractive, but it lacks a reputation for illicit use. Dependence can develop.

Drug interactions. People using a monoamine oxidase inhibitor (MAOI, found in some antidepressants and other medicines) are supposed to stop taking any such drug two weeks before using benzphetamine. Tricyclic antidepressants may reduce benzphetamine's effectiveness. The drug may interfere with the blood pressure medicine guanethidine, causing pressure to rise.

Cancer. The digestive system can convert benzphetamine into methylbenzylnitrosamine, a substance identified as causing cancer.

Pregnancy. Benzphetamine is considered to have high potential for causing birth defects if used by a pregnant woman. The drug may pass into breast milk.

Additional scientific information may be found in:

Chait, L.D., and C.E. Johanson. "Discriminative Stimulus Effects of Caffeine and Benzphetamine in Amphetamine-Trained Volunteers." *Psychopharmacology* (Berlin) 96 (1988): 302–8.

Chait, L.D., E.H. Uhlenhuth, and C.E. Johanson. "Reinforcing and Subjective Effects of Several Anorectics in Normal Human Volunteers." *Journal of Pharmacology and Experimental Therapeutics* 242 (1987): 777–83.

Patel, N., D.C. Mock, Jr., and J.A. Hagans. "Comparison of Benzphetamine, Phenmetrazine, D-Amphetamine, and Placebo." *Current Pharmacology and Therapeutics* 4 (1963): 330–33.

Poindexter, A. "Appetite Suppressant Drugs: A Controlled Clinical Comparison of Benzphetamine, Phenmetrazine, D-Amphetamine and Placebo." *Current Therapeutic Research: Clinical and Experimental* 2 (1960): 354–63.

Veldkamp, W., et al. "Some Pharmacologic Properties of Benzphetamine Hydrochloride." *Toxicology and Applied Pharmacology* 6 (1964): 15–22.

Boldenone

Pronunciation: BOHL-duh-nohn

Chemical Abstracts Service Registry Number: 846-48-0. (Undecylenate form 13103-34-9)

Formal Names: Dehydrotestosterone, Equipoise, Parenabol, Vebonol

Type: Anabolic steroid. *See* page 24

Federal Schedule Listing: III (DEA no. 4000)

USA Availability: Prescription

Uses. Boldenone has had experimental use to explore whether it is beneficial in the treatment of persons suffering from osteoporosis. This disease not only makes bones fragile, but it also causes pain and loss of appetite. Patients in the study reported feeling better, but scientific measurements failed to confirm improvement.

The drug has been given to pigeons, greyhounds, and horses in order to enhance their racing abilities. Boldenone can promote weight gain in horses.

Drawbacks. A research study administering the drug to stallions found their testes to be smaller than those of stallions receiving a placebo, and the boldenone animals had less sperm production. Mares receiving the drug in an experiment had a shortened breeding season and abnormal sexual behavior (mounting and male-like conduct), though they seemed to recover several weeks after drug cessation. The drug has been used illegally to increase cattle growth, usage that might harm consumers of the meat.

Horses can become aggressive after receiving the drug, a trait that may continue for weeks after administration stops. A human case is reported in which a pleasant and easygoing person became rageful after using the drug at a dosage 20 times higher than an amount sufficient to make horses aggressive.

Abuse factors. A case report notes that someone taking boldenone and other anabolic steroids for bodybuilding suffered serious temporary depression after the supply was cut off. Until then the person had been psychologically normal.

Drug interactions. Not enough scientific information to report.

Cancer. Not enough scientific information to report.

Pregnancy. Female rats on boldenone showed lower fertility, and their offspring had a higher than normal death rate.

Additional information. The substance is banned from sporting competitions.

Additional scientific information may be found in:

Cowan, C.B. "Depression in Anabolic Steroid Withdrawal." *Irish Journal of Psychological Medicine* 11 (1994): 27–28.

Dalby, J.T. "Brief Anabolic Steroid Use and Sustained Behavioral Reaction." *American Journal of Psychiatry* 149 (1992): 271–72.

Melick, R.A., and C.W. Baird. "Effect of Parenabol on Patients with Osteoporosis." *Medical Journal of Australia* 2 (1970): 960–62.

Melloni, R.H., et al. "Anabolic-Androgenic Steroid Exposure during Adolescence and Aggressive Behavior in Golden Hamsters." *Physiology and Behavior* 61 (1997): 359–64.

Moss, H.B., and G.L. Panzak. "Steroid Use and Aggression." *American Journal of Psychiatry* 149 (1992): 1616.

Bufotenine

Pronunciation: boo-foh-TEN-een
Chemical Abstracts Service Registry Number: 487-93-4
Formal Names: Chan Su, Mappine, N,N-dimethylserotonin
Informal Names: Cohoba
Type: Hallucinogen. *See* p. 25
Federal Schedule Listing: Schedule I (DEA no. 7433)
USA Availability: Illegal to possess
Pregnancy Category: None

Uses. This drug occurs naturally in a number of plants and animals, apparently including trace amounts in humans. Rainforests in the Amazon and deserts in the U.S. Southwest have been key regions for natural sources of the drug, although plants and animals with the substance are found elsewhere as well. Accounts about natural products containing bufotenine reach back to ancient times. **Amanita** mushrooms containing the substance are believed to have been available to ancient Vikings, and some students of the topic wonder if the drug powered the Vikings' famed Berserker rage, in which they would descend upon opponents and attack them (just as modern soldiers sometimes take drugs to improve performance in battle). Native American religious use of a bufotenine snuff called cohoba was reported in 1496. Although bufotenine gained notoriety from research conducted by the U.S. military and Central Intelligence Agency in hopes that the substance would be effective in brainwashing efforts, the drug is perhaps best known for its presence in skins of certain toads. This source is speculated as the origin of fairy tales about wondrous experiences that happen when a woman kisses a frog. Such toads were a traditional component of witches' brews.

A tropical aphrodisiac compounded from the dried venom of toads has been found to contain bufotenine. A traditional Chinese medicine called Chan Su is rubbed on a spot of the body to numb the area and is also used for heart ailments and to fight nosebleeds; Chan Su is prepared from toads and contains bufotenine. Other toad venom preparations have been used to relieve toothache, to help bleeding gums, to promote urination, and to help people cough up phlegm.

Drawbacks. When scientists administered bufotenine to some individuals they showed alarming physical symptoms ranging from faces turning purple to production of so much saliva that medical observers intervened to prevent the person from breathing it into her lungs and drowning. Other physical effects can include high blood pressure and a feeling that one's air supply is inadequate. Researchers who gave the substance to dogs reported that they howled in an unnerving manner for hours.

Although bufotenine lowers pulse rate, it has been described as a heart stimulant. Overdose from products with the substance can cause death from heart failure, although the fatal poisoning may be from chemicals other than bufotenine in the products.

Abuse factors. Stories claim that licking bufotenine toads can produce hallucinations. Some persons familiar with the animals scoff at those tales, but there is a known case of a child being poisoned from licking one. Controversy arose when an Australian horse won a race and tested positive for bufotenine, a substance banned from the sport. Lacking any other explanation, bewildered observers at first jokingly speculated that the horse had eaten a toad, but investigators later focused on a variety of pasture grass containing bufotenine.

Typically toad venom is harvested, dried, and smoked. One authority says that swallowing enough venom to cause hallucinations would be fatal. Smokers, however, are apparently not automatically poisoned by the product, although reportedly some persons have instantly passed out upon inhaling the smoke. Smokers have reported altered consciousness and hallucinations involving sight, sound, smell, and touch. In research studies volunteers who took bufotenine have experienced psychedelic effects, such as mild visual hallucinations (seeing geometric shapes), distortions of time and space, and intense emotional experiences.

One authority notes that analysis of seeds used by Argentine shamans reveals bufotenine as their sole alkaloid, a finding suggesting that bufotenine is indeed psychedelic. Nonetheless, scientific research has not confirmed that the pure drug, as opposed to natural products containing this drug along with many other chemicals, is a psychedelic. For example, some toad venom having bufotenine is also a source of a hallucinogen called 5-MeO-DMT, and a person who uses this venom may be experiencing effects from 5-MeO-DMT rather than bufotenine. (Not everyone finds 5-MeO-DMT pleasant. Scientist A. McDonald, who engaged in self-experimentation, reported "an intense feeling of unease quite unlike the effects of **DMT**. My scientific curiosity has not yet proved sufficient to try it a second time.")

Although news media stories have described bufotenine as more powerful than **LSD**, researchers find that the substance does not readily cross from the bloodstream into brain tissue. Evidence also exists that a person's physical condition might affect bufotenine's hallucinogenic impact. Some authorities say the drug's apparent hallucinogenic qualities are caused instead by its ability to lower heart rate enough to produce oxygen starvation in the optic nerves, causing a person to "see stars." Some natural products containing bufotenine (such as some kinds of seeds and toads) are unquestionably psychedelic, but no scientific consensus exists about the psychedelic qualities of pure bufotenine.

Drug interactions. Not enough scientific information to report.

Cancer. Not enough scientific information to report.

Pregnancy. Not enough scientific information to report.

Additional information. Studies have found that levels of the substance are often elevated in the urine of schizophrenics, in some types of autistic individuals, and in depressed persons but rarely in psychologically normal people. Although cause and effect is by no means established, a study found higher bufotenine levels in urine of paranoid persons convicted of violent crimes than in urine from nonparanoid violent offenders.

Additional scientific information may be found in:

"Deaths Associated with a Purported Aphrodisiac—New York City, February 1993–May 1995." *Morbidity and Mortality Weekly Report* 44 (1995): 853–55, 861.

Fabing, H.D., and J.R. Hawkins. "Intravenous Bufotenine Injection in the Human Being." *Science* 123 (1956): 886–87.

Horgan, J. "Bufo Abuse: A Toxic Toad Gets Licked, Boiled, Teed up and Tanned." *Scientific American* 263 (August 1990): 26–27.

Lyttle, T. "Misuse and Legend in the 'Toad Licking' Phenomenon." *The International Journal of the Addictions* 28 (1993): 521–38.

Lyttle, T., D. Goldstein, and J. Gartz. "Bufo Toads and Bufotenine: Fact and Fiction Surrounding an Alleged Psychedelic." *Journal of Psychoactive Drugs* 28 (1996): 267–90.

McBride, M.C. "Bufotenine: Toward an Understanding of Possible Psychoactive Mechanisms." *Journal of Psychoactive Drugs* 32 (2000): 321–31.

McDonald, A. "Mushrooms and Madness. Hallucinogenic Mushrooms and Some Psychopharmacological Implications." *Canadian Journal of Psychiatry* 25 (1980): 586–94.

Sandroni, P. "Aphrodisiacs Past and Present: A Historical Review." *Clinical Autonomic Research* 11 (2001): 303–7.

Siegel, D.M., and S.H. McDaniel. "The Frog Prince: Tale and Toxicology." *American Journal of Orthopsychiatry* 61 (1991): 558–62.

Buprenorphine

Pronunciation: boo-preh-NOHR-feen

Chemical Abstracts Service Registry Number: 52485-79-7. (Hydrochloride form 53152-21-9)

Formal Names: Buprenex, Subutex, Temgesic, Tidigesic

Type: Depressant (opiate class). *See* page 22

Federal Schedule Listing: Schedule V (DEA no. 9064). In 2002 a rescheduling to III was underway.

USA Availability: Prescription

Pregnancy Category: C

Uses. This pain reliever is produced from **thebaine** and is both longer lasting than **morphine** and 25 to 50 times stronger. Buprenorphine is given to persons suffering from conditions causing great discomfort, such as cancer, pancreatitis, and surgery. Experimental use of the drug to treat depression and schizophrenia has had promising results.

Drawbacks. Typical unwanted effects are sedation, nausea, constipation, dizziness, sweating, and low blood pressure. Impairment of breathing can occur. The drug can interfere with skills needed to operate a car or other dangerous machinery; volunteers in one experiment still had trouble eight hours after a dose. Visual or auditory hallucinations are possible. A medical case report tells of a heart attack after someone inhaled powder from a pulverized oral buprenorphine tablet. Heart trouble has also been noted when the drug is used medically, but in a therapeutic context, such difficulty is very unusual. Long-term administration of the drug in mice can change their blood composition, including a drastic decline in the number of white blood cells, but these changes clear up after administration of buprenorphine stops.

Abuse factors. Although the drug produces sensations likened to those of morphine, when this book was written, buprenorphine was a Schedule V controlled substance, a classification reserved for drugs with the lowest addictive potential. Research conducted on behalf of the National Institute on Drug Abuse and published in 2001 found no illicit buprenorphine use in the United States but described the drug as having appeal to street markets. Such a market may develop; in an experiment testing opiate users' ability to detect differences among drugs, the volunteers misidentified buprenorphine as **heroin**.

Buprenorphine abuse is well documented in other countries, ranging from Scotland and France to India and New Zealand.

People can become addicted to buprenorphine; one study found no difference other than age between buprenorphine addicts and heroin addicts, suggesting the two drugs appeal to the same kinds of people. Given that finding, it is unsurprising that buprenorphine's experimental use as an alternative to **methadone** has been successful in switching heroin addicts to buprenorphine. Various studies note that buprenorphine may create euphoria, an effect that is normally considered a drawback if a drug is used for treating addiction. Some researchers feel that buprenorphine has large potential for abuse. Treating **cocaine** addiction with buprenorphine has had mixed success. Indeed, an experiment indicated that buprenorphine increases pleasurable effects from cocaine.

After a certain point, buprenorphine's effects no longer increase as much when dosage size increases; this characteristic may deter addicts from taking too much buprenorphine and thereby make it a relatively safe substitute for heroin. An experiment demonstrated that persons lacking dependence with opiates could receive 70 times the normal medical dose of buprenorphine without harm, a safety factor of significance in addiction treatment programs, particularly since dependent persons (such as those in addiction treatment) normally can withstand even higher opiate doses than nondependent persons can. A statistical analysis of drug abuser fatalities in France concluded that the death rate from buprenorphine is far less than the rate from methadone. Another advantage to buprenorphine is that maintenance doses can be given less often than with methadone. Still another advantage is that, unlike most opiates, buprenorphine can provoke withdrawal symptoms when taken with another opiate. Thus addicts may be deterred from continuing to take heroin or other opiates while using buprenorphine. Some addicts, however, are able to take both heroin and buprenorphine simultaneously.

Tolerance does not necessarily develop with long-term use, although evidence of tolerance exists among buprenorphine addicts. Animals that are dosed on buprenorphine develop little or no dependence, a finding duplicated in a study of heroin addicts receiving maintenance doses of buprenorphine. Experiments show, however, that when buprenorphine addicts receive a drug that counteracts opiate actions, subjects experience classic symptoms of withdrawal from opiate dependence: yawning, muscle ache, and general uneasiness.

Drug interactions. An experiment showed that buprenorphine further accelerates pulse rates that are already raised by cocaine. Another human study and a monkey experiment found no significant interaction between cocaine and buprenorphine, but still another primate study showed buprenorphine as boosting cocaine effects. Researchers operating a rat study concluded that buprenorphine boosts cocaine actions, but mice studies found that buprenorphine diminished some cocaine effects; such varying results from different animal species indicate the difficulty of applying those results to humans. A human experiment showed that blood flow damage in the brain caused by cocaine can improve after taking buprenorphine.

People using buprenorphine have suffered collapse of breathing and blood circulation when also taking **diazepam**. Taking a monoamine oxidase inhibitor (MAOI—a component in some antidepressants and other medication) may be risky when using buprenorphine. Evidence exists that the drug may promote bleeding under the skin when taken with the anti–blood clot medicine phenprocoumon. Adverse interaction is also reported between buprenorphine and **flunitrazepam**. Antihistamines can add to buprenorphine's general depressant effects. Another possible drug interaction involves **nicotine**; people using buprenorphine tend to increase their tobacco cigarette consumption. Buprenorphine should be used with particular carefulness if a person suffers from enlarged prostrate, urination difficulty, alcoholism, thyroid gland deficiency, or adrenal gland deficiency.

Cancer. Animal experiments have not indicated that the compound produces cancer.

Pregnancy. Pregnant rats receiving 1,000 times the normal human dose have had difficulty when giving birth. Early pregnancy failure and fetal deaths occurred when rats received 10 to 100 times the normal human dose, but not if they had 1,000 times the standard dose. No birth defects were seen at any of those dose levels. More experimentation shows that buprenorphine alters brain development in fetal rats, but the practical effects of those changes are unclear. Results from other research demonstrate long-term effects on behavior of offspring if pregnant rats receive high doses of buprenorphine; those measurements do not indicate what the human outcome would be but nonetheless serve as a warning. Malformations occurred when pregnant rabbits received 1,000 times the recommended human dose. A case report says no malformations occurred when a pregnant heroin addict was switched to daily doses of buprenorphine for several months; the infant showed mild dependence but quickly got through the withdrawal symptoms. One group of researchers who gave daily doses of the drug to pregnant women observed no withdrawal symptoms in the infants, and offspring also had normal weight. Another group of researchers found no adverse effect on fetal development and no harm in infants born to pregnant women who were also using nicotine and **marijuana** in addition to buprenorphine. Buprenorphine has been given to premature newborns with no apparent ill effect.

Milk production declined after nursing rats received buprenorphine, and the same effect has been observed in women who received the drug during Caesarean section. The drug passes into human milk, but a case report indicates the amount is not enough to cause dependence in the infant.

Additional scientific information may be found in:

Agar, M., et al. "Buprenorphine: 'Field Trials' of a New Drug." *Qualitative Health Research* 11 (2001): 69–84.

Bedi, N.S., et al. "Abuse Liability of Buprenorphine—A Study among Experienced Drug Users." *Indian Journal of Physiology and Pharmacology* 42 (1998): 95–100.

Hammersley, R., T. Lavelle, and A. Forsyth. "Predicting Initiation to and Cessation of Buprenorphine and Temazepam Use amongst Adolescents." *British Journal of Addiction* 87 (1992): 1303–11.

Heel, R.C. "Buprenorphine: A Review of Its Pharmacological Properties and Therapeutic Efficacy." *Drugs* 17 (1979): 81–110.

Lewis, J.W. "Buprenorphine." *Drug and Alcohol Dependence* 14 (1985): 363–72.

Pickworth, W.B. "Subjective and Physiologic Effects of Intravenous Buprenorphine in Humans." *Clinical Pharmacology and Therapeutics* 53 (1993): 570–76.

Zacny, J.P., K. Conley, and J. Galinkin. "Comparing the Subjective, Psychomotor and Physiological Effects of Intravenous Buprenorphine and Morphine in Healthy Volunteers." *Journal of Pharmacology and Experimental Therapeutics* 282 (1997): 1187–97.

Butalbital

Pronunciation: byoo-TAL-bi-tall

Chemical Abstracts Service Registry Number: 77-26-9

Formal Names: Esgic, Fioricet, Fiorinal, Phrenilin, Sedapap

Type: Depressant (barbiturate class). *See* page 20

Federal Schedule Listing: Schedule III (DEA no. 2100)

USA Availability: Prescription

Pregnancy Category: C

Uses. The drug is a potent sedative. Butalbital's primary medical use is for headache relief, and a product containing butalbital has also been found effective in treating pain of oral surgery.

Drawbacks. In excessive amounts butalbital can interfere with breathing and induce coma. The drug can increase body temperature, cause reddening of the skin, slow manual dexterity, and bring on confusion and glumness, all rather reminiscent of what **alcohol** can do. Compared to other barbiturates butalbital is rather short acting, which can have the advantage of lessening the time that users experience unwanted effects.

Abuse factors. Excessive use can cause problems both when actively taking the drug and when the drug is stopped. A case is reported when butalbital was suspected of promoting periods of wandering with the person having no recollection of what happened during those times. A single dose of one thousand milligrams (mg) is considered a poisonous dose, and a woman who took 900 mg daily for more than two years developed hallucinations, seizures, and delirium when she stopped the drug; hospitalization was needed to cure those symptoms. Two individuals taking 1,500 mg daily for months became confused, experienced hallucinations, and needed medical help to wean themselves from the drug. Persons taking butalbital for migraine have had grand mal brain seizures upon stopping the drug. Some medical practitioners feel that drug abuse is a cause of chronic headache, a belief that may make prescribing a controlled substance such as butalbital a touchy issue if a patient complains of daily headache.

Drug interactions. Monoamine oxidase inhibitors (MAOIs) can boost the effects of butalbital. Like other barbiturates, butalbital can increase the effects of alcohol and tranquilizers. Butalbital is suspected of decreasing the blood levels of imipramine, so persons taking tricyclic antidepressants such as imipramine may need to have blood levels monitored.

Cancer. Not enough scientific information to report.

Pregnancy. Animal experiments apparently do not indicate butalbital's potential for causing birth defects, but a large study of human pregnancy outcomes found no link between the drug and birth defects. In one case when a pregnant woman using butalbital gave birth, the child experienced seizures identified as butalbital withdrawal symptoms. Those symptoms disappeared when the infant received another barbiturate on a gradually decreasing dose that weaned the child off the drug.

Combination products. Fiorinal is a headache remedy that has had several formulations but is typically butalbital, aspirin, and **caffeine**. The product has been found useful for pain relief among women who have recently given birth, apparently more effective than **propoxyphene**. Also oral surgery patients have received good pain relief from Fiorinal and **codeine**. Fiorinal is known to produce a false positive for **phenobarbital** in body fluid testing. Abuse of the butalbital, aspirin, and caffeine (BAC) combination headache remedy can in itself cause rebound headaches. Although most persons feel no particular attraction to that combination when they take it, a minority of users experience elevation of physical energy and psychic mood, which makes the tablets attractive. Persons have been known to take from 150 to 420 BAC tablets a month for years, habits requiring hospitalization and psychological help to overcome. Substituting acetaminophen for aspirin in this combination has been found to be just as good for treating headache and less likely to cause unwanted effects. This latter combination, under the brand name Fioricet, has been found to have the additional effect of relieving tension.

Sedapap and Phrenilin (both with butalbital and acetaminophen) are remedies for headaches produced by tension or muscle contraction. The combination is not recommended for preadolescents or for persons suffering from porphyria, a condition involving disturbances in body chemistry and abnormal sensitivity to light. Potential for causing cancer or birth defects is unknown, and the combination is assigned to Pregnancy Category C. The combination passes into the milk supply of nursing mothers with unknown effect.

Additional scientific information may be found in:

Forbes, J.A. "Analgesic Effect of an Aspirin-Codeine-Butalbital-Caffeine Combination and an Acetaminophen-Codeine Combination in Postoperative Oral Surgery Pain." *Pharmacotherapy* 6 (1986): 240–47.

Friedman, A.P., and F.J. DiSerio. "Symptomatic Treatment of Chronically Recurring Tension Headache: Placebo-Controlled, Multicenter Investigation of Fioricet and Acetaminophen with Codeine." *Clinical Therapeutics* 10 (1987): 69–81.

Good, M.I. "Organic Dissociative Syndrome Associated with Antimigraine Pharmacotherapy." *Canadian Journal of Psychiatry* 36 (1991): 597–99.

Preskorn, S.H., R.L. Schwin, and W.V. McKnelly. "Analgesic Abuse and the Barbiturate Abstinence Syndrome." *Journal of the American Medical Association* 244 (1980): 369–70.

Raja, M. "Severe Barbiturate Withdrawal Syndrome in Migrainous Patients." *Headache* 36 (1996): 119–21.

Butane

Pronunciation: BYOO-tain

Chemical Abstracts Service Registry Number: 106-97-8

Formal Names: Butyl Hydride, Liquefied Petroleum Gas, Methylethylmethane, Pyrofax

Type: Inhalant. *See* page 26

Federal Schedule Listing: Unlisted

USA Availability: Nonprescription chemical

Pregnancy Category: None

Uses. Some recreational use is for psychic effects: During butane intoxication, time may appear to pass more slowly, and thoughts may seem to come faster. Other recreational usage has nothing to do with altered consciousness: Some persons ingest butane to perform the stunt of fire breathing, appearing to exhale flames by filling the mouth with butane and then exhaling over a flame source.

Drawbacks. Inhaling butane to achieve euphoria, hallucinations, and sensory distortion is one of the riskier forms of substance abuse. The amount required for hallucinatory action can be close to a lethal dose, making a slight miscalculation fatal.

Users have complained of headache and coughing. Lung injury is reported, ranging from fluid build-up and congestion to impaired breathing function and lung collapse. Unwanted effects can also include cardiac arrest, from which persons can seldom be resuscitated. A case report tells of a 14-year-old male who suffered a heart attack due to inhaling butane. Another case report describes a teenager who became paralyzed on one side of the body due to butane inhalation. Explosion is a common misadventure; one hospital in South Korea found that 1.6% of all flame burn patients had been abusing butane. Most were teenagers. Accidents often happened in a group setting in bedrooms or motel rooms. Burns typically covered more than 25% of the body: face, hands, arms, midsection. About half the victims required skin grafts, and the overall death rate was just over 10%. An American case study noted how treacherous treatment can be for such injuries. A female was hospitalized after striking a match in a closed vehicle while inhaling butane. She was released after a couple of days but died a week later. In addition to external burns, the explosion had burned interior airways into the lungs, an injury that gradually destroyed her ability to breathe. Medical caregivers emphasize the importance of victims honestly describing circumstances of a butane injury so that their lung condition will be properly examined in detail. Caregivers also emphasize that a person who experiences seemingly minor burns in a butane explosion should always seek immediate medical examination of the lungs, because breathing distress may not occur until several days later, when successful treatment is less likely.

Butane is suspected of causing liver damage and is suspected of making users ill-tempered.

Some recreational butane sniffers use sources also containing other ingredients. Those other substances can be harmful as well. For example, a case report notes problems encountered by someone who inhaled spray from oven cleaner that contained butane. Butane spray from aerosol cans and other pressurized containers can be cold enough to cause frostbite. Cases have been seen of skin burns from the severe cold, also frostbite damage to the throat, lungs, and esophagus. Associated inflammation of stomach lining is also known. The instant severe cold can affect the vagus nerve, which influences voice quality and affects heartbeat; such impact on the vagus nerve can produce heart failure.

A case report notes a habitual practitioner of the fire breathing stunt who developed stomach inflammation and a bleeding esophagus from irritation caused by repeated exposure to butane. Another case report tells of severe lung damage caused by exposure to unignited fumes. Judging from the expected progress of such disease and from autopsy findings, such lung damage can be fatal. Because butane is heavier than air, it can flow into the lungs even if a person is trying to hold butane in the mouth without inhaling. One fire breather routinely swallowed some of the butane, numbing the rear of the mouth.

Abuse factors. Authorities have described butane's effects as weaker and having less addictive appeal than those of **toluene**. Tolerance and dependence are reported. Withdrawal may involve several days of nausea, perspiration, crankiness, troubled sleep, abdominal cramps, and general shakiness.

Drug interactions. Not enough scientific information to report.

Cancer. Potential for causing cancer is unknown.

Pregnancy. Potential for causing birth defects is unknown.

Additional scientific information may be found in:

Evans, A.C., and D. Raistrick. "Patterns of Use and Related Harm with Toluene-Based Adhesives and Butane Gas." *British Journal of Psychiatry* 150 (1987): 773–76.

Evans, A.C., and D. Raistrick. "Phenomenology of Intoxication with Toluene-Based Adhesives and Butane Gas." *British Journal of Psychiatry* 150 (1987): 769–73.

Gomibuchi, K., T. Gomibuchi, and H. Kurita. "Treatment and 9-Year Outcome of Butane-Induced Psychotic Disorder in a Butane-Dependent Japanese Male Adolescent." *Psychiatry and Clinical Neurosciences* 55 (2001): 163.

Gray, M.Y., and J.H. Lazarus. "Butane Inhalation and Hemiparesis." *Journal of Toxicology: Clinical Toxicology* 31 (1993): 483–85. Hemiparesis is paralysis on one side of a person's body.

Marsh, W.W. "Butane Firebreathing in Adolescents: A Potentially Dangerous Practice." *Journal of Adolescent Health Care* 5 (1984): 59–60.

Oh, S.J., et al. "Explosive Burns during Abusive Inhalation of Butane Gas." *Burns* 25 (1999): 341–44.

Rieder-Scharinger, J., et al. "Multiorganversagen nach Butangasinhalation: Ein Fallbericht [Multiple Organ Failure Following Inhalation of Butane Gas: A Case Report]." *Wiener Klinische Wochenschrift* 112 (2000): 1049–52. Abstract in English.

Rohrig, T.P. "Sudden Death Due to Butane Inhalation." *American Journal of Forensic Medicine and Pathology* 18 (1997): 299–302.

Butorphanol

Pronunciation: byoo-TOR-fa-nohl

Chemical Abstracts Service Registry Number: 42408-82-2. (Tartrate form 58786-99-5)

Formal Names: Dorphanol, Stadol, Stadol NS, Torbugesic

Type: Depressant (opioid class). *See* page 24

Federal Schedule Listing: Schedule IV (DEA no. 9720)

USA Availability: Prescription

Pregnancy Category: C

Uses. This pain reliever is a narcotic agonist/antagonist, meaning that it acts like an opioid when used by itself but counteracts other opioids if given simultaneously with them; the counteraction can be significant enough to provoke a withdrawal syndrome if a person is dependent on the other opioids.

Butorphanol is used to control pain in conditions ranging from cancer and surgery to migraine headache and dental work. Women seem to achieve better pain control from butorphanol than men. The drug also suppresses coughs, and researchers have found that it improves appetite. The substance has been used illicitly by the type of bodybuilders who take **nalbuphine** and for the same reasons (to reduce pain from workouts and in hopes of promoting muscle mass).

Experiments show butorphanol to be about 4 to 7 times stronger than **morphine**, 20 to 30 times stronger than **pentazocine**, and 30 to 50 times stronger than **meperidine**. Butorphanol is powerful enough that it has been used to help sedate rhinoceroses. The substance has other veterinary uses as well, including illicit doping of racehorses to improve performance (at certain dosages opioids can both excite the animals and mask pain).

Drawbacks. Unwanted effects include uneasy feelings, ill temper, sleepiness, dizziness, nausea, vomiting, blood pressure changes (up or down), and impaired breathing. Reports of hallucinations and psychoses exist. People using the drug can feel faint if they suddenly stand up. The drug can make people woozy and cloud their thinking, impeding their ability to operate dangerous machinery. Illicit users who inject butorphanol into muscles can cause damage that is long-lasting, if not permanent.

Abuse factors. Tolerance and dependence can develop. Withdrawal symptoms are characterized as minor. Addiction is possible but is not commonly reported in scientific literature. Two investigators say, however, that dependency and addiction were the most frequent adverse reaction reports about the drug received by the U.S. Food and Drug Administration in the early 1990s. **Heroin** users who received butorphanol in an experiment described butorphanol as unpleasant. Former opioid addicts have said it reminded them of pentazocine. At one time in the United States butorphanol was not a controlled substance, but instances of addiction prompted government authorities to change the drug's status to Schedule IV in 1997.

Drug interactions. Some recreational users combine butorphanol with the common cold and allergy remedy diphenhydramine to produce a typical opiate-type stupor. Users of that combination sometimes report loss of interest in other drugs. Unwanted results can include emotional flip-flops, dizziness, nausea, vomiting, breathing difficulty, and general reduction of mental and physical abilities. Withdrawal symptoms from the combination may involve impaired concentration, mental restlessness and unease, and emotional instability and peevishness.

In a mice experiment butorphanol and acetaminophen (Tylenol and similar products) boosted each other's pain relieving effects.

Cancer. Laboratory tests and two-year animal experiments have not indicated that butorphanol causes cancer.

Pregnancy. Research using rats, mice, and rabbits has not yielded evidence of birth defects caused by butorphanol, but some of the experiments produced fetal death. The drug passes from a pregnant woman into the fetus and can cause abnormal fetal heartbeat. When used in childbirth, impact on newborns is similar to that of meperidine; respiratory distress can occur in the infant. One study found the average drug level in newborns to match the maternal level at time of birth. The amount of drug that passes into milk is believed unharmful to nursing infants.

Additional scientific information may be found in:

Fisher, M.A., and S. Glass. "Butorphanol (Stadol): A Study in Problems of Current Drug Information and Control." *Neurology* 48 (1997): 1156–60.

Gillis, J.C., P. Benfield, and K.L. Goa. "Transnasal Butorphanol: Review of Its Pharmacodynamic and Pharmacokinetic Properties, and Therapeutic Potential in Acute Pain Management." *Drugs* 50 (1995): 157–75.

Rosow, C.E. "Butorphanol in Perspective." *Acute Care* 12 (1988, Suppl. 1): 2–7.

Smith, S.G., and W.M. Davis. "Nonmedical Use of Butorphanol and Diphenhydramine." *Journal of the American Medical Association* 252 (1984): 1010.

Vogelsang, J., and S.R. Hayes. "Butorphanol Tartrate (Stadol): A Review." *Journal of Post Anesthesia Nursing* 6 (1991): 129–35.

Zacny, J.P., et al. "Comparing the Subjective, Psychomotor and Physiological Effects of Intravenous Butorphanol and Morphine in Healthy Volunteers." *Journal of Pharmacology and Experimental Therapeutics* 270 (1994): 579–88.

Zacny, J.P., et al. "The Effects of Transnasal Butorphanol on Mood and Psychomotor Functioning in Healthy Volunteers." *Anesthesia and Analgesia* 82 (1996): 931–35.

Caffeine

Pronunciation: KAFF-een

Chemical Abstracts Service Registry Number: 58-08-2

Type: Stimulant. *See* page 11

Federal Schedule Listing: Unlisted

USA Availability: Prescription and nonprescription drug; also in food

Pregnancy Category: C

Uses. This drug is responsible for the stimulating jolt that coffee drinkers get. Many drinkers would probably be surprised to see caffeine listed as an ingredient in medicines they take. Caffeine is so widely used (typically in coffee, tea, soda, and chocolate) that it is scarcely considered a drug. Yet an overdose can be fatal.

Caffeine makes people more alert, and experimentation finds that it can help persons function more effectively during sleep deprivation. Caffeine is commonly used in the workplace to increase employees' energy and output. Laboratory measurements indicate that a single dose of 250 mg to 400 mg at the beginning of a night work shift is more effective than several smaller doses spread out during the work period. Some studies find that caffeine helps extroverts perform simple physical assignments but overstimulates introverts and thereby worsens their performance. Scientific measurements prove that caffeine, by itself or in combination with **ephedrine**, improves athletic performance.

Like some amphetamine class stimulants, caffeine has reduced hyperactivity in children when they received 600 mg daily, but it has been found ineffective for attention deficit hyperactivity disorder (ADHD).

Studies demonstrate caffeine can mildly help asthma sufferers. Theophylline, a drug commonly used to widen airways and help asthmatics breathe, is related to caffeine. Caffeine is a standard drug to help premature infants that have interruptions in breathing.

Rat experiments indicate that caffeine can promote weight loss. In humans a combination of caffeine and ephedrine has been used for that purpose. A study found that caffeine increased women's energy outlay and body temperature but that the temperature change correlated with smaller weight and waistlines only in younger women.

Caffeine has been suspected of promoting osteoporosis, a disease causing loss of bone density in older women; studies controlling other factors (such as cigarettes and drugs promoting calcium loss) found that caffeine had no tendency to reduce bone density, but one study published in 2000 and tracking almost 35,000 postmenopausal women found a slight correlation of caffeine usage to broken bones—a correlation implying loss of density. Coffee drinking is associated with loss of density. In contrast, examination of over 1,200 older women in England showed that tea drinkers were less likely to have osteoporosis, leading investigators to wonder if something in tea, other than caffeine, affects bone density.

Investigators examining caffeine consumption in a group of 8,000 men who were tracked for three decades discovered that the more caffeine someone ingested over the years, the less likely the person was to come down with Parkinson's disease. In a group of 46,000 men tracked for a decade, increased consumption of caffeinated coffee was linked to decreased likelihood of having gallstones; consumption of decaffeinated coffee did not have such a link. As one analyst pointed out, such associations are interesting but do not prove cause and effect; for example, perhaps some physical aspect leading to Parkinson's disease also makes caffeine beverages unappealing—thus persons without the disease would consume more caffeine beverages than sufferers do, but that consumption would not mean that caffeine prevents the affliction.

Mice experiments demonstrate that if caffeine is administered in the right amount and at the right time before exposure to radiation, the drug will allow mice to survive otherwise lethal amounts of radiation.

Drawbacks. In the 1990s, 20% of the U.S. population was believed to be using over 700 mg of caffeine each day. That is enough to produce behavior mimicking an anxiety neurosis. If a person only ingests caffeine through pharmaceutical preparations or food products with labels listing caffeine amounts, intake can easily be measured. The amount in a restaurant cup of coffee is more difficult to measure; one rule of thumb says 100 mg to 150 mg.

The substance can accelerate pulse rate; it can also make people more peevish and jumpy (even promote panic attacks) and interfere with getting good sleep. Caffeine can cause heartburn and increase urine output. Experimentation has confirmed that the drug's tendency to promote loss of body fluid will dry the vocal cords and affect voice quality.

Analysis of over 30 years of reports about caffeine and blood pressure found that the drug reliably increased blood pressure when persons began using it but that the effect did not persist in all users. Investigators measuring blood pressure among medical students found caffeine raising the readings far enough that anyone at risk for high blood pressure should avoid the drug during times of stress. Persons with coronary artery disease may be at significant risk for sudden cardiac arrest if they drink more than 10 cups of coffee a day.

Excessive doses can dangerously reduce blood potassium levels, damage muscles, produce extremely rapid heartbeat, and cause delirium and seizures. As the twenty-first century began a case report associated caffeine with retina damage in several persons.

Abuse factors. Coffee was formerly treated as an illicit drug. Centuries ago possession was a death penalty offense in Spain and the Near East. In the early twentieth century one standard medical textbook warned of coffee addiction peril, and another medical volume described coffee as a gateway to opiate addiction. In a modern study volunteers showed no particular desire for caffeine but did find that 300 mg mimicked some effects of **dextroamphetamine**. Although caffeine is not a scheduled substance, users can develop a physical dependence on the drug that results in withdrawal symptoms including weariness and headache. Such symptoms are not inevitable nor are they necessarily troubling to persons experiencing them. In 2000 an international panel of experts convened by European drug regulation agencies described caffeine's potential for dependence as low. Tolerance can develop to some of caffeine's effects.

Drug interactions. Caffeine itself can reduce headache, and an experiment involving hundreds of participants showed caffeine to substantially improve ibuprofen's ability to relieve headache. Phenylpropanolamine is a drug commonly found in remedies for colds. It seems to increase caffeine levels in a person using both drugs, and together the two can produce mood elevation, hyperactivity and manic behavior, confusion, high blood pressure, and stroke. In rat experiments, caffeine boosts the effects of **cocaine** and amphetamine, enough to transform normally tolerable doses into fatal ones. Human observations show that cocaine users tend to take lower doses of that drug if they also use caffeine. Perhaps the most common drug taken with caffeine is **nicotine**. Animal experiments find that interactions of that combination may make cigarette smoking more pleasurable. Cigarette smoking increases the body's rate of metabolizing caffeine, which decreases the influence from a given amount of caffeine; British researchers found that smokers tend to use more caffeine than nonsmokers. Birth control pills can double the time that a given amount of caffeine lasts in the body. The drug can reduce drowsiness produced by **pentobarbital**, and it can reduce **diazepam**'s interference with cognitive function. Caffeine is a traditional remedy for alcohol intoxication, but in fact it does not speed alcohol's elimination from the body, although caffeine's stimulant properties may help a drunken person function better. Estrogen replacement therapy appears to interfere with women's ability to metabolize caffeine.

Cancer. Caffeine does not seem to produce cancer in animal experiments. Indeed, green and black tea reduce development of cancer in mice, an effect in which caffeine is believed to play a part. In humans, however, caffeine is suspected of promoting premenopausal ovarian cancer and also cancer of the pancreas and bladder.

Pregnancy. Experiments examining caffeine's influence on pregnancy yield conflicting results, which may indicate the question is particularly complex or may simply mean that caffeine is an "invalid variable" having no effect. Here are examples. A 1994 survey of 259 women in the Netherlands found that caffeine raised the likelihood of becoming pregnant, but when the same subject was examined in the 1980s among almost 2,000 women in Connecticut, caffeine was found to suppress fertility. During the 1990s a study of farm couples in Canada found that caffeine had no effect on fertility but that coffee-drinking women and tea-drinking men had lower birthrates, suggesting involvement of something besides caffeine in the natural products' effect. Rat experimentation shows that caffeine reduces female fertility, produces smaller than usual offspring, and may affect brain development.

Research in Yugoslavia indicates that pregnant women who do not smoke cigarettes but do take more than 71 mg of caffeine daily have smaller infants. A British study found the opposite; slightly smaller infants came from cigarette-smoking women who used 1,000 mg or more of caffeine a week, but the effect was not seen in nonsmokers. Still other studies find no connection between caffeine and either birthweight or prematurity.

Caffeine affects vital signs in a human fetus even when the dose is so low as to have no influence on the pregnant woman.

Question has arisen about whether caffeine promotes spontaneous abortion; a study published in 1994 found 140 mg to 280 mg a day to pose a significant risk; a rigorous study published in 1999 was unable to find such a hazard among moderate caffeine users; and a study published in 1993 saw caffeine as reducing the incidence of spontaneous abortion. Still another study found that women who drank decaffeinated coffee were even more likely to experience a spontaneous abortion than women who drank caffeinated coffee. Research in New Zealand indicated that sudden infant death syndrome (SIDS) was more likely if a woman had ingested more than 400 mg of caffeine daily during pregnancy, but an examination of SIDS in Scandinavia found no correlation with caffeine use during or after pregnancy.

Instant coffee can damage DNA, but implications for general health or birth defects are unclear. Testing caffeine on mice produced birth defects in limbs, and tests on chicken embryos produced heart deformities. Chicken embryos, however, are so sensitive to various chemicals that such results are not considered a warning of human danger. Indeed, a substantial body of research indicates that caffeine causes no human birth defects.

Evidence does exist that caffeine can increase the likelihood of birth defects caused by **alcohol** and tobacco. An Egyptian study found that caffeine increases alcohol birth defects in rats.

A statistical study showed that women who use more than 300 mg of caffeine daily around the time of conception and who do not smoke are less likely to have infants with Down syndrome.

Given all the uncertainties, pregnant women are advised to use caffeine "moderately"—no more than 200 mg to 300 mg daily (150 mg or less is considered "minimal").

Caffeine increases milk production in nursing mothers and passes into the milk but appears unharmful to infants if the women are moderate users. On occasions when mothers use a lot of caffeine, however, their nursing infants may be fussier and have more trouble sleeping. A dose lasts longer in infants than in older persons.

Additional scientific information may be found in:

Anderson, M.E., et al. "Improved 2000-Meter Rowing Performance in Competitive Oarswomen after Caffeine Ingestion." *International Journal of Sport Nutrition and Exercise Metabolism* 10 (2000): 464–75.
Eskenazi, B. "Caffeine—Filtering the Facts." *New England Journal of Medicine* 341 (1999): 1688–89.

Golding, J. "Reproduction and Caffeine Consumption—A Literature Review." *Early Human Development* 43 (1995): 1–14.

Marsden, G., and J. Leach. "Effects of Alcohol and Caffeine on Maritime Navigational Skills." *Ergonomics* 43 (2000): 17–26.

Nurminen, M.-L., et al. "Coffee, Caffeine and Blood Pressure: A Critical Review." *European Journal of Clinical Nutrition* 53 (1999): 831–39.

Reyner, L.A., and J.A. Horne. "Early Morning Driver Sleepiness: Effectiveness of 200 Mg Caffeine." *Psychophysiology* 37 (2000): 251–56.

Smit, H.J., and P.J. Rogers. "Effects of Low Doses of Caffeine on Cognitive Performance, Mood and Thirst in Low and Higher Caffeine Consumers." *Psychopharmacology* (Berlin) 152 (2000): 167–73.

Tanda, G., and S.R. Goldberg. "Alteration of the Behavioral Effects of Nicotine by Chronic Caffeine Exposure." *Pharmacology, Biochemistry, and Behavior* 66 (2000): 47–64.

Chloral Hydrate

Pronunciation: KLOHR-ul HIGH-drait
Chemical Abstracts Service Registry Number: 302-17-0
Formal Names: Aquachloral, Chloradorm, Chloralex, Felsules, Noctec, Somnos
Informal Names: Jelly Beans, Knockout Drops, Mickey Finn, Mickeys
Type: Depressant. *See* page 19.
Federal Schedule Listing: Schedule IV (DEA no. 2465)
USA Availability: Prescription
Pregnancy Category: C

Uses. This substance is the first synthetic central nervous system depressant, created in the 1830s. After that creation, however, several decades passed before chloral hydrate's medical usage as a sleep inducer began. The anesthetic chloroform is produced from it. Chloral hydrate has also been used against pain of rheumatism. In the nineteenth century the drug was popular among middle-class women and middle-aged men for reducing anxiety.

In former times chloral hydrate was routinely administered to produce anesthesia, but such use is tricky; the difference between an effective dose and a poisonous one is so close that the drug has been replaced by other substances for human anesthesia, although chloral hydrate is still used for that purpose in animals. The substance has been largely superseded by barbiturates but still has medical applications as a sedative and to induce sleep. Chloral hydrate is also used to treat seizures caused by fever and is a secondary choice for controlling the seizures of status epilepticus (an emergency in which persons keep having epileptic seizures, one after another, with little or no letup). Medical caregivers sometimes administer chloral hydrate to help withdrawal from **heroin** and **GHB** dependence and to help **alcohol** addicts withstand delirium tremens during withdrawal. The famed "Mickey Finn" drug used by criminals to knock out victims was a combination of chloral hydrate and alcohol, but animal and human experiments have failed to demonstrate that the combination worked as advertised.

Drawbacks. Chloral hydrate users may act drunken and confused. An experiment found reduction in abilities needed to drive an automobile. The same research, however, also showed that if the product was taken to induce sleep the night before, persons performed better the next day after the drug had worn off, presumably because they were better rested than usual. At normal doses gastrointestinal distress may occur, and persons suffering from stomach irritation are supposed to avoid the compound. A case report notes a deliberate overdose that destroyed part of a patient's stomach. Heart attack has occurred from chloral hydrate overdose, but that is unusual. In high quantities the compound interferes with heart rhythm and reduces blood pressure and breathing; seizures are possible. Experiments using chloral hydrate on rats and mice have injured the liver, and inhaling the drug's vapor has caused lung damage in mice. Human physical contact with the compound can irritate the skin, lungs, and eyes. The substance is suspected of causing kidney damage and colon cysts and of aggravating a disease called porphyria. Reduction may occur in the number of white blood cells. Although the substance is a depressant, some persons are stimulated by the drug.

Abuse factors. In the 1800s a number of prominent persons became addicted to chloral hydrate: English poet and painter Dante Gabriel Rossetti, German literary figure Karl Ferdinand Gutzkow, and renowned German philosopher Friedrich Wilhelm Nietzsche. Such addiction grew uncommon in the twentieth century as the drug itself grew less common. As is so often the case with drug abuse, chloral hydrate addicts were typically polydrug abusers, often using alcohol, **opium**, or **morphine** as well. Today chloral hydrate does not seem to be a popular recreational intoxicant, quite possibly because the kind of person who would enjoy chloral hydrate may instead be attracted to barbiturates, a type of drug that was unavailable in the nineteenth century.

No dependence developed after experimenters gave chloral hydrate to monkeys twice a day for six weeks, but tolerance and dependence can develop in humans. The most common origin of dependence is medical usage. Chloral hydrate withdrawal symptoms include tremors, worry, sleeping difficulty, confusion, delirium, hallucinations, and convulsions. Some authorities describe the syndrome as delirium tremens. Withdrawal may have a fatal outcome.

Drug interactions. Actions of anti–blood clotting medicines may be temporarily boosted by chloral hydrate, but the amount of change and its medical significance are disputed. The drug may reduce blood levels of the epilepsy medicine phenytoin, thereby impeding phenytoin's therapeutic actions. In mice experimentation chloral hydrate had inconsistent impact on alcohol blood level (sometimes raising it, sometimes reducing it) but extended the time that intoxication lasted. In humans the combination produces changes in heart rate and blood pressure that might harm cardiac patients (the face and neck of one volunteer turned reddish purple from the combination). Alcohol and chloral hydrate are both depressants, and taking them together is like taking an extra dose of one or the other. Injecting **marijuana**'s main active ingredient THC (tetrahydrocannabinol) into animals increases chloral hydrate's potency.

Cancer. Lab tests of chloral hydrate's potential for causing cancer have produced mixed results. The compound has increased the liver cancer rate in mice, but skepticism exists about human relevance of those mice results because dosage was long term and so high as to be poisonous—circumstances not at all similar to an occasional normal therapeutic dose. Experimenters administered the substance to hundreds of rats every day for over two years without evidence developing that the drug causes cancer. The cancer-causing potential in humans is uncertain.

Pregnancy. Chloral hydrate passes from a pregnant woman into the fetus but is not considered a cause of birth defects. Infants born to such women are, however, more likely to have a condition called hyperbilirubinemia, which can lead to jaundice. Some investigators also believe that administering the drug to infants after birth causes hyperbilirubinemia. The compound passes into the milk of a nursing mother, enough to slightly sedate the infant.

Additional scientific information may be found in:

Butler, T.C. "The Introduction of Chloral Hydrate into Medical Practice." *Bulletin of the History of Medicine* 44 (1970): 168–72.

Miller, R.R., and D.J. Greenblatt. "Clinical Effects of Chloral Hydrate in Hospitalized Medical Patients." *Journal of Clinical Pharmacology* 19 (1979): 669–74.

Robinson, J.T. "A Case of Chloral Hydrate Addiction." *International Journal of Social Psychiatry* 12 (1966): 66–71.

Sellers, E.M., et al. "Interaction of Chloral Hydrate and Ethanol in Man. II. Hemodynamics and Performance." *Clinical Pharmacology and Therapeutics* 13 (1972): 50–58.

Sourkes, T.L. "Early Clinical Neurochemistry of CNS-Active Drugs. Chloral Hydrate." *Molecular and Chemical Neuropathology* 17 (1992): 21–30.

Steinberg, A.D. "Should Chloral Hydrate Be Banned?" *Pediatrics* 92 (1993): 442–46.

Chlordiazepoxide

Pronunciation: klor-dye-az-uh-POX-ide

Chemical Abstracts Service Registry Number: 58-25-3. (Hydrochloride form 438-41-5)

Formal Names: Libritabs, Librium, Limbitrol

Informal Names: Libs

Type: Depressant (benzodiazepine class). *See* page 21

Federal Schedule Listing: Schedule IV (DEA no. 2744)

USA Availability: Prescription

Pregnancy Category: D

Uses. Chlordiazepoxide was the first benzodiazepine tranquilizer and has been commonly used since 1960. It is considered one of the safer psychiatric drugs and has actions comparable to those of barbiturates and **alcohol**.

This classic benzodiazepine is used mainly for calming anxiety and for treating symptoms of alcohol withdrawal, including delirium tremens. Studies have found, however, that alcoholics receiving this drug to help them through withdrawal are about three times more likely to resume drinking than alcoholics who receive a placebo. The substance is also used to overcome convulsions and to treat insomnia, migraine headache, gastric ulcers, and irritable bowel syndrome (persistent cramps and diarrhea). Actions from a dose of this drug take longer to appear than actions from a dose of **lorazepam** or **diazepam**, so those latter substances are sometimes preferred when faster results are needed.

Researchers have used rats and mice to demonstrate partial cross-tolerance between **pentobarbital**, alcohol, and chlordiazepoxide, and that relationship may contribute to the latter's therapeutic role in treating alcohol withdrawal. An argument has been made that when clinical signs of alcohol withdrawal can be treated as well with chlordiazepoxide as with lorazepam, the former is preferable because of cheaper cost. Chlordiazepoxide can be substituted for **alprazolam** to wean someone from that drug, although one study found chlordiazepoxide to be about 86 times weaker than alprazolam (consistent with animal experiments, where large doses of chlordiazepoxide are needed to produce dependence). Chlordiazepoxide can be used in place of most benzodiazepines if someone who stops taking one of those drugs is troubled by withdrawal. An experiment found chlordiazepoxide to be as effective as **methadone** in easing opiate withdrawal symptoms experienced by **heroin** addicts.

Drawbacks. Chlordiazepoxide is one of the longer-lasting benzodiazepines, which can have advantages—but it can also have disadvantages; for example, the drug is associated with higher chance of hip fractures in older persons, perhaps because it makes them unsteady longer and more likely to fall.

Blood disorders can be an unusual unwanted effect, and a case is reported in which long-term use produced purpura, tiny purple spots in the skin caused by bleeding under the skin surface. Although the drug is used to relieve anxiety, studies conflict on whether it increases users' hostility. The drug reduces aggression in animal experiments, and human aggression is certainly not a typical result of a dose; perhaps lowered anxiety among resentful persons also lowers inhibitions, allowing those angry individuals to engage in aggression they had been afraid to attempt. That outcome is more likely when a person using chlordiazepoxide has also been drinking alcohol, and alcohol definitely can lower inhibitions. Chlordiazepoxide can make people weary, degrade verbal communication ability, and raise or lower interest in sex. Among alcoholics, measurements find that chlordiazepoxide reduces rapid eye movement (REM) sleep and delta (deep) sleep; those types are considered important for maintaining normal mental functioning. A case report indicates that the substance may worsen symptoms of Parkinson's disease, possibly due to untoward reaction with the Parkinson's drug levodopa. Another case report notes a diabetic whose blood sugar levels rose substantially while taking chlordiazepoxide. An instance is known of continual hiccups starting soon after a person started taking the drug and stopping soon after the drug dosage stopped. Still another case report associated the drug with gout.

Persons who receive chlordiazepoxide by injection should avoid hazardous activity (such as driving a car) for several hours; a test of the oral format showed that it lowered driving ability as well. Drivers can be unaware that chlordiazepoxide is affecting them. A study of bronchitis patients found that the drug worsened their breathing, and in general the compound impairs respiration. Chlordiazepoxide is also suspected of worsening porphyria, a disease involving body chemistry and that makes a person extremely sensitive to light. Porphyria caused the madness of George III, king of Great Britain during the American Revolution.

Abuse factors. Sudden stoppage of chlordiazepoxide dosage can produce symptoms similar to those of alcohol or barbiturate withdrawal: tremors and cramps, vomiting, perspiring, and even convulsions.

Drug interactions. When delta-9-tetrahydrocannabinol (also called THC, the main psychoactive chemical in **marijuana**) was given to pregnant mice in an experiment, administering chlordiazepoxide along with THC raised the blood level of THC. Another mice experiment showed an increase in THC's cataleptic effect when chlordiazepoxide was administered. In mice chlordiazepoxide can increase potency of the anticancer drug ifosfamide, and in both mice and humans alcohol can boost chlordiazepoxide's potency (though a rat experiment did not find that effect). In humans monoamine oxidase inhibitors (MAOIs) boost chlordiazepoxide actions, and the antacid-heartburn medicine cimetidine lengthens the effect of a chlordiazepoxide dose. Cigarette smoking reduces chlordiazepoxide actions, and **morphine** and **meperidine** each make oral dosage of chlordiazepoxide less effective. The drug is suspected of affecting blood clotting and is known to constrain the healing abilities of the anticoagulant medicine warfarin.

Cancer. Chlordiazepoxide has produced DNA damage in experiments designed to reveal potential for such defects. Under certain laboratory conditions the drug can promote DNA damage in rats, which theoretically might encourage development of cancer, but that outcome has not been observed in practice.

Pregnancy. "Nitrosatable" drugs, of which chlordiazepoxide is one, cause birth defects in animal experiments. Some studies suggest that using chlordiazepoxide during pregnancy may cause human birth defects, but confirmation is elusive. For example, a study of 50,000 pregnancies published in 1975, including many women who used chlordiazepoxide, found no difference in outcome regardless of whether women used the drug. In contrast, a study of almost 20,000 pregnancies (published in 1974) compared women who took chlordiazepoxide to those who took assorted other antianxiety drugs or none at all in early pregnancy. In the chlordiazepoxide group birth defects were more than two times as frequent compared to the "other drugs" group and over four times as frequent compared to the "no drug" group. Some researchers believe chlordiazepoxide may cause infant skull deformities if a pregnant woman uses the drug.

Combination products. Limbitrol is a combination product using chlordiazepoxide to reduce anxiety and amitriptyline as a tricyclic antidepressant. Taking a tricyclic antidepressant along with an MAOI can be fatal. Tricyclics are not recommended for persons with glaucoma or urinary difficulties. An experiment with hamsters showed that the drug combination is more likely to produce birth defects than either drug alone. Amitriptyline is Pregnancy Category C and passes into a nursing mother's milk supply.

Additional scientific information may be found in:

Giri, A.K. and S. Banerjee. "Genetic Toxicology of Four Commonly Used Benzodiazepines: A Review." *Mutation Research* 340 (1996): 93–108.

Harmatz, J.S., et al. "Differential Effects of Chlordiazepoxide and Oxazepam on Hostility in a Small Group Setting." *American Journal of Psychiatry* 132 (1975): 861–63.

Palva, E.S., and M. Linnoila. "Effect of Active Metabolites of Chlordiazepoxide and Diazepam, Alone or in Combination with Alcohol, on Psychomotor Skills Related to Driving." *European Journal of Clinical Pharmacology* 13 (1978): 345–50.

Salzman, C., et al. "Chlordiazepoxide-Induced Hostility in a Small Group Setting." *Archives of General Psychiatry* 31 (1974): 401–5.

Sternbach, L.H. "The Discovery of Librium." *Agents and Actions* 43, nos. 3–4 (1994): 82–85.

Clonazepam

Pronunciation: kloh-NA-zuh-pam

Chemical Abstracts Service Registry Number: 1622-61-3

Formal Names: Iktorivil, Klonopin, Lansden, Rivotril

Type: Depressant (benzodiazepine class). *See* page 21

Federal Schedule Listing: Schedule IV (DEA no. 2737)

USA Availability: Prescription

Pregnancy Category: D

Uses. Clonazepam is considered one of the more powerful benzodiazepine class drugs. Primary medical uses are against some kinds of convulsions, particularly in certain kinds of epilepsy, and against panic attacks. For persons suffering from panic attacks, measurements indicate the drug improves both quality of life and work productivity. The drug is also used as an antidepressant and to treat anxiety, catatonia, obsessive-compulsive disorder, the manic phase of manic-depressive behavior, and social phobia in general. A two-year follow-up study of persons receiving brief clonazepam treatment for social phobia found their improvement to be sustained after dosage stopped, and at the two-year mark they were doing better than a control group that had received a placebo. Clonazepam is sometimes preferred over **alprazolam** in treating anxiety because that condition seems less likely to reappear between doses of clonazepam than between doses of alprazolam. Clonazepam can be substituted for alprazolam in order to withdraw persons who have dependence with the latter drug. Clonazepam has been used to fight tics and also to treat muscle control diseases such as akathisia and tardive dyskinesia. Among children with attention deficit hyperactivity disorder (ADHD) who also have tics, a study found clonazepam could help suppress tics without harming the psychiatric effect of ADHD medicine. Although clonazepam is not a multiple sclerosis medicine, it is administered to relieve the affliction's symptoms. Clonazepam has helped reduce fainting spells. It is prescribed to relieve insomnia and to reduce a disorder in which sleeping persons thrash about. The substance has promoted cure of sleepwalking, including a documented extreme case in which a sleeping person would drive a car and engage in violence involving knives. The drug can relieve pain caused by jaw trouble and has been given to cancer patients to reduce vomiting from chemotherapy. Clonazepam and the antimania medicine lithium have been experimentally administered together as a successful treatment for cluster headaches. Clonazepam has eased burning mouth syndrome, a self-descriptive sensation that can persist for years. The drug has been used experimentally with limited success to treat ringing in the ears.

Drawbacks. Clonazepam is not recommended for persons suffering from narrow-angle glaucoma. The compound may worsen respiratory disease. The substance increases saliva production. It often makes people tired, interferes with muscular coordination, and can impede decision making; such effects hinder ability to operate dangerous machinery. Dozens of less common adverse effects are described, ranging from skin rash to painful gums. One case report concludes that clonazepam may promote porphyria, a body chemistry disorder that can make a person violent and supersensitive to light, but such a result is virtually unheard of. A review of medical records of men being treated for posttraumatic stress disorder suggested that the drug may commonly inhibit sexual performance in such a population. Some persons suffer from a disquieting affliction called apnea in which they temporarily stop breathing; case reports say clonazepam can cause apnea attacks. An experiment noted a rebound effect when people stop taking the drug for insomnia, meaning the condition is not cured but instead returns worse than ever, at least for awhile.

Contrary to normal expectations, the drug has occasionally been reported to bring on mania and even aggression. One case report noted that if panic attacks act as a warning against certain behavior, clonazepam's ability to reduce or eliminate panic attacks can also remove a person's inhibitions against the behavior. A small study suggests that clonazepam may reduce inhibitions in children, and case reports exist about the same effect in children, teenagers, and adults. Researchers curious about whether clonazepam especially reduces inhibitions examined medical records of 323 persons institutionalized for psychiatric disturbance, a population in which such a clonazepam effect might be particularly evident; although the study was not designed to demonstrate cause and effect, the records were consistent with a low risk of reduced inhibition from clonazepam and other benzodiazepine class drugs.

Abuse factors. Clonazepam has a withdrawal syndrome similar to **alcohol**'s: cramps and tremors, convulsions, hallucinations, and general mental distress. The syndrome can be avoided if a person reduces dosage gradually. Suddenly halting the drug after taking it for an extended period of time can cause epileptic seizures.

Drug interactions. Clonazepam's actions can be boosted by alcohol, barbiturates, opiates, tricyclic antidepressants, and monoamine oxidase inhibitors (MAOIs). A case report suggests that effects may also be boosted by the heart medicine amiodarone. Another case report indicates that clonazepam reduces blood levels of the epilepsy medicine phenytoin. Taking clonazepam with the antidepressant paroxetine is suspected of causing a dangerous reaction called serotonin syndrome, a serious condition which can involve confusion, tremors, and high body temperature. Combining clonazepam with the antimania medicine lithium is suspected of causing muscular discoordination, including muscles used for speech. A case report noted delirium brought on by simultaneously taking clonazepam and the schizophrenia medicine clozapine.

Cancer. Not enough scientific information to report.

Pregnancy. No increase in birth defects was noted when pregnant rats and mice received many times the recommended human dose while embryos were in the organ-forming stage. Pregnant rabbits receiving clonazepam during the same stage, however, have produced offspring with birth defects such as limb malformations and cleft palate. Because other drugs in the benzodiazepine class are assumed to have potential for causing human birth defects, clonazepam is considered inadvisable for pregnant women unless they and their physicians have considered the issue. Among 51 infants whose mothers took clonazepam during pregnancy, almost 10% had "major malformations"; although that small sample did not compare outcomes in matched women who took no such drug, the study's finding nonetheless raises a caution. A much larger study said that clonazepam taken in combination with other epilepsy drugs increased the chance of birth defects but said nothing about using clonazepam alone. Clonazepam may disturb fetal heartbeat. Offspring with fetal exposure may be sedated, show poor muscle tone, and have low body temperature. Infants can be born with dependence to the drug. Clonazepam passes into human milk at levels high enough to affect infants, and breastfeeding mothers are counseled to avoid clonazepam.

Additional scientific information may be found in:

Cohen, L.S., and J.F. Rosenbaum. "Clonazepam: New Uses and Potential Problems." *Journal of Clinical Psychiatry* 48 (1987, Suppl.): 50–56.

Commander, M., S.H. Green, and M. Prendergast. "Behavioural Disturbances in Children Treated with Clonazepam." *Developmental Medicine and Child Neurology* 33 (1991): 362–63.

Davidson, J.R., and G. Moroz. "Pivotal Studies of Clonazepam in Panic Disorder." *Psychopharmacology Bulletin* 34 (1998): 169–74.

Davidson, J.R., et al. "Treatment of Social Phobia with Clonazepam and Placebo." *Journal of Clinical Psychopharmacology* 13 (1993): 423–28.

Morishita, S., S. Aoki, and S. Watanabe. "Clonazepam as a Therapeutic Adjunct to Improve the Management of Psychiatric Disorders." *Psychiatry and Clinical Neurosciences* 52 (1998): 75–78.

Rosenbaum, J.F., G. Moroz, and C.L. Bowden. "Clonazepam in the Treatment of Panic Disorder with or without Agoraphobia: A Dose-Response Study of Efficacy, Safety, and Discontinuance." *Journal of Clinical Psychopharmacology* 17 (1997): 390–400.

Worthington, J.J., III, et al. "Long-term Experience with Clonazepam in Patients with a Primary Diagnosis of Panic Disorder." *Psychopharmacology Bulletin* 34 (1998): 199–205.

Clorazepate

Pronunciation: klor-AZ-uh-pait

Chemical Abstracts Service Registry Number: 23887-31-2. (Dipotassium form 57109-90-7)

Formal Names: Tranxene

Type: Depressant (benzodiazepine class). *See* page 21

Federal Schedule Listing: Schedule IV (DEA no. 2768)

USA Availability: Prescription

Pregnancy Category: D

Uses. Clorazepate dipotassium is a "prodrug" related to **diazepam**. A prodrug is a substance that may have little effect itself but that the body metabolizes into another chemical that does have a drug effect. For example, one metabolite of clorazepate dipotassium is desmethyldiazepam, which in turn transforms into **oxazepam**. Prodrugs are prescribed when direct administration of the desired chemical does not work, such as when the chemical would degrade before it has time to build up in the part of the body where it is needed or when the normal dosage form cannot be given (perhaps a substance that can be absorbed through the skin is needed rather than giving an injection). Although metabolites of clorazepate dipotassium generally create the medical actions, for simplicity this discussion usually refers only to the prodrug clorazepate dipotassium and calls it a drug.

This long-acting drug's primary medical uses are for anxiety, for convulsions, and as a muscle relaxant. The substance can be taken on a long-term basis for successful control of epilepsy but is described as a "second-line" medication, meaning it is not used unless other drugs have been tried without success. Clorazepate dipotassium's long-term effectiveness against anxiety is unclear. A common short-term use is to reduce nervousness in surgery patients shortly before an operation. The drug is also given to ease withdrawal from **zolpidem** and **alcohol** (including delirium tremens). An injection can quickly calm a bellicose individual.

Weight, age, and gender can affect dosage. A study found that an active metabolite (desmethyldiazepam) from a dose of clorazepate dipotassium lasts almost three times as long in overweight persons compared to normal weight persons, apparently due to accumulation in body fat. Another study noted that the older a male was, the longer the same metabolite from a dose lasted, but that effect was not seen in women.

Although clorazepate dipotassium is used against anxiety, the drug is generally considered unsuitable for depressed or psychotic persons. It has nonetheless been given with success for treating depression (even though sometimes the drug can instead worsen that condition). The drug has helped reduce nightmares caused by other pharmaceuticals and has helped alleviate psychosomatic complaints. It has also been used against tetanus.

Drawbacks. People with severe breathing trouble or acute narrow-angle glaucoma should avoid clorazepate dipotassium. Loosening of the nails has been attributed to the drug in a case report, but that is unusual. Somewhat less surprising is a case report of jaundice, less surprising because many drugs add a burden to the liver. Oral overdose can provoke rage.

The drug routinely makes people sleepy, and users are cautioned against operating dangerous machinery. In experiments the drug increases reaction time and decreases attention. Nonetheless, a laboratory simulation of driving showed no effect on operating a motor vehicle. One authority contends that the substance should not impair driving performance but acknowledges that trouble arises if a driver does not use the drug as medically directed or uses alcohol simultaneously. Other unwanted effects occur less often: peevishness, headache, stomach irritation, dry mouth, rashes, double vision, and unclear speech. Therapeutic advantage sometimes comes from the drowsiness factor, with patients instructed to take the drug at bedtime to help reduce insomnia, a technique that then also allows them to obtain the long-lasting antianxiety effect during daytime hours the next day. In one study people reported more restful sleep, and measurements after they awoke showed little drug impact on performance tests (illustrating the difference a few hours can make on how well someone performs after taking a substance).

Abuse factors. If usage continues for a long time and suddenly stops, a withdrawal syndrome can occur. Withdrawal symptoms can include trouble with sleeping and memory, jitteriness and crankiness, sore muscles, and loose bowels. Those discomforts are similar to what happens in alcohol or barbiturate withdrawal. Researchers suspect the problem may be worsened if a person has taken some other benzodiazepine class drug off and on. The withdrawal problem may be avoided by gradual discontinuation of clorazepate dipotassium. Experiments with dogs and rabbits also show withdrawal symptoms. A canine test demonstrated that abrupt clorazepate dipotassium withdrawal can cause fatal seizures. The kinds of well-documented dependence mentioned above involve relatively brief withdrawal. Reportedly human withdrawal symptoms may continue for months, which is an unusual persistence of dependence. Long-term signs of withdrawal, however, are described as reappearance of anxiety, sometimes accompanied by psychosis and convulsions. Such long-term "withdrawal symptoms" sound much like conditions for which the drug is prescribed, raising a question of whether the victim is experiencing long-term dependence or simply reemergence of conditions formerly controlled by the now-absent drug.

A group of recreational drug abusers was tested to determine their likings, and the group declared clorazepate dipotassium to be less attractive than diazepam or **lorazepam**.

Drug interactions. Members in a group of recreational drug abusers reported that alcohol boosted clorazepate dipotassium's effect and that the combination made their mood bleaker, but when subjects in another study took that combination they felt happier than alcohol normally made them. Another experiment found that the combination impaired memory, although still another study found that clorazepate alone did not affect memory. In testing how long the desmethyldiazepam metabolite lasts from a clorazepate dipotassium dose, conflicting results have come from experiments comparing cigarette smokers to nonsmokers. Opiates, barbiturates, and monoamine oxidase inhibitors (MAOIs) found in some antidepressants may boost actions of clorazepate dipotassium. Clorazepate dipotassium may boost alcohol's effects.

Cancer. Animal studies have failed to find evidence of any cancer-causing potential in clorazepate dipotassium.

Pregnancy. Experiments with pregnant rats and rabbits revealed no impairment of fertility and failed to produce any birth defects attributable to clorazepate dipotassium. One rat study also found no behavioral consequences from prenatal exposure to the drug, but another rat study discovered that offspring walked more slowly than normal and also had some learning difficulty. The drug's potential for creating human birth defects is unknown. A case report associates it with fatal lung collapse in a newborn whose mother had used the drug during pregnancy, and another case report associates the drug with fatal birth defects. "Association" may mean caution is appropriate, but it does not demonstrate cause and effect. Breast-feeding mothers are warned to avoid the drug because its metabolite nordiazepam (which is also a metabolite of diazepam) passes into the milk and into the infant. The metabolite desmethyldiazepam also passes into milk, as does clorazepate dipotassium itself.

Additional scientific information may be found in:

Fabre, L.F., and H.P. Putman III. "Depressive Symptoms and Intellectual Functioning in Anxiety Patients Treated with Clorazepate." *Journal of Clinical Psychiatry* 49 (1988): 189–92.

Fujii, T., et al. "Clorazepate Therapy for Intractable Epilepsy." *Brain and Development* 9 (1987): 288–91.

Henderson, J.G. "Value of a Single Night-time Dose of Potassium Clorazepate in Anxiety: A Controlled Trial Comparison with Diazepam." *Scottish Medical Journal* 27 (1982): 292–96.

Moodley, P., S. Golombok, and M. Lader. "Effects of Clorazepate Dipotassium and Placebo on Psychomotor Skills." *Perceptual and Motor Skills* 61 (1985): 1121–22.

Zung, W.W. "Effect of Clorazepate on Depressed Mood in Anxious Patients." *Journal of Clinical Psychiatry* 48 (1987): 13–14.

Coca

See also **Cocaine**

Pronunciation: KOH-kuh

Chemical Abstracts Service Registry Number: None

Formal Names: *Erythroxylum coca*

Informal Names: Cocaine Plant, Cocaine Tree, Cuca

Type: Stimulant (cocaine class). *See* page 17

Federal Schedule Listing: Schedule II (DEA no. 9040)

USA Availability: Prescription (due to Schedule II status, but not a standard medical drug)

Pregnancy Category: None

Uses. The coca bush is native to the Andes, where it has been harvested since ancient Inca days. Use in that era has been confirmed through analysis of hair from ancient corpses and from examination of artwork. At first only upper-class Incas and select individuals were permitted to use coca, but usage spread to Inca society as a whole after the Spanish conquest. In modern times the plant has been cultivated in India and Sri Lanka as well as Formosa, Indonesia, and Malaysia. During the 1960s Malaysia was the world's primary source of coca. Its leaves are the natural product from which **cocaine** is refined, and blood measurements confirm that coca users receive cocaine from the leaves. Cocaine content is commonly 0.6% to 1.5% of the leaves by weight. Cocaine is not the only drug component of coca, but relatively little exploration has been made of other components. Some investigators suspect that these other drugs are more important than cocaine in producing coca's effects.

Traditionally coca has enjoyed wide use and social acceptance in the Andes, although leaf chewing (as opposed to taking coca in tea) is associated with lower social classes. Persons from middle and higher social classes who do not engage in physical labor may use coca recreationally. Short-term mental effects of coca leaves have been likened to those of coffee. Usage is much more common among persons living at high altitudes than at sea level. Coca can be a social lubricant, much in the way that **khat** is traditionally utilized. As with wine, coca leaves produced in different regions under different conditions can have flavor characteristics making some varieties more sought after than others even if the drug content is virtually identical. Veins are stripped from the leaves, which typically are then chewed or sucked upon in a small quantity for hours, much like chewing gum. Coca is a local anesthetic and numbs the mouth when a person chews coca leaves. Lime (the mineral, not the fruit) may be added to improve the body's absorption of cocaine from the leaves. Habitual leaf chewers routinely receive a daily cocaine dose of 0.25 grams spread over several hours. Coca tea or the leaves themselves are used to aid digestion, reduce gastrointestinal colic, fight asthma, soothe vocal cords (laryngitis), relieve stress and elevate mood, alleviate cold and thirst, produce sweat, and fight motion sickness. Milk with coca has been used against colic and diarrhea in babies. Coca cigarettes have been used to treat both asthma and colds. Proposals have been made to produce coca lozenges and chewing gum to make the natural product available in formats more familiar to persons coming from a European heritage.

Habitual coca chewing interferes with the body's insulin and thereby tends to raise blood sugar levels. That finding should interest diabetic chewers but is also relevant to persons using leaves at high altitudes (common in the Andes) because the reduced oxygen supply at upper elevations tends to lower blood sugar. Habitual coca use apparently compensates for that effect. Blood sugar tends to decline during exercise; coca can prevent that decline, and scientists suspect that coca can increase the body's effective use of blood sugar during exercise.

Coca leaves improve a person's access to stored energy sources in the human body and thereby increase capacity for physical labor. During the nineteenth century such qualities attracted notice in Europe, but suggestions that coca be used in industrial and military labor were apparently ignored. In the 1970s a sample of Argentine miners showed that 65% chewed coca leaves every day, and another 14% used leaves less often. The more physical power and endurance required for a particular job, the more likely that a miner used coca leaves each day. One study of coca found the typical stimulant actions of raising pulse rate and blood pressure but also found that coca had a more unusual effect of decreasing the volume of blood plasma—a condition normally associated with bleeding or with not drinking enough fluids. This condition interferes with proper blood circulation during physical exercise, but centuries of experience suggest that coca-chewing laborers get along well enough nonetheless. The study just referred to involved habitual chewers of coca; occasional chewers may not experience the same results. For example, in another study scientists concluded that regular chewers had more access to energy stored in body fat but that occasional chewers did not and also concluded that occasional chewers would not show the same improved endurance during physical exercise that is demonstrated by habitual chewers. One investigator has concluded that coca improves endurance but does not otherwise help physical labor (a person cannot lift more or run faster).

Like many stimulants, coca reduces feelings of hunger and can thereby reduce food intake. The appetite suppressant effect is slight, however, simply helping a person to get by more comfortably when food is scarce. Coca chewers exhibit robust appetites when victuals are plentiful, and coca preparations can even be an element of meal-taking. Some research suggests that under low atmospheric pressure coca can improve the body's metabolism of carbohydrates and thereby improve nutrition of users. Coca itself is a good source of vitamins, iron, and phosphorus; and lime used with coca can provide almost a gram of calcium per day—important supplements where diet is often deficient in such factors. Malnourishment exhibited by rural coca chewers seems related more to poor food supply than to use of coca. Rat experiments, however, indicate that coca slows growth rate if used in mountainous altitudes.

Drawbacks. Although individuals have to work hard to abuse coca enough to create problems, persons who succeed at that task can experience the kinds of hallucinations and other mental afflictions associated with stimulant abuse. That outcome is very unusual among persons who use coca in traditional ways. Contrary to what one would expect from a stimulant, scientific tests show that coca (like khat) retards reaction time and increases errors in work performance. Long-term mental effects of habitual coca usage decrease thinking abilities in ways that are seldom noticeable in rural village life but that are clearly documented through scientific tests. Such decline would put persons at a disadvantage in coping with modern urban conditions, on or off the job. The decline is presumed to be evidence of organic brain damage.

Coca depresses the immune system, presumably making users more susceptible to disease. Coca chewing is suspected of promoting spread of cholera, not from coca itself but from lime or other alkali substances chewed with the leaves, having the result of lowering the stomach's acid content and thereby providing an excellent environment for growth of microscopic cholera organisms. Coca is suspected of causing liver damage. Archeologists examining ancient human remains have concluded that coca chewing may cause tooth decay and loss. In contrast, modern-day chewers claim that the habit promotes dental health and makes users less susceptible to disease in general. Coca's effects on general physical health remain uncertain. Differing backgrounds of users and abstainers hinder efforts to measure effects; factors other than coca may be affecting health.

Abuse factors. Tolerance to the drug effect (resulting in a need to keep increasing the dose) is not observed among coca chewers; lack of that classic indication of addiction is evidence of coca's low addictive potential. Heavy coca users may exhibit mild signs of physical dependence with the drug if they stop using it, but any such transitory illness is too slight to be a factor in choosing to continue using the drug.

Drug interactions. Not enough scientific information on the natural product to report.

Cancer. Mouths of habitual chewers show tissue abnormalities but no precancerous conditions. Nonetheless, coca is considered a probable cause of cancer.

Pregnancy. Coca is considered a probable cause of fetal injury.

Additional information. In the 1970s a lift of all legal controls over coca was proposed on the theory that the natural product was far less harmful than pharmaceutical stimulants and might be just as attractive to persons who were damaging themselves through stimulant abuse. The proposal was rejected.

Cocaine and ecgonine can be removed from coca leaves, and such "decocainized" leaves are legal to possess without a prescription. Not all leaves marketed as decocainized have undergone such treatment, and urine tests of persons drinking tea steeped from such leaves may be positive for cocaine use.

Coca paste. This substance is made from coca leaves but has the same sort of relationship to them that 100 proof alcohol has to 3.2 beer. Paste is yielded midway in the process of refining cocaine from coca; by volume the paste is anywhere from about 40% to 90% cocaine, thus as potent as typical street varieties of cocaine itself. Some persons desiring cocaine sensations prefer paste, which can be smoked without the heat destroying cocaine's drug effects. Such persons routinely add the paste to tobacco or **marijuana**. Because of coca paste's high potency, a user basically receives the same impact as with using cocaine. Descriptions of coca paste smoking and crack smoking are similar: euphoria, insomnia, compulsive use. Adverse effects duplicate those of cocaine (even including "coke bugs"—a hallucination of vermin crawling under the skin). Using coca paste is very different from using coca leaves. The difference can be inferred from a 1996 report that combined surveys involving over 24,000 persons in several countries of the Andes region. In 1965 about 13% of Peru's population apparently used coca leaves, but only 0.8% to 3% of persons in the 1996 multicountry survey reported "lifetime" coca paste or cocaine use—meaning people had tried them at least once; the percentage of regular users would be lower yet. Direct comparison of those 1965 and 1996 figures would be invalid because of difference in dates and survey designs, but the huge gap between their percentages is consistent with a general rule that the stronger a drug is, the less popular it is. Also, the kinds of persons who use coca leaves and coca paste differ. The 1965 figure included over half the laborers in Peru's countryside. The 1996 survey found coca paste and cocaine to be used predominantly by educated middle-class urbanites. A 1992 study of hospitalized coca paste smokers also found most to be middle class, but almost as many were from a low-income background.

Additional scientific information may be found in:

Favier, R., et al. "Effects of Coca Chewing on Hormonal and Metabolic Responses during Prolonged Submaximal Exercise." *Journal of Applied Physiology* 80 (1996): 650–55.

Grinspoon, L., and J.B. Bakalar. "Coca and Cocaine as Medicines: An Historical Review." *Journal of Ethnopharmacology* 3 (1981): 149–59.

Hamner, J.E., III, and O.L. Villegas. "The Effect of Coca Leaf Chewing on the Buccal Mucosa of Aymara and Quechua Indians in Bolivia." *Oral Surgery, Oral Medicine, and Oral Pathology* 28 (1969): 287–95.

Heath, D.B. "Coca in the Andes: Traditions, Functions and Problems." *Rhode Island Medical Journal* 73 (1990): 237–41.

Jeri, F.R., et al. "The Syndrome of Coca Paste." *Journal of Psychoactive Drugs* 24 (1992): 173–82.

Negrete, J.C. "Coca Leaf Chewing: A Public Health Assessment." *British Journal of Addiction to Alcohol and Other Drugs* 73 (1978): 283–90.

Weil, A.T. "Coca Leaf as a Therapeutic Agent." *American Journal of Drug and Alcohol Abuse* 5 (1978): 75–86.

Zapata-Ortiz, V. "The Chewing of Coca Leaves in Peru." *International Journal of the Addictions* 5 (1970): 287–94.

Cocaine

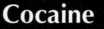

See also **Coca**

Pronunciation: koh-KAIN

Chemical Abstracts Service Registry Number: 50-36-2. (Hydrochloride form 53-21-4)

Formal Names: Methylbenzoylecgonine

Informal Names: All-American Drug, Angie, Apple Jacks, Aunt Nora, Baby T, Bad, Badrock, Ball, Barbs, Base, Baseball, Basuco, Bazooka, Bazulco, Beam, Beamer, Beans, Beat, Beautiful Boulders, Bebe, Beemer, Bernice, Bernie, Bernie's Flakes, Bernie's Gold Dust, Big Bloke, Big C, Big Flake, Big Rush, Bill Blass, Billie Hoke, Bings, Birdie Powder, Biscuit, B.J., Black Rock, Blanca, Blanco, Blast, Blotter, Blow, Blowcaine, Blowout, Blue, Bobo, Bolivian Marching Powder, Bollo, Bolo, Bomb, Bone, Bonecrusher, Boost, Botray, Boubou, Boulder, Boulya, Bouncing Powder, Boy, Bubble Gum, Bullia Capital, Bullyon, Bump, Bunk, Burese, Burnese, Bush, Butler, Butter, C, Cabello Cadillac, Caine, Cakes, California Cornflakes, Came, Canamo, Candy, Candy C, Cap, Capsula, Carnie, Carrie, Carrie Nation, Casper, Casper the Ghost, C-Dust, Cecil, C-Game, Chalk, Charlie, Chemical, Chewies, Chippy, Chocolate Ecstasy, Choe, Cholly, Climax, Cloud, Cloud 9, Coca, Coconut, Coco Rocks, Coke, Cola, Combol, Cookies, Coolie, Corine, Corrine, Corrinne, Crack, Crank, Crib, Crimmie, Croak, Crumbs, Crunch & Munch, Crystal, Cube, Dama Blanca, Demolish, Devil, Devil Drug, Devil's Dandruff, Devilsmoke, Dice, Dip, DOA, Double Bubble, Double Ups, Double Yoke, Dove, Dream, Duct, Dust, Eastside Player, Egg, Eightball, Esnortiar, Everclear, Eye Opener, Famous Dimes, 51, Fish Scales, Flake, Florida Snow, Foo Foo, Foolish Powder, Freeze, French Fries, Fries, Friskie Powder, Garbage Rock, Geek (with **marijuana**), Gift of the Sun, Gift of the Sun God, Gimmie (with marijuana), Gin, Girl, Girlfriend, Glad Stuff, Glo, Gold, Gold Dust, Golf Ball, Goofball (with **heroin**), Gravel, Green Gold, Gremmies (with marijuana), Grit, Groceries, G-Rock, H & C (with heroin), Hail, Half Track, Hamburger Helper, Happy Dust, Happy Powder, Happy Trails, Hard Ball, Hard Line, Hard Rock, Have a Dust, Haven Dust, Heaven, Heaven Dust, Hell, Henry VIII, Her, Hit, Hooter, Hotcakes, Hubba, Hunter, Ice, Ice Cube, Icing, Inca Message, Issues, Jam, Jejo, Jelly, Jelly Beans, Johnson, Joy Powder, Junk, King, King's Habit, Kokayeen, Kokomo, Kryptonite, Lady, Lady Caine, Lady Snow, Late Night, Leaf, Line, Love, Love Affair, Ma'a, Mama Coca, Marching Dust, Marching Powder, Mayo, Merck, Merk, Mixed Jive, Mojo, Monkey, Monster, Mosquitos, Movie Star Drug, Mujer, Murder 1 (with heroin), New Addition, Nieve, Nose, Nose

Candy, Nose Powder, Nose Stuff, Nuggets, Number 3, 151, Onion (quantity), Oyster Stew, Paradise, Paradise White, Parlay, Paste, Patico, Pearl, Pebbles, Pee Wee, Percia, Perico, Peruvian, Peruvian Flake, Peruvian Lady, P-Funk (crack cocaine mixed with **PCP**), Piece, Piedra, Piles, Pimp, Pimp's Drug, Pipero, Polvo Blanco, Pony, Potato Chips, Powder, Powder Diamonds, Press, Prime Time, Primo, Product, Quill, Racehorse Charley, Rane, Raw, Ready Rock, Red Caps, Regular P, Rest in Peace, Roca, Rock, Rock Attack, Rocks of Hell, Rooster, Rox, Roxanne, Roz, Rush, Schmeck, Schoolboy, Schoolcraft, Scorpion, Scottie, Scotty, Scrabble, Scramble, Scruples, Serpico 21, 7-Up, Shabu, She, Sherm, Sightball, Slab, Sleet, Sleigh Ride, Smoke, Smoking Gun (with heroin), Snowball (with heroin), Snow Bird, Snowcone, Snow Seals (with amphetamine), Snow White, Society High, Soda, Space Base (crack mixed with PCP), Space Cadet (crack with PCP), Space Dust (crack with PCP), Speed, Speedball (with heroin), Speedboat (crack with PCP and marijuana), Square Time Bob, Squirrel (crack with PCP and marijuana), Star, Star Dust, Star-Spangled Powder, Stones, Studio Fuel, Sugar, Sugar Block, Sweet Stuff, Swell Up, T, Talco, Tardust, Teenager, Teeth, Tension, Thing, Tissue, Toot, Top Gun, Topo, Tornado, Toss Up, Tragic Magic (crack with PCP), Trails, Troop, Turkey, Tweaks, 24–7, 20 Rock, Ultimate, Wave, Whack, White Ball, White Dragon, White Ghost, White Girl, White Horse, White Lady, White Mosquito, White Powder, White Sugar, White Tornado, Whiz Bang, Wicky Stick (crack with marijuana and PCP), Wild Cat (with **methcathinone**), Wings, Witch, Wooly (crack with marijuana), Wrecking Crew, Yahoo, Yale, Yayoo, Yeaho, Yeah-O, Yeyo, Yimyom, Zip

Type: Stimulant (cocaine class). *See* page 17

Federal Schedule Listing: Schedule II (DEA no. 9041)

USA Availability: Prescription

Pregnancy Category: C

Uses. The drug was first isolated from **coca** plants in the mid-1800s. Cocaine apparently functions as an insecticide in the plants, but the substance has had no commercial agricultural use for that purpose. Early medical applications included administration to treat addiction to **alcohol** and opiates, but persons addicted to those drugs did not better on cocaine. Like many stimulants, cocaine has anorectic (weight-reducing) properties that decline as usage stretches over time; but the drug's main medical use has been as a local anesthetic, particularly in ear, nose, and mouth surgery. Experimental use as an antidepressant has been unsuccessful. Cocaine has been used to treat tonsillitis, earache, toothache, burns, skin rash, hay fever, asthma, hemorrhoids, nerve pain, nausea, and vomiting. It makes the body's immune system more active. For medical purposes cocaine has been largely superseded by drugs having less potential for abuse, but it is still called an excellent anesthetic for nose and throat surgery, has been used for gynecological surgery in modern times, and still has ophthalmological use as eye drops, although the latter employment must be cautious in order to prevent corneal damage. Due to hazards of cocaine injections, since the 1920s medical usage of cocaine has been largely limited to topical (applying it directly to a body surface).

Like other stimulants, cocaine may improve mood, self-confidence, and so-ciability. Taking the drug for such purposes may be recreational or for self-medication of psychological distress; for example, a strong association exists between posttraumatic stress disorder and cocaine use. Cocaine can tempo-rarily enhance work performance whether the task be manual labor or intel-lectual concentration. A century ago railroad engineers, dock workers, and cotton pickers were reported to be using the drug for that purpose, and it also received experimental military use in that pre-amphetamine era. On an oc-casional basis cocaine can help accomplish intense intellectual effort, such as staying awake all night to finish a piece of writing, and on a regular basis, cocaine can help accomplish dull repetitive tasks requiring close mental atten-tion. As with other stimulants, steady use can eventually worsen work ability as a person's physical reserves are exhausted and as a person becomes emo-tionally strung out.

For over a century the most popular ways of taking cocaine were by injec-tion or by inhaling the drug as a snuff. The latter technique inherently pro-duces sensations of lesser strength than injection does, but a person desiring more can simply inhale larger quantities of powder.

Drawbacks. Habitually inhaling cocaine powder can cause a runny or con-gested nose and nosebleeds. Too much inhalation can bring on nasal ulcers and in exceptional cases can kill tissue and pierce the cartilage in the middle of the nose. Snorting can cause headaches. Abuse can also damage muscles (including heart), kidneys, and liver. Cases of heart attack and stroke are known, as are cases of serious intestinal damage related to problems with blood flow. Preexisting asthma can be worsened. Rupture of pulmonary air sacs and lung collapse are possible, though uncommon, results from cocaine smoking. The drug may bring on a type of glaucoma.

Some undesired effects are similar to those of amphetamine abuse: peevish-ness, nervousness, combativeness, paranoia, insomnia, and (after a dose wears off) depression. Typical afflictions include repetitions in movement or speech. Males may engage in sexual intercourse far longer than usual. Abusers may cut themselves off from other persons and become suspicious of them. As-sorted hallucinations may occur, the classic one being "coke bugs" crawling under the skin. Psychological problems produced by unwise use of cocaine are so similar to those from other stimulants that some scientists believe sim-ilar mechanisms must cause the problems. Psychosis can be induced by co-caine but, as with other stimulants, generally does not continue after the drug use stops. Smoking cocaine can produce respiratory difficulties reminiscent of tobacco smoking—difficulties that develop faster than with tobacco because lungs must deal not only with the "air pollution" but with powerful drug effects as well. Particles of crack smoke floating in the air and landing on someone's eye can damage the cornea.

The amount of drug needed to kill a person varies; depending on a person's condition a dose that provides pleasure one day can kill on another. The same goes for persons sharing a supply: What satisfies one user can cause serious trouble for another. In rat experiments females are more sensitive to cocaine than males. Immediate problems in humans may include high blood pressure, irregular heartbeat, and seizures. The drug promotes rises in pulse rate and body temperature, which can be problems if a person engages in strenuous physical activity such as wild dancing.

Abuse factors. Before the 1970s cocaine smoking was never popular because the necessary heat destroyed much of the drug's potency. In that decade, however, the practice of freebasing cocaine began. That process allowed the drug's potency to be retained when smoking it, thereby allowing a route of administration providing the same intense impact formerly available only through intravenous injection. Freebasing, however, involves volatile chemicals that can explode in a flash fire if they are mishandled. In the 1980s illicit chemists discovered a much safer way to modify cocaine into a smokable format. The resultant product was known as crack cocaine and became the most notorious illicit drug since **heroin**.

A few seconds after inhaling crack smoke a user can experience a sense of well-being and joy accompanied by what has been described as a total body orgasm, followed by a few minutes of afterglow.

Tolerance is reported. Debate exists about whether a cocaine addict experiences physical withdrawal symptoms upon giving up the drug. A consensus holds that any physical consequences caused by the initial phase of abstinence can be less serious than those that develop when withdrawing from opiates and far less serious than withdrawing from alcohol or barbiturates.

Drug interactions. Cocaine masks some effects of alcohol, encouraging drinkers to ingest larger quantities of beverages. Alcohol's effects are longer lasting than cocaine, however, so a person functioning adequately under both drugs can suddenly become very drunk as the cocaine intoxication ends. If that transition happens while a person is operating dangerous machinery (such as a car), for example, the consequences may be disastrous. Cocaine's influence on the heart and liver seem increased by alcohol. **Mazindol** boosts the elevation that cocaine causes in pulse rate and blood pressure and makes those changes last longer. Mice experiments indicate possible fatal interaction if a cocaine-using asthmatic is treated with aminophylline (a combination of ethylenediamine and theophylline). Cocaine abusers also tend to be extra susceptible to the benzodiazepine class of depressant drugs. In animal experiments **caffeine** and **nicotine** boost cocaine effects. Naloxone, a drug used to counteract opiate actions, can boost cocaine effects in humans. For many years some medical practitioners have mixed adrenalin with topical applications of cocaine in order to make anesthetic effects last longer. The reason adrenalin interacts in that way with cocaine is unclear, and the custom is disputed. What works when applying cocaine to a body surface for anesthesia does not necessarily work in other contexts. Seeking to stretch out effects of recreational cocaine with various substances can be so unsuccessful as to require hospitalization for unexpected interactions. In some manipulations of a rat experiment the tricyclic antidepressant amitriptyline reduced cocaine actions.

Cancer. Cocaine's potential for causing cancer is uncertain.

Pregnancy. The drug's potential for causing birth defects is uncertain. Some animal experiments produce birth defects; some do not. In the 1980s and 1990s cocaine was widely reported to have devastating impact on mental ability of infants whose mothers used the drug during pregnancy. Scientists have been unable to verify those reports. Evidence is growing that offspring tend to perform at the lower end of the normal range, but pregnant women who use cocaine also typically use hefty amounts of tobacco cigarettes and beverage alcohol while failing to get proper nutrition and prenatal care. Such confounding factors hinder scientists' ability to measure what cocaine does to a fetus, although persistent investigators are beginning to separate cocaine's influence from other factors. Even so, despite excellent theoretical reasons to suspect that cocaine damages fetal development, those suspicions have not been confirmed. Nonetheless, cocaine is not considered safe for a pregnant woman to use. Apparently cocaine enters human milk and can be passed to infants via that route. A case report tells of an infant hospitalized for cocaine overdose received from the mother's milk.

Additional scientific information may be found in:

Brain, P.F., and·G.A. Coward. "A Review of the History, Actions, and Legitimate Uses of Cocaine." *Journal of Substance Abuse* 1 (1989): 431–51.

Gay, G.R., et al. "Cocaine: History, Epidemiology, Human Pharmacology, and Treatment. A Perspective on a New Debut for an Old Girl." *Clinical Toxicology* 8 (1975): 149–78.

Johnson, B., et al. "Effects of Acute Intravenous Cocaine on Cardiovascular Function, Human Learning, and Performance in Cocaine Addicts." *Psychiatry Research* 77 (1998): 35–42.

Lester, B.M., L.L. LaGasse, and R. Bigsby. "Prenatal Cocaine Exposure and Child Development: What Do We Know and What Do We Do?" *Seminars in Speech and Language* 19 (1998): 123–46.

Magura, S., and A. Rosenblum. "Modulating Effect of Alcohol Use on Cocaine Use." *Addictive Behaviors* 25 (2000): 117–22.

Middleton, R.M., and M.B. Kirkpatrick. "Clinical Use of Cocaine. A Review of the Risks and Benefits." *Drug Safety: An International Journal of Medical Toxicology and Drug Experience* 9 (1993): 212–17.

Rawson, R., et al. "Methamphetamine and Cocaine Users: Differences in Characteristics and Treatment Retention." *Journal of Psychoactive Drugs* 32 (2000): 233–38.

Siegal, H.A., et al. "Crack-Cocaine Users as Victims of Physical Attack." *Journal of the National Medical Association* 92 (2000): 76–82.

Siegel, R.K. "Cocaine and the Privileged Class: A Review of Historical and Contemporary Images." *Advances in Alcohol and Substance Abuse* 4 (1984): 37–49.

Codeine

Pronunciation: KOH-deen

Chemical Abstracts Service Registry Number: 76-57-3. (Phosphate hemihydrate form 41444-62-6)

Formal Names: BRON, Methylmorphine

Informal Names: AC/DC, Barr, C, Captain Cody, Co-Dine, Cody, Coties, Cough Syrup, Down, Homebake, Karo, Lean, Lean & Dean, Nods, Schoolboy, Syrup, T-3s. *With **glutethimide***: Doors & 4, 4 Doors, Hits, Loads, Packets, Pancakes & Syrup, Sets, 3s & 8s

Type: Depressant (opiate class). *See* page 22

Federal Schedule Listing: Schedule II, III, V controlled substance, depending on product formulation (DEA no. 9050)

USA Availability: Prescription and nonprescription

Pregnancy Category: C

Uses. Codeine was discovered in 1832 by French chemist Pierre-Jean Robiquet. Typically it is derived from the more potent drug **morphine**, which, depending on dosage route (oral, injection), is considered about 3 to 12 times stronger than codeine. After codeine is administered, body chemistry transforms it back into morphine; thus employer drug screens on someone who used a codeine cough remedy can be positive for morphine. Basically codeine is a prodrug, a substance having little medicinal effect itself but that the body transforms into a useful drug—in this case, morphine. Although scientists have long believed that codeine's therapeutic effects come from morphine, as the twenty-first century began, one group of researchers reported that persons whose bodies cannot properly convert codeine into morphine can nonetheless experience medical benefit from codeine itself.

Codeine is administered for sedation and to stop diarrhea, coughs, and pain. The substance is considered one of the best cough medicines, although research in the 1990s indicated the drug has little ability to control coughs from colds. Some people take the drug regularly to diminish chronic pain. One study of the drug's ability to ease pain after tonsillectomy found its effectiveness comparable to morphine, but another tonsillectomy study found codeine no more effective than acetaminophen (Tylenol and similar products). Research examining pain from a wide variety of causes, ranging from cancer to backache, found no more discomfort relief from a combination dose of codeine and acetaminophen than from combining **hydrocodone** and ibuprofen. Such findings probably indicate simply that various kinds of pain relievers work adequately for various discomforts, with codeine often being as good as the other drugs.

Some regular codeine users take it to reduce anxiety, and some simply find the substance's effects pleasant. A clinical test of codeine found no antidepressant action, but people who use codeine for a long time tend to be depressed and may be taking that drug to medicate themselves for depression—so if they have access to antidepressants they may have less interest in codeine. Codeine cough syrups may include stimulants and other ingredients that persons find pleasant, increasing the syrups' appeal.

Drawbacks. Codeine can promote sleepiness, abdominal cramps, constipation, urinary retention, nausea, and breathing impairment. A case report tells of a massive dose followed by several days of hallucinations and paranoia in a person already prone to psychiatric problems. After taking a dose, people should avoid operating dangerous machinery until they know the drug is not hindering their ability to do so. When 70 professional army drivers in Finland were tested in a driving simulator after taking 50 mg of codeine, they ran off the roadway more frequently than when they were under the influence of **alcohol**. Elderly persons who take codeine have an increased likelihood of hip fracture, presumably because the substance makes them woozy and more likely to fall. Codeine has been known to cause pancreatitis, particularly if the victim's gallbladder has been surgically removed, but this effect is considered unusual. Medical personnel refrain from administering the drug through intravenous injection because that route can lower blood pressure and blood oxygen to fatal levels.

In two studies researchers found that people taking codeine felt few sensations from the drug and had normal performance on assorted tests of physical and mental functioning. Those findings, however, may be related to dosages given by experimenters; higher dosages might well produce different results.

Abuse factors. Codeine abuse can be troublesome enough that persons need treatment to break the addiction. Some cases have required hospitalization. Nonetheless, prevalence of codeine addiction was disputed in 1989 by two authorities who carefully examined past reports of addiction: Little scientific research had been done on the topic, and most had involved persons already addicted to morphine. As morphine addicts will use codeine as a stopgap to hold off a withdrawal syndrome when their main drug is unavailable, their responses to codeine are not necessarily representative of a general population's reactions. In addition, codeine cough syrups may contain a substantial percentage of alcohol, so heavy use of such a product can involve a further confounding factor of alcoholism. The 1989 authorities concluded that verifiable accounts of people being addicted primarily to codeine (rather than mainly to some other drug, with codeine on the side) were unusual.

Dependence with codeine can develop; withdrawal symptoms are like those of morphine withdrawal, but milder. A study of rheumatism patients receiving codeine found that quite a few needed higher doses to control pain as months went by, but the increase was caused by decline of their physical condition rather than development of tolerance.

The same study noted that almost no patients abused the drug, and of those few who did, all abused other substances as well. That finding is consistent with many observations of other drugs having abuse potential; only a small minority of users misuse them, and this minority is prone to problems with more than one substance. People having a bad relationship with codeine tend to have bad relationships with alcohol, **marijuana**, and (less commonly) **heroin**. One study found that almost half the patients requesting treatment for codeine cough syrup addiction engaged in sexual conduct putting them at risk for AIDS, conduct illustrating a multiproblem lifestyle in which codeine abuse was simply one aspect. Background checks of deceased Los Angeles–area codeine abusers revealed almost 66% had attempted suicide, had a prior overdose on some drug, had been hospitalized for psychiatric problems, had been in physical fights, and had an alcohol problem (87% had an alcohol-related arrest record). So codeine may be only one of several problems in such lives.

Not all drug abuse is illicit. Sometimes people develop an abusive relationship with a drug that is supplied to them through legitimate medical channels. Swedish researchers compared the use of codeine in that country to the use of **propoxyphene**, an opioid related to **methadone**. Those investigators found that doctors in two of Sweden's largest cities typically tended to prescribe codeine to middle-aged females and that in one of those cities codeine was used the most in poor areas of town and was often associated with taking benzodiazepines frequently (in experiments the benzodiazepine **diazepam** lengthened the time that a codeine dose lasted, while codeine interfered with diazepam—suggesting that a codeine user would have to take more diazepam to get benzodiazepine sensations, consistent with the Swedish findings of increased benzodiazepine consumption among codeine users). Those kinds of codeine usage characteristics were not found for propoxyphene in the Swedish research even though both drugs would have opiate-type effects; the difference in usage suggests that physicians' customs may have been promoting codeine abuse.

In drug abuse treatment programs codeine has been used successfully to shift addicts from other opiates—so successfully that one group of researchers suggests that codeine maintenance programs might be an alternative to methadone maintenance, particularly because codeine produces fewer unwanted effects than methadone.

Drug interactions. The antidepressants fluoxetine (Prozac) and paroxetine interfere with the body's transformation of codeine into morphine; therefore, persons taking those antidepressants are considered less likely to develop codeine abuse (because they would experience fewer effects from codeine). Although codeine is weaker than morphine, similarities between the two drugs mean that interactions occurring with morphine can be expected to occur with codeine.

Cancer. Laboratory tests find no evidence that the drug causes cell mutations that might lead to cancer. Experimenters gave codeine to rats and mice for two years and looked for evidence of cancer caused by the drug but found none. Although no direct observations have noted codeine causing cancer in rats or mice, computer analysis of data from some experiments indicates that the drug may cause cancer in rodents. The human body produces very small amounts of codeine naturally, and researchers suspect this naturally occurring codeine may deter development of lung cancer; but those natural processes do not mean that doses of the drug would help prevent cancer.

Pregnancy. Whether codeine causes birth defects is unknown. It produced no evidence of malformations when given to pregnant rats and rabbits. Codeine reduced fetal weight in mice and hamsters in one experiment but did not increase the normal rate of defects in mice, nor was a statistically significant change in malformation rate observed in hamsters. Investigators running another mice experiment, however, concluded that codeine does cause assorted malformations. Researchers seeking evidence about various human birth defects examined medical records of 100 to 199 women who used a cough remedy containing codeine and found that none of the offspring had any of the congenital abnormalities being investigated. Suspicion exists that codeine may cause cleft palate and cleft lip in humans, but birth defects are considered unlikely if the drug is used during pregnancy. A pregnant woman who takes codeine can produce an infant who is dependent on that drug and who undergoes a withdrawal syndrome upon birth.

Codeine passes into the milk of nursing mothers, but researchers find its level and that of its metabolite morphine to be acceptable if the woman is using codeine moderately. Nonetheless, nursing mothers are advised to avoid codeine because mechanisms that break down codeine in the body are incompletely formed in newborns, causing them to react more strongly to the drug than older children or adults.

Additional scientific information may be found in:

Eggen, A.E., and M. Andrew. "Use of Codeine Analgesics in a General Population. A Norwegian Study of Moderately Strong Analgesics." *European Journal of Clinical Pharmacology* 46 (1994): 491–96.

Mattoo, S.K., et al. "Abuse of Codeine-Containing Cough Syrups: A Report from India." *Addiction* 92 (1997): 1783–87.

Romach, M.K., et al. "Long-Term Codeine Use Is Associated with Depressive Symptoms." *Journal of Clinical Psychopharmacology* 19 (1999): 373–76.

Rowden, A.M., and J.R. Lopez. "Codeine Addiction." *DICP: The Annals of Pharmacotherapy* 23 (1989): 475–77.

Sproule, B.A., et al. "Characteristics of Dependent and Nondependent Regular Users of Codeine." *Journal of Clinical Psychopharmacology* 19 (1999): 367–72.

DET

Pronunciation: dee-ee-tee

Chemical Abstracts Service Registry Number: 61-51-8

Formal Names: Diethyltryptamine

Type: Hallucinogen. *See* page 25

Federal Schedule Listing: Schedule I (DEA no. 7434)

USA Availability: Illegal to possess

Pregnancy Category: None

Uses. In rats DET actions resemble some of **bufotenine**'s, but DET effects in humans are likened to those of **mescaline** and **LSD**. Volunteers report major changes in body perception, such as feeling porous or having an empty chest or absent hands. Sometimes users feel they are outside of their bodies. Hallucinations may seem real; typically they are visual, but sometimes sounds and smells are perceived as well. Users have reported that faces of individuals around them look different, taking on a masklike or caricature quality. Barriers between senses may erode, for example, allowing sounds to be seen. Altered perception of time is common. Perception of space can also change; a room's size may appear to grow, with walls getting further away or becoming curved, or motionless objects may appear to keep coming closer. Typically consciousness becomes fuzzy, with persons reporting they feel partially asleep.

Reactions to such experiences differ. A researcher who engaged in self-experimentation, once a more common procedure in science but now uncommon, reported that his mood flipped back and forth between happiness and anxiety. He also reported temporary autism while intoxicated by the drug. Another self-experimenting scientist noted a need to avoid interacting with people. A group of artists and professional colleagues of researchers who wanted to explore creative possibilities with the drug were ecstatic about what happened to them. Some had spiritually moving experiences; afterward some felt impelled to begin creating artwork they had never attempted before. The substance can promote meditation, allowing repressed concerns to emerge. For that reason the drug was considered to have potential in psychotherapy. One research team reported examples of reticent schizophrenics becoming communicative while under DET's influence, revealing honest information that benefitted therapy. In a setting where users feel safe they may become more sensitive to one another's emotions and have genial interactions.

Drawbacks. If persons want to stay in control of what happens to them, they may become upset if they are unable to stop DET's effects. One group of volunteers found DET unpleasant, and some said the experience was so negative that they would depart the research center if a repeat performance was expected. These were unemployed laborers who had no particular interest in the drug. Some users in another study compared the experience to delirium caused by typhus or pneumonia. DET typically raises blood pressure, causes dizziness and perspiration, and may cause tremors and burning sensations. Rapid heartbeat has been reported. In addition to those symptoms, schizophrenics have routinely experienced shakiness, nausea, and vomiting. Some persons feel agitated and have a need to move around. The drug makes people more open to suggestion and therefore more susceptible to exploitation. In a research environment, normal subjects often become suspicious of persons managing the experiment. Performance declines on tests of reaction time and intelligence. A technically accomplished artist drew with less proficiency during DET intoxication, but at the time she seemed unaware of decline in performance. After the drug has worn off, users may feel a little depressed and suffer from headache; they may be tired but have difficulty sleeping. These problems clear up in a day's time.

Abuse factors. Not enough scientific information to report about tolerance, dependence, withdrawal, or addiction.

Drug interactions. Not enough scientific information to report.

Cancer. Not enough scientific information to report.

Pregnancy. Not enough scientific information to report.

Additional scientific information may be found in:

Böszörményi, Z. "Creative Urge as an After Effect of Model Psychoses." *Confina Psychiatrica* 3 (1960): 177–26.

Böszörményi, Z., P. Dér, and T. Nagy. "Observations on the Psychotogenic Effect of N-N Diethyltryptamine, a New Tryptamine Derivative." *Journal of Mental Science* 105 (1959): 171–81.

Szára, S. "The Comparison of the Psychotic Effect of Tryptamine Derivatives with the Effects of Mescaline and LSD-25 in Self-Experiments." In *Psychotropic Drugs*, ed. S. Garattini and V. Ghetti. New York: Elsevier, 1957. 460–67. Szára refers to DET as T-9.

Szára, S., et al. "Psychological Effects and Metabolism of N,N-Diethyltryptamine in Man." *Archives of General Psychiatry* 15 (1966): 320–29.

Dextroamphetamine

Pronunciation: DEK-stroh am-FET-uh-meen

Chemical Abstracts Service Registry Number: 51-64-9. (Sulphate form 51-63-8)

Formal Names: Adderall, Amsustain, Biphetamine, D-Amphetamine, Dexamphetamine, Dexedrine, Dexidrine, DextroStat, Sympamin

Informal Names: Beans, Black Beauties, Brownies, Christmas Trees, Dexies, Fastballs, Orange Hearts, Oranges, Purple Hearts

Type: Stimulant (amphetamine class). *See* page 12

Federal Schedule Listing: Schedule II (DEA no. 1100)

USA Availability: Prescription

Pregnancy Category: C

Dextroamphetamine is often called amphetamine. To reduce potential confusion, remember that in this book "amphetamine" refers to a class of stimulants, and "dextroamphetamine" refers to a specific drug in that class.

Uses. The substance stimulates the central and sympathetic nervous systems and is comparable to **methamphetamine**. Dextroamphetamine is typically used to treat narcolepsy, to treat attention deficit hyperactivity disorder (ADHD) in adults and children, and to help reduce a person's weight—in rhesus monkey experiments it is one of the most effective appetite suppressants. Some use has been made to help epileptics. The drug can be given in combination with scopolamine as an anti–motion sickness medicine; astronauts have used this combination during missions in outer space and consider it effective.

Dextroamphetamine has been found more effective than standard antidepressants in alleviating depression among HIV (human immunodeficiency virus) patients and can also increase their energy. The drug has successfully treated depression among non-HIV hospital patients and among other persons as well. The drug has helped restore physical vigor and positive mental outlook to institutionalized elderly persons, so that older individuals who had been unable to take care of themselves were able to go home. Experimenters in the 1970s and 1990s found that the drug could accelerate work rate without multiplying mistakes in performing tasks. Those laboratory results cannot be extrapolated to the workplace in general but nonetheless remind us of the original welcome that employers gave to the first amphetamines. Dextroamphetamine can help persons maintain satisfactory job performance while being deprived of sleep. In the Persian Gulf War of 1991, U.S. aviators used the drug. Some pilots called the substance crucial for top performance of responsibilities. Outside evaluation concluded that efficiency and safety improved when pilots were under the drug's influence. Athletic performance may be enhanced by the drug, but amphetamine class substances are generally banned by sports regulatory authorities.

Drawbacks. Tests on healthy volunteers found that taking enough dextroamphetamine to produce euphoria was also enough to produce mania. The drug may cause stroke and is normally avoided if patients have heart disease, hardening of the arteries, high blood pressure, glaucoma, hyperthyroidism, restlessness, and former or current drug abuse. Heart trouble has been attributed to several years' abuse of the drug, and brain damage has been noted.

Abuse factors. Lack of dependency has been noted among juveniles receiving medical doses of dextroamphetamine. Another study found that adults with medical authorization to use dextroamphetamine for obesity or depression often found it no more appealing than a placebo. These results are consistent with the fact that any drug's potential for abuse depends on the needs it satisfies in a user; if a medical need is the only one satisfied, then the person will have no interest in continuing the drug once the affliction is cured. Among persons inclined toward abuse, that inclination can be increased by taking dextroamphetamine with **morphine**. Those two substances can cancel out some of each other's unpleasant physical sensations while retaining the psychological pleasures of both drugs. Abusers may interpret the situation as "gain without pain," but combining stimulants with depressants can give the human body quite a beating. Moreover, researchers find that abusers can acquire tolerance to the psychological effects of dextroamphetamine while effects on blood pressure remain strong. Therefore, boosting the dose to maintain the level of psychic high may pose as much danger to a habituated user as to someone unaccustomed to the drug.

Drug interactions. Although the antimania medicine lithium reduces central nervous system stimulation caused by amphetamine, experiments have not shown lithium reducing either mania or heart rate and blood pressure increases caused by dextroamphetamine. Dextroamphetamine is to be avoided if persons have taken a monoamine oxidase inhibitor (MAOI—in some antidepressants and other medicine) within the past 14 days. Particular hazard arises when combining an MAOI and dextroamphetamine while eating foods containing tyramine. Such foods include beer, some wines, cheese, chocolate, bananas, raisins, avocados, salami, and soy sauce. Although an experimental study found that dextroamphetamine could enhance the beneficial effects of MAOIs, using the two drugs together can be fatal. Tricyclic antidepressants make a dose of dextroamphetamine last longer and can increase amphetamine blood levels produced by dextroamphetamine.

Although extrapolation of animal studies to human conditions must always be cautious, it is known that dextroamphetamine's effects become stronger in rats if they take **caffeine** at the same time. Rat and human experiments also indicate that dextroamphetamine will improve pain relief provided by morphine. Animal experiments indicate that dextroamphetamine interferes with **alcohol** absorption, suggesting that achieving alcohol intoxication might require a dextroamphetamine user to drink more than normal. Upon taking dextroamphetamine, tobacco cigarette smokers use more cigarettes and report greater pleasure from smoking.

Combining **marijuana** smoking with dextroamphetamine does not seem to affect physical coordination (walking and the like) more than just using marijuana alone. Each of those two drugs raises heart rate and blood pressure but do not seem to have a multiplier effect when used together—the increase in cardiac effects is simply the amount caused by dextroamphetamine plus the amount caused by marijuana; one does not make cardiac effects of the other more potent.

Cancer. Potential for causing cancer is unknown.

Pregnancy. As with many drugs, effect on fetal development is unknown. One instance of serious birth defects is reported from a woman who used dextroamphetamine in the first trimester, but the meaning of that one instance is uncertain because she also used lovastatin (a drug for reducing cholesterol in persons at serious risk of heart attack), and lovastatin by itself is considered highly dangerous to fetal development. A statistical association has been reported between maternal dextroamphetamine use and infant heart defects. Dextroamphetamine has been prescribed for use in pregnancy without apparent ill effect on infants but is considered potentially hazardous. Possible consequences merit full discussion between doctor and pregnant patient.

Combination products. Adderall contains several active ingredients: dextroamphetamine saccharate, amphetamine aspartate, dextroamphetamine sulfate USP, and amphetamine sulfate USP (the latter substance formerly marketed as Benzedrine).

Biphetamine, like other dextroamphetamines, is medically used to treat obesity, narcolepsy, and ADHD. Biphetamine is used recreationally to boost mental quickness and physical activity and to create euphoria. The compound can facilitate hallucinations, raise blood pressure, and prevent sleep.

Dexedrine's oral capsule is designed to deliver some of the drug immediately, followed by gradual delivery of the remaining drug. Capsule and tablet products both contain "inactive" ingredients. In this context "inactive" means an ingredient that does not promote a drug's medical purpose, not that the ingredient has no pharmaceutical effect. Inactive ingredients in the tablet include FD&C Yellow No. 5 (tartrazine), a substance to which some persons are allergic, particularly if they are abnormally sensitive to aspirin. Their reactions can include bronchial asthma. When used against ADHD in children Dexedrine can curtail growth, but that effect is believed to be temporary. Dexedrine can raise body temperature. Experimenters found that the product can allow satisfactory performance by airplane pilots on continuous simulator flight duty for 64 hours straight without sleep.

DextroStat tablets include FD&C Yellow No. 5 (tartrazine).

Additional scientific information may be found in:

Brauer, L.H., J. Ambre, and H. De Wit. "Acute Tolerance to Subjective But Not Cardiovascular Effects of D-Amphetamine in Normal, Healthy Men." *Journal of Clinical Psychopharmacology* 16 (1996): 72–76.
Caldwell, J.A., et al. "Efficacy of Dexedrine for Maintaining Aviator Performance dur-

ing 64 Hours of Sustained Wakefulness: A Simulator Study." *Aviation, Space, and Environmental Medicine* 71 (2000): 7–18.

Domino, E.F., et al. "Effects of D-Amphetamine on Quantitative Measures of Motor Performance." *Clinical Pharmacology and Therapeutics* 13 (1972): 251–57.

Emonson, D.L., and R.D. Vanderbeek. "The Use of Amphetamines in U.S. Air Force Tactical Operations during Desert Shield and Storm." *Aviation, Space, and Environmental Medicine* 66 (1995): 260–63.

Graybiel, A. "Space Motion Sickness: Skylab Revisited." *Aviation, Space, and Environmental Medicine* 51 (1980): 814–22.

Griffith, J.D., et al. "Dextroamphetamine." *Archives of General Psychiatry* 26 (1972): 97–100.

Jacobs, D., and T. Silverstone. "Dextroamphetamine-Induced Arousal in Human Subjects as a Model for Mania." *Psychological Medicine* 16 (1986): 323–29.

Jasinski, D.R., and K.L. Preston. "Evaluation of Mixtures of Morphine and D-Amphetamine for Subjective and Physiological Effects." *Drug and Alcohol Dependence* 17 (1986): 1–13.

Ward, A.S., et al. "Effects of D-Amphetamine on Task Performance and Social Behavior of Humans in a Residential Laboratory." *Experimental and Clinical Psychopharmacology* 5 (1997): 130–36.

Dextromethorphan

Pronunciation: dex-troh-meth-OR-fan

Chemical Abstracts Service Registry Number: 125-71-3

Formal Names: Benylin, Cosylan, Creo-Terpin, Demorphan Hydrobromide, Dexylets, Drixoral, DXM, Medicon, Mediquell, MorphiDex, Pertussin CS, Robitussin-DM

Informal Names: Bromage, Brome, Cough Syrup, Dex, Dextro, DM, Drix, K (with alcohol), Mega-Perls, Pole (with heroin), Polo (with heroin), Robe, Robo, Rojo, Sky, Syrup, Triple C, Tussin, Velvet

Type: Depressant (opioid class). *See* page 22

Federal Schedule Listing: Unlisted

USA Availability: Nonprescription

Pregnancy Category: C

Uses. This cough and cold medicine has been used in the United States since the 1950s. Because the drug is an opiate analogue and is related to **levorphanol**, for convenience this book lists dextromethorphan as an opioid. Naloxone, a chemical used to provoke withdrawal symptoms in persons who have dependence with opiates and opioids, can bring forth those symptoms in addicts who have switched from **methadone** to dextromethorphan. That finding is consistent with dextromethorphan being an opioid; nonetheless, the substance is not generally classified as an opioid.

The drug resembles **codeine** but is considered weaker in humans, although a cat experiment measured dextromethorphan as three times stronger than codeine. Body processes break down dextromethorphan into other substances including **dextrorphan**.

Urinalysis comparing the amounts of dextromethorphan and its breakdown product dextrorphan can identify a person's susceptibility to lung cancer. Case reports tell of dextromethorphan's success in treating infants' brain seizures. One experiment found the substance to be a useful supplement in treating older epileptics, but another study detected no improvement. Parkinson's disease patients have shown encouraging response to treatment with the drug, but using it against Huntington's disease and Lou Gehrig's disease has brought disappointment. Animal research suggests that the substance may be useful in treating stroke. A mice experiment in France tested whether dextromethorphan can protect against the effects of the chemical warfare agent soman, but the results were negative. A U.S. Army experiment with guinea pigs also found dextromethorphan to have little value as protection against soman poisoning.

Dextromethorphan is considered ineffective as a general pain reliever but does reduce certain kinds of pain: Experiments show the drug can relieve pain from diabetes, and researchers speculate that the drug may also provide similar benefit to AIDS (acquired immunodeficiency syndrome) sufferers.

Drawbacks. Most persons find the drug unpleasant if the medically recommended dosage is exceeded, with unwanted effects such as easy excitability, memory trouble, nausea, itching, interference with male sexual function, slurred speech, trouble with thinking, and difficulty with moving arms and legs. Some persons become tired and woozy even on normal doses. Nonetheless, one study of cough medicines found that volunteers preferred dextromethorphan to other remedies that were effective, leading the researchers to speculate that the drug was providing pleasure unrelated to effectiveness in relieving cough. Indeed, some users feel more sociable and report euphoria and hallucinations. Cases of mania are known, likened to the kind of stereotypical behavior popularly associated with **PCP**. In one instance, the compound allowed a lawyer to work industriously for weeks with little sleep, followed by mental collapse requiring hospitalization. This individual had engaged in manic episodes and drug abuse in the past, however. A patient in another mania case report also had a medical history of drug abuse. Persons without such a history may well be susceptible to manic reactions from overuse of dextromethorphan, but the examples just cited raise the question of whether persons prone to drug abuse are particularly susceptible.

Investigators examining dextromethorphan's potential for treating juvenile bacterial meningitis called off the experiment when patients began developing diabetes after receiving high doses of the drug (possibly because of action on the pancreas inhibiting insulin production), and reports exist about other instances of juveniles developing diabetes when being treated with the compound.

Abuse factors. Accounts of persons abusing dextromethorphan began appearing in science journals during the 1960s. In the 1990s news media reports described the substance as popular among teenagers, who sometimes referred to this drug use as "robo-copping." Usage by persons of that age group is not limited to the United States. For example, authorities in Korea have expressed concern about fatal overdoses among young illicit users, particularly when they combine dextromethorphan with another drug to intensify effects.

In the 1960s human addiction to dextromethorphan was dismissed as highly unlikely. Subsequently, researchers who documented behavior of rats exposed to drug combinations concluded that dextromethorphan has abuse potential. Human addiction has indeed been reported, although this is described as unusual. Scientists have not found dependence or withdrawal symptoms. A rat study determined that dextromethorphan can reduce **alcohol** withdrawal symptoms, and experiments with rats and mice show that dextromethorphan can reduce **morphine** withdrawal symptoms. One human study found that dextromethorphan by itself did not relieve methadone abstinence, but different research shows that in combination with other substances dextromethorphan can relieve abstinence symptoms experienced by **heroin** addicts. Such results do not demonstrate whether dextromethorphan has cross-tolerance with all the drugs just named, allowing it to be substituted for any of them; their withdrawal syndromes all include elements mimicking the common cold and flu, and dextromethorphan may simply be able to relieve flulike symptoms regardless of cause.

Rats that dose themselves with intravenous **cocaine** have shown less interest in that drug after receiving dextromethorphan, but the meaning of that reduced interest is unclear: Does dextromethorphan promote abandonment of drug use, or do the animals find dextromethorphan so preferable that cocaine cannot compete?

Drug interactions. Dextromethorphan can boost pain relief actions of morphine, allowing patients to use less of that opiate. Research has also found that dextromethorphan does not boost euphoria or dependence produced by morphine, leading one investigator to conclude that morphine's illicit attractions are not increased by dextromethorphan.

Dangerous interactions may occur if dextromethorphan is taken along with **MDMA**, with monoamine oxidase inhibitors (MAOIs, found in some antidepressants and other medicine), or with serotonin uptake reinhibitors (a type of antidepressant). When taken with dextromethorphan the latter substances could provoke the "serotonin syndrome," a potentially fatal emergency involving muscle tremors, heartbeat and blood pressure abnormalities, changes in mental state, and loss of consciousness. In rats the drug reduces effects produced by PCP. Dextromethorphan can cause false positives for PCP in urine tests, but an experiment failed to produce positives for opioids.

Cancer. Not enough scientific information to report.

Pregnancy. The drug has been widely used for decades without report of congenital malformations. After chicken embryo experiments in the 1990s suggested that dextromethorphan might cause birth defects, a study in Canada compared women who used the drug during pregnancy with those who did not and found no increase of congenital defects in the drug group. A study looking for birth malformations in Spain found none that could be attributed to dextromethorphan and concluded that normal medical used of the drug did not produce birth defects. Those negative findings have not surprised experts familiar with drawbacks in using chicken embryos to test for birth defects; chicken development can be harmed by conditions having no effect on humans, and chicken embryo tests are no longer accepted as indicating human risk of birth defects. Several human studies, however, have found a slight increase in risk of birth defects among pregnant women using dextromethorphan. The risk is close to negligible, but, as one authority points out, that is not the same as zero risk. The small chance can be reduced to zero by avoiding the drug during pregnancy.

Additional scientific information may be found in:

Darboe, M.N. "Abuse of Dextromethorphan-Based Cough Syrup as a Substitute for Licit and Illicit Drugs: A Theoretical Framework." *Adolescence* 31 (1996): 239–45.
Einarson, A., D. Lyszkiewicz, and G. Koren. "The Safety of Dextromethorphan in Pregnancy: Results of a Controlled Study." *Chest* 119 (2001): 466–69.

Hinsberger, A., V. Sharma, and D. Mazmanian. "Cognitive Deterioration from Long-Term Abuse of Dextromethorphan: A Case Report." *Journal of Psychiatry and Neuroscience* 19 (1994): 375–77.

Martínez-Frias, M.L., and E. Rodríguez-Pinilla. "Epidemiologic Analysis of Prenatal Exposure to Cough Medicines Containing Dextromethorphan: No Evidence of Human Teratogenicity." *Teratology* 63 (2001): 38–41.

Pender, E.S., and B.R. Parks. "Toxicity with Dextromethorphan-Containing Preparations: A Literature Review and Report of Two Additional Cases." *Pediatric Emergency Care* 7 (1991): 163–65.

Polles, A., and J.L. Griffith. "Dextromethorphan-Induced Mania." *Psychosomatics* 37 (1996): 71–74.

Rammer, L., P. Holmgren, and H. Sandler. "Fatal Intoxication by Dextromethorphan: A Report on Two Cases." *Forensic Science International* 37 (1988): 233–36.

Dextromoramide

Pronunciation: deks-troh-MOHR-a-meyed

Chemical Abstracts Service Registry Number: 357-56-2. (Tartrate form 2922-44-3)

Formal Names: Alcoid, Dauran, Dimorlin, Jetrium, Linfadol, Moramide, Narcolo, Palfium, Troxilan

Type: Depressant (opioid class). *See* page 24

Federal Schedule Listing: Schedule I (DEA no. 9613)

USA Availability: Illegal to possess

Pregnancy Category: None

Uses. This drug was first identified in the 1950s. It has no officially sanctioned medical role in the United States but is used elsewhere for pain control in conditions such as kidney stone attacks, cancer, surgery, or injury. A case report tells of a person who used this drug to diminish pain during self-mutilation. Dextromoramide can provide relief when standard opiates fail. Although generally classified as an opioid (a synthetic chemical) the drug is produced from unripened **opium** seeds and is 2 to 70 times stronger than **morphine**, depending on the animal species being tested and the effect being measured. Dextromoramide acts quickly; authorities disagree on how long its effects last.

Drawbacks. Unwanted effects can include nausea, vomiting, perspiration, rapid pulse, breathing impairment, urinary difficulty, lowered body temperature and blood pressure, and dizziness. Compared to morphine, dextromoramide is less likely to cause constipation or sleepiness. Euphoria can occur. Persons taking dextromoramide are generally warned against driving cars or running other dangerous machinery. A case report mentions a drug abuser's serious, but curable, heart damage caused by injecting crushed oral tablets of dextromoramide.

Abuse factors. Dextromoramide is chemically related to **methadone**, and some researchers believe that dextromoramide could be a useful supplemental drug for addicts being treated in methadone maintenance programs. Morphine and dextromoramide have enough cross-tolerance to prevent morphine withdrawal symptoms. Dextromoramide itself is addictive; around 1990 a survey of 150 methadone patients in London found that 7 were being treated for dextromoramide addiction. At one time some medical observers doubted that dextromoramide is addictive, but negative results in their research were probably due to the medical context in which the drug was being used. In rats the development of dextromoramide tolerance is so much slower than with morphine that one group of investigators doubted the phenomenon was really occurring. Researchers have disagreed about how fast tolerance appears in humans, but it does occur, as does dependence. Disagreement about how quickly tolerance emerges in humans may be related to which drug effects are being examined; tolerance does not necessarily develop to all of a drug's effects at the same rate. For example, tolerance to pain relief properties might emerge at a different point of treatment than tolerance to nausea or sleepiness caused by a drug.

Drug interactions. Taking this drug with antihistamines or depressants (such as **alcohol**) can be risky. Monoamine oxidase inhibitors (MAOIs, found in some antidepressants and other medicine) are particularly dangerous to take with dextromoramide. Persons with breathing difficulty or poor thyroid activity should be careful about taking this drug.

Cancer. Not enough scientific information to report.

Pregnancy. The drug produces massive birth defects in mice, but its ability to cause human malformations at normal medical dosage levels is unknown. Dextromoramide has been used to ease childbirth, but if pregnant women receive the drug shortly before giving birth, their infants may have trouble breathing. One medical authority has called the substance too dangerous to use during labor. Dextromoramide passes into milk of nursing mothers.

Additional scientific information may be found in:

De Vos, J.W., et al. "Craving Patterns in Methadone Maintenance Treatment with Dextromoramide as Adjuvant." *Addictive Behaviors* 24 (1999): 707–13.

Jurand, A., and Martin, L.V. "Teratogenic Potential of Two Neurotropic Drugs, Haloperidol and Dextromoramide, Tested on Mouse Embryos." *Teratology* 42 (1990): 45–54.

La Barre, J. "The Pharmacological Properties and Therapeutic Use of Dextromoramide." *Bulletin on Narcotics* 11, no. 4 (1959): 10–19.

Newgreen, D.B. "Dextromoramide: Review and Case Report." *Australian Journal of Pharmacy* 61 (1980): 641–44.

Dextrorphan

Pronunciation: dex-TROR-fan
Chemical Abstracts Service Registry Number: 125-73-5
Type: Depressant (opioid class). *See* page 24
Federal Schedule Listing: Unlisted

Uses. This substance is closely related to **levorphanol** and can produce a false positive for levorphanol in drug screen tests. The human body will transform part of a **dextromethorphan** dose into dextrorphan. The same transformation occurs in rats; when comparing results in males and females, researchers found that a given amount of dextrorphan lasts twice as long in female rats.

Dextrorphan can fight coughs and reduce epileptic seizures, although test results differ about how well it diminishes seizures. Mice research has found that the drug helps mice recover from strokes, and in humans the drug appears useful for treating minor strokes. Some research indicates that the substance has potential for treating various human neurological afflictions, but such potential has yet to be fulfilled. A rat experiment found dextrorphan ineffective in preventing brain damage caused by the chemical warfare agent soman. A rat study testing dextrorphan's potential as an antidote for **methcathinone** poisoning had limited success.

Drawbacks. Unwanted side effects may include nausea, vomiting, sleepiness, high or low blood pressure, uncontrollable eye movement, and hallucinations. Rat experiments show that high enough does can impair memory and learning. When one group of researchers tested dextrorphan's ability to prevent some types of brain damage, the scientists found instead that dextrorphan caused damage in rats.

Abuse factors. At one time dextrorphan was a Schedule I substance, but eventually it was removed from any schedule of controlled substances. Such a journey is most unusual; assorted drugs have been moved from one schedule to another over the years, but the direction is almost always to put the drugs under more controls rather than fewer. Scientists describe dextrorphan as producing effects similar to **PCP**. At sufficiently high levels, dextrorphan can make people feel as if they are intoxicated with **alcohol**.

Drug interactions. Dextrorphan has reduced **cocaine** effects in mice.

Cancer. Not enough scientific information to report.

Pregnancy. After male mice received dextrorphan in an experiment, they produced offspring having lower weight, delays in maturation, and abnormal swimming behavior. Whether the drug passes into a human fetus or the milk supply of a nursing mother is unknown.

Additional scientific information may be found in:

Aylward, M., et al. "Dextromethorphan and Codeine: Comparison of Plasma Kinetics and Antitussive Effects." *European Journal of Respiratory Diseases* 65 (1984): 283–91.

Dematteis, M., G. Lallement, and M. Mallaret. "Dextromethorphan and Dextrorphan in Rats: Common Antitussives—Different Behavioural Profiles." *Fundamental and Clinical Pharmacology* 12 (1998): 526–37.

"Safety, Tolerability and Pharmacokinetics of the N-Methyl-D-Asparate Antagonist Ro-01-6794/706 in Patients with Acute Ischemic Stroke." *Annals of the New York Academy of Sciences* 765 (1995): 249–61, 298.

Schutz, C.G., and M. Soyka. "Dextromethorphan Challenge in Alcohol-Dependent Patients and Controls." With reply by Drystal and Petrakis. *Archives of General Psychiatry* 57 (2000): 291–92.

Szekely, J.I., L.G. Sharpe, and J.H. Jaffe. "Induction of Phencyclidine-Like Behavior in Rats by Dextrorphan But Not Dextromethorphan." *Pharmacology, Biochemistry, and Behavior* 40 (1991): 381–86.

Diazepam

Pronunciation: dye-AZ-e-pam

Chemical Abstracts Service Registry Number: 439-14-5

Formal Names: Alupram, Atensine, Diastat, Diazemuls, Evacalm, Solis, Stesolid, Tensium, Valium, Valrelease, Vival

Informal Names: Blues, Drunk Pills, Ludes, Mother's Little Helper, V, Val

Type: Depressant (benzodiazepine class). *See* page 21

Federal Schedule Listing: Schedule IV (DEA no. 2765)

USA Availability: Prescription

Pregnancy Category: D

Uses. By the end of the twentieth century diazepam was one of the best-known antianxiety agents in America. Other medical uses of this fast-acting and long-lasting drug include treatment of insomnia, migraine, facial pain, muscle spasms, convulsions, vomiting, malaria, rattlesnake bite, **alcohol** and **heroin** withdrawal syndromes, cardiac difficulty created by **cocaine**, and muscle stiffness from tetanus and other causes. In children the drug is used to combat seizures caused by fever. Diazepam is commonly administered to calm patients just before surgery. The body converts the drug into other chemicals, including **temazepam** and **oxazepam**.

Drawbacks. Unwanted actions of diazepam include weariness and weakness and occasionally headache, dizziness and vertigo, nausea, fuzzy or double vision, urinary control problems, and depressed mood. A case report tells of the drug bringing on an attack of gout. Diazepam is not recommended for persons with acute narrow-angle glaucoma.

The compound can make users tired and impair vigilance, judgment, reaction times, and movement. A person using diazepam should be cautious about operating dangerous machinery; simulated driving tests demonstrate reduced ability after a dose. The drug can cause memory problems. A study of newborn rats receiving the drug found that it slowed learning, but their learning capacity was normal even though the rats needed more time to learn something. Diazepam can interfere with the ability to recognize an angry expression on someone's face—a disability with distinct potential for social consequences—and a laboratory experiment demonstrated the drug's ability to make people more aggressive if they are provoked.

Diazepam is given to treat epileptic seizures, but long-term use can increase epileptic seizures. Among epileptics the drug can also cause status epilepticus, a potentially fatal condition in which seizures occur back to back.

Injecting diazepam into an artery is perilous. This mishap has been known to occur even when medical professionals administer the drug, and most recreational users lack training in anatomy. This mistake can cause gangrene, leading to amputation of appendages. Intravenous injection of diazepam can stop breathing and heart action; when administering the drug intravenously hospitals are prepared for such emergencies, but most street users are not. Intravenous injection can also lower muscle strength and blood pressure. In a small percentage of human volunteers (5% or less), rectal administration has produced euphoria, breathing difficulty, skin rash, runny nose, or diarrhea.

Diazepam is one of the few drugs that can cause flat brain wave readings in a living person. Such readings are a classic sign of death, and medical personnel seeing such readings might decide to stop efforts that are keeping a patient alive.

Abuse factors. Among illicit drug users in the 1990s diazepam was the most common benzodiazepine. When researchers supplied recreational drug users with several benzodiazepine class substances, diazepam was rated as having the most abuse potential. In testing of the drug's appeal, volunteers reported that the higher the dose, the higher the attractiveness. Researchers evaluating results of an experiment involving recreational drug users judged diazepam to be even more effective in producing pleasure than in producing medical effects.

In one experiment with recreational drug users over one third of them described diazepam's effects as reminiscent of barbiturates, which produce effects similar to alcohol. Perhaps such effects explain why tests of drug preference show diazepam to be popular among moderate alcohol drinkers. Research indicates that euphoria from diazepam is more likely in a person with a family history of alcoholism. Moderate drinkers find diazepam more appealing than light drinkers do, but that may be due less to alcohol per se than due to a personality that finds drugs generally attractive.

A rat experiment measured development of diazepam tolerance in those animals. Humans can develop dependence with diazepam, causing a withdrawal syndrome if dosage ceases all at once instead of gradually. Depending on how much of the drug has been used for how long, withdrawal symptoms can be mild or strong. Mild cases may simply involve trembling, reduced appetite, and trouble falling asleep. In bad cases a person can experience perspiration, muscle cramps and tremors, vomiting, and convulsions. Sudden stoppage of long-term diazepam dosage can provoke seizures, so doses need to be tapered off instead.

Drug interactions. Alcohol and diazepam can boost each other's actions. Diazepam effects can also be intensified by barbiturates, opiates, and monoamine oxidase inhibitors (MAOIs—found in some antidepressants). Those interactions can be fatal. Effect of a diazepam dose can be lengthened by **propoxyphene** and by the ulcer drugs omeprazole and cimetidine. One study found that a dose tends to last for a shorter time among alcoholics. In a dog experiment **phenobarbital** decreased diazepam levels in the animals. In mice diazepam has boosted toxic effects from the cancer medicine ifosfamide. The more tobacco cigarettes people smoke, the less drowsy diazepam makes them. Body weight also affects diazepam actions, with drug build-up and elimination taking longer in bodies of fatter people. Experimenters have even found that drug effects can vary by time of day; at night diazepam prolongs the presence of an ibuprofen dose.

Cancer. Experimentation shows diazepam to have potential for causing cancer in mice, results causing researchers to suspect the same possibility in humans. Tests with rats, gerbils, and hamsters produced no cancer risk. Examination of medical records from almost 13,000 diazepam users found no link to a higher cancer rate. Several other investigations found no connection between the drug and assorted human cancers, but results have been mixed on association with ovarian cancer.

Pregnancy. Hamsters receiving the drug during pregnancy can produce offspring with cleft palate and other skull abnormalities. Similar results are seen in mice, particularly if cocaine is used as well. Chicken embryos exposed to diazepam develop malformations. Diazepam experiments with rats have resulted in fewer pregnancies and higher death rates for pups. Some rat experiments produce birth defects and some do not; size of dose may be important. If pregnant mice receive the drug, their male offspring may have difficulty with sexual functioning as adults. (In contrast, the drug is used for treating impaired male sexual functioning in humans.) Rodent offspring may suffer from compromised immune systems. They also may act more nervous than pups who lack fetal exposure, although rats that have no fetal exposure, but instead receive multiple doses soon after birth, act less uneasy in later life after dosage has stopped. A number of rodent studies find that prenatal exposure to diazepam may produce assorted behavioral effects that do not appear until adolescence or adulthood. Those effects are measured by various tests (running mazes and the like) that are difficult to extrapolate to human experience, but the point is that diazepam's effects may be unapparent in newborns and take years to emerge.

A study of 689 pregnant women taking assorted antidepressants was unable to attribute any birth defects to diazepam, and the same results came from a smaller study; but nonetheless the drug is suspected of causing malformations. Measurements from pregnant women indicate that diazepam passes to the fetus and builds up there; blood levels of the drug in newborns can be higher than the mother's. Some researchers find that the drug slows fetal brain development. A case report notes severe multiple malformations in an infant whose mother used diazepam during pregnancy but does not establish cause and effect. Researchers tracked medical histories of several thousand women whose babies had major malformations and found an association between diazepam and cleft lip, the association becoming even stronger if women had smoked while taking diazepam during pregnancy. Additional research has associated diazepam with birth defects involving the heart, stomach obstruction, and hernia. Association, however, does not prove cause and effect. Indeed, other research has found no association between diazepam and cleft lip or any other congenital malformation. One study found that newborns with fetal exposure to diazepam tend to weigh less than normal, but they soon gain weight and reach a normal level. Infants have exhibited withdrawal symptoms if their mothers used diazepam during pregnancy; those symptoms may not appear immediately after birth.

Nursing mothers are advised to avoid the drug, which can continue to pass into breast milk long after drug use is halted. The drug can build up in babies, enough that they can be sedated by milk from mothers using diazepam, and the infants may lose weight while nursing.

Additional information. **Methaqualone** and diazepam each have the nickname "Ludes," but the drugs are different substances.

Additional scientific information may be found in:

Clarke, C.H., and A.N. Nicholson. "Immediate and Residual Effects in Man of the Metabolites of Diazepam." *British Journal of Clinical Pharmacology* 6 (1978): 325–31.

Giri, A.K., and S. Banerjee. "Genetic Toxicology of Four Commonly Used Benzodiazepines: A Review." *Mutation Research* 340 (1996): 93–108.

Gotestam, K.G., and B.E. Andersson. "Subjective Effects and Vigilance after Diazepam and Oxazepam in Normal Subjects." *Acta Psychiatrica Scandinavica* 19, no. 274 (1978, Suppl.): 117–21.

Griffiths, R.R., et al. "Comparison of Diazepam and Oxazepam: Preference, Liking and Extent of Abuse." *Journal of Pharmacology and Experimental Therapeutics* 229 (1984): 501–8.

Griffiths, R.R., et al. "Relative Abuse Liability of Diazepam and Oxazepam: Behavioral and Subjective Dose Effects." *Psychopharmacology* (Berlin) 84 (1984): 147–54.

Juergens, S. "Alprazolam and Diazepam: Addiction Potential." *Journal of Substance Abuse Treatment* 8 (1991): 43–51.

Sutton, L.R., and S.A. Hinderliter. "Diazepam Abuse in Pregnant Women on Methadone Maintenance. Implications for the Neonate." *Clinical Pediatrics* 29 (1990): 108–11.

Willumeit, H.P., H. Ott, and W. Neubert. "Simulated Car Driving as a Useful Technique for the Determination of Residual Effects and Alcohol Interaction after Short- and Long-Acting Benzodiazepines." *Psychopharmacology*, no. 1 (1984, Suppl.): 182–92.

Diethylpropion

Pronunciation: dye-eth-ill-PROH-pee-on

Chemical Abstracts Service Registry Number: 90-84-6. (Hydrochloride form 134-80-5)

Formal Names: Adiposan, Amfepramone, Anfamon, Apisate, Bonumin, Brendalit, Dietic, Dietil-Retard, DIP, Dobesin, Frekentine, Lineal-Rivo, Linea-Valeas, Lipomin, Liposlim, Magrene, Moderatan, M-Orexic, Nobesine, Nulobes, Prefamone, Propion, Regenon, Regibon, Slim-plus, Tenuate, Tenuate Dospan, Tepanil

Informal Names: Blues

Type: Stimulant (anorectic class). *See* page 15

Federal Schedule Listing: Schedule IV (DEA no. 1610)

USA Availability: Prescription

Pregnancy Category: B

Uses. Humans find the drug's effects similar to those of **dextroamphetamine** but at a weaker level. One experiment found dextroamphetamine 6 to 11 times stronger than diethylpropion when given orally, 10 to 20 times stronger when given by subcutaneous injection. Although diethylpropion was created in the 1920s, this amphetamine derivative was not marketed for weight loss until around 1960. The drug then achieved great popularity. Over 30 million persons around the globe had taken the drug by 1978. That year 1.5 billion prescriptions were written, but the number dropped to just one-fourth that amount by 1988 as the medical world became more aware of the drug's drawbacks.

Occasional short-term usage rather than continual use has been recommended. The compound breaks up sleep and interferes with dreaming but has fewer stimulant effects than some other anorectics. Users feel less fatigue than with **fenfluramine**, and undesirable effects of diethylpropion disappear faster than those of fenfluramine when the drug is stopped. Studies of weight loss patients using diethylpropion found only trivial impact on heart rate or blood pressure, and the compound is considered a good choice for patients with high blood pressure.

Diethylpropion has been used experimentally to reduce craving for **cocaine**, with some success. Some researchers question that finding, however, pointing out that craving for cocaine diminishes in a hospital setting regardless of whether patients receive diethylpropion or a placebo. In a two-week study, former crack cocaine users receiving diethylpropion showed no change in tests of thinking abilities. That result is interpreted as meaning that short-term use of diethylpropion may cause no measurable harm to brain function.

Another experimental use of the drug has been for relief of arthritis pain. Patients experienced increase of comfort but no increase in ability to use affected joints.

Drawbacks. Minor unwanted actions may include dizziness, dry mouth, and constipation. In a study of 132 patients taking the drug, about 3% had experiences such as euphoria, muscle tremors, or trouble with sleeping. Assorted scientific reports indicate the drug rarely has untoward physical effects; the medical literature mentions an addict who ingested 30 to 100 times the recommended amount each day without major impact. Exceptions to the drug's relative safety do occur. Diethylpropion is suspected of being involved in a case where someone suffered minor strokes (transient ischemic attacks), is suspected of contributing to a case of heart trouble, and is known to cause heart trouble if an overdose is taken. A rare affliction ascribed to the drug is overdevelopment of the vestigial male mammary glands.

The drug may bring on psychosis, especially when taken along with a monoamine oxidase inhibitor (MAOI, found in some antidepressants and other medicine). One user felt under assault from persons using mental telepathy; another heard voices; another thought a television set was observing her; another began worrying about someone using the "evil eye" to kill a child. In some cases those problems ceased after the diet drug stopped; in others the affliction reappeared. A therapist reporting on the latter type of cases suspected that the persons would have developed psychosis regardless of whether they used diethylpropion. The typical sufferer is a female 25 to 40 years old, leading a troubled life with a history of mental instability and drug abuse. Drugs abused by these women often include amphetamines, an important factor because a former amphetamine abuser who later takes another stimulant can quickly shift back into the old abuse mode. Often such persons begin taking diethylpropion to help them lose weight but afterward continue taking it for pleasurable psychic effect. That special group's experience, however, is not commonplace among users in general.

Abuse factors. The drug's amphetamine-type effects are strong enough to have produced an illicit market for diethylpropion in the 1960s, but large surveys determining levels of abuse for various drugs yielded no mention of diethylpropion during the drug's peak of popularity in the mid-1970s. In that era analysis of 5,204 street drug samples found 1 containing diethylpropion. Because the compound is described as producing effects resembling those of amphetamine, diethylpropion is not recommended for persons who have suffered from psychological illness or drug abuse. Binge abusers report that pleasant sensations can be obtained for one to three days, but then nervousness and restlessness predominate if dosing continues. Tolerance develops to the drug's stimulant actions.

Drug interactions. Experiments with mice show that **alcohol** and diethylpropion produce more locomotor activity than either drug alone. Researchers in Brazil speculate that combining the two substances may increase other stimulation sensations, perhaps explaining why using alcohol and anorectic drugs together is allegedly so popular in that country. How popular is that practice? In the latter 1980s the total distribution of diethylpropion and other anorectics was compared to Brazil's population, yielding enough drugs to supply a daily dose to about 1.4% of the population that could afford to buy it, which is the same as saying 0.7% of that wealthier population could be taking two doses a day. The percentage of users becomes one third of those totals if doses are divided among the entire population rather than just among those with enough money to buy the drugs. By using a survey other researchers measured use of anorectics as totaling 1.3% of the population in one area of southern Brazil in 1994, confined mostly to women from higher classes using the drugs under medical prescription. Those percentages lump together usage of diethylpropion with other anorectics, so usage of diethylpropion would be a fraction of those percentages. And recreational usage of diethylpropion together with alcohol would be smaller yet.

Cancer. The drug's potential for causing cancer is unknown.

Pregnancy. Tests with rabbits, mice, and rats produced no birth defects. A case in which a pregnant woman taking diethylpropion gave birth to a malformed infant raised fear that it may cause fetal damage, but studies of pregnant women taking the drug attribute no birth defects to it. Nonetheless, potential for human birth defects is unknown. The drug passes into breast milk.

Additional scientific information may be found in:

Bolding, O.T. "Diethylpropion Hydrochloride: An Effective Appetite Suppressant." *Current Therapeutic Research: Clinical and Experimental* 16 (1974): 40–48.

Carney, D.E., and E.D. Tweddell. "Double Blind Evaluation of Long Acting Diethylpropion Hydrochloride in Obese Patients from a General Practice." *Medical Journal of Australia* 1 (1975): 13–15.

Carney, M.W.P., and M. Harris. "Psychiatric Disorder and Diethylpropion Hydrochloride." *Practitioner* 223 (1979): 549–52.

Cohen, S.D. "Diethylpropion (Tenuate): An Infrequently Abused Anorectic." *Psychosomatics* 18 (1977): 28–33.

"Diethylpropion Psychosis." *Medical Journal of Australia* 2 (1970): 1052–53.

Glazer, G. "Long-Term Pharmacology of Obesity 2000: A Review of Efficacy and Safety." *Archives of Internal Medicine* 161 (2001): 1814–24.

Hoffman, B.F. "Diet Pill Psychosis: Follow-up after 6 Years." *Canadian Medical Association Journal* 129 (1983): 1077–78.

Silverman, M., and Ronald O. "The Use of an Appetite Suppressant (Diethylpropion Hydrochloride) during Pregnancy." *Current Therapeutic Research: Clinical and Experimental* 13 (1971): 648–53.

Dihydrocodeine

Pronunciation: dye-high-droh-KOH-deen

Chemical Abstracts Service Registry Number: 125-28-0

Formal Names: BRON, DHC Continus, Drocode, Fortuss, Paracodin, Synalgos

Type: Depressant (opiate class). *See* page 22

Federal Schedule Listing: Schedule II, III, or V, depending on product formulation (DEA no. 9120)

USA Availability: Prescription and nonprescription

Uses. Cough suppression is a standard medical use for dihydrocodeine, and it can also improve sleep in chronic coughers by reducing the number of times that coughing wakes them. Although a dose may briefly impede breathing, in a successful experiment the drug improved breathing in persons having chronic airflow obstruction, allowing them to engage in more exercise such as walking. The compound has also helped respiration of emphysema patients. Dihydrocodeine has allowed persons with chronic heart failure to become more physically active. The substance is a standard pain reliever but has been found ineffective in helping some kinds of discomfort from surgical and dental procedures, and excessive amounts of the drug can have the paradoxical effect of increasing pain. Dihydrocodeine has at least the same pain relieving strength as **codeine**, perhaps more. **Morphine** is considered about seven times stronger than dihydrocodeine.

Drawbacks. Typical unwanted effects include sleepiness, nausea, and constipation. Euphoria, dizziness, and abnormal dreams are occasionally reported. Excessive dihydrocodeine dosage can cause muscle damage that is known to clear up if the drug is discontinued. Hallucinations may occur. An unusual case report tells of a person developing Alice in Wonderland Syndrome and Lilliputian hallucinations after routinely drinking a dihydrocodeine cough syrup for several years. In the Alice Syndrome people may see real objects as far smaller than they actually are; the Lilliputian situation (named for an episode in *Gulliver's Travels*) involves seeing tiny imaginary objects. Such conditions have also been associated with migraine, fevers, and mononucleosis. In the apparently drug-induced case just mentioned, Lilliputian hallucinations persisted despite psychiatric treatment.

Abuse factors. Although dihydrocodeine addiction rarely arises from medical use, tolerance and dependence can develop if a person uses the substance long enough. Drug maintenance programs, in which addicts are weaned off one drug of abuse and switched to one that treatment authorities consider preferable, have used dihydrocodeine to switch addicts from **heroin** and other opiates. Those programs have also used **methadone** and dihydrocodeine to substitute for each other: Methadone addicts have been switched to dihydrocodeine and vice versa, substitution indicating that drug abusers find the two substances to be similar. Body chemistry converts dihydrocodeine into dihydromorphine, a Schedule I controlled substance. Although an illicit market exists for dihydrocodeine, some physicians believe illegal diversion of prescriptions is discouraged by the nature of the drug: Dissolving oral tablets for injection is difficult, and intravenous injection typically produces discontentment rather than euphoria.

Drug interactions. The drug may boost actions of the anti–blood clotting medicine warfarin.

Cancer. Not enough scientific information to report.

Pregnancy. Many pregnant women have used dihydrocodeine with no apparent harm to fetal development. Nonetheless, the compound is not recommended during pregnancy, and excessive quantities can produce an infant who is dependent at birth. Although researchers are uncertain if the substance passes into breast milk, they believe the amount would be too small to noticeably affect nursing infants.

Additional scientific information may be found in:

Frame, J.W., et al. "A Comparison of Ibuprofen and Dihydrocodeine in Relieving Pain Following Wisdom Teeth Removal." *British Dental Journal* 166 (1989): 121–24.

Johnson, M.A., A.A. Woodcock, and D.M. Geddes. "Dihydrocodeine for Breathlessness in Pink Puffers." *British Medical Journal* 286 (1983): 675–77.

Marks, P., H. Ashraf, and T.R. Root. "Drug Dependence Caused by Dihydihydrocodeine." *British Medical Journal* 1 (1978): 1594.

Palmer, R.N., et al. "Incidence of Unwanted Effects of Dihydrocodeine Bitartrate in Healthy Volunteers." *Lancet* 17 (1966): 620–21.

Takaoka, K., and T. Takata. " 'Alice in Wonderland' Syndrome and Lilliputian Hallucinations in a Patient with a Substance-Related Disorder." *Psychopathology* 32 (1999): 47–49.

Wotherspoon, H.A., G.N. Kenny, and C.S. McArdle. "Analgesic Efficacy of Controlled-Release Dihydrocodeine. A Comparison of 60, 90 and 120 Mg Tablets in Cold-Induced Pain." *Anaesthesia* 46 (1991): 915–17.

Diphenoxylate

Pronunciation: dye-fen-OCK-see-lait

Chemical Abstracts Service Registry Number: 915-30-0. (Hydrochloride form 3810-80-8)

Formal Names: Diarphen, Eldox, Logen, Lomotil, Lonox, Protector, Reasec, Retardinr, Topergan

Type: Depressant (opioid class). *See* page 24

Federal Schedule Listing: Schedule II or V, depending on product formulation (DEA no. 9170)

USA Availability: Prescription and nonprescription

Pregnancy Category: C

Uses. Diphenoxylate was developed in the 1950s but did not see much use until the next decade. The drug is related to **meperidine**. When used alone at high dosage levels, diphenoxylate produces effects reminiscent of **morphine**, although pain relief capability is nil. Experimental rubbing of diphenoxylate on patches of psoriasis has helped that skin condition. The drug is a standard remedy for diarrhea and is commonly combined with atropine for that purpose. Another purpose of the combination format is to deter recreational use of the controlled substance, by forcing a would-be misuser to experience the simultaneous unpleasant actions of atropine (such as dry mouth, fever, excited behavior, and fuzzy eyesight).

Drawbacks. Diphenoxylate can reduce alertness and speed of movements, making operation of dangerous machinery (such as cars) inadvisable. Other effects of normal doses may include nausea, vomiting, dizziness, numbness, despondency, or euphoria. The drug should be avoided by persons who are prone to intestinal blockage because the compound can aggravate that condition. Pancreatitis is associated with the drug, but a cause and effect relationship is unconfirmed. Because diphenoxylate is available in a nonprescription format, some people do not realize how dangerous an overdose can be; breathing trouble leading to brain injury and death can occur; those consequences mostly involve accidental overdose in children. Overdose on the atropine component of a diphenoxylate combination product is also possible; atropine poisoning can include fever, agitation, irregularity in heartbeat and breathing, and psychosis involving hallucinations and delirium.

Abuse factors. Addiction to the diphenoxylate-atropine combination is unusual, but a case report tells of someone who used dozens of tablets every day for years. Under medical supervision the individual gradually reduced and finally stopped dosage over a two-week period; dependence was only slight, with mild flulike symptoms. A case is also reported of a drug addict using diphenoxylate-atropine tablets to hold off withdrawal symptoms when the person's abused drug was unavailable. Medical personnel have administered the diphenoxylate-atropine combination in order to wean addicts off **methadone** maintenance. When the combination was used in that context, recipients showed no signs of tolerance or addiction to it, an intriguing finding because that population of recipients would be particularly susceptible to such effects. Diphenoxylate has also been used to help addicts withdraw from **heroin**.

Drug interactions. The drug may interact dangerously with monoamine oxidase inhibitors (MAOIs, a component of some antidepressants and other medication). Tranquilizers, **alcohol**, or barbiturates should not be mixed with diphenoxylate.

Cancer. Diphenoxylate's potential for causing cancer is unknown, although animal experiments with the drug have found no tendency for the disease to appear.

Pregnancy. Fertility of female rats was impaired when they were dosed daily throughout a three-litter cycle at 50 times the recommended human level. Litter sizes declined when the females daily received 10 times the human dose. Tests on rats, mice, and rabbits revealed no birth defects, but results were not conclusive. A small survey of human medical records found "no strong associations" between the drug and various congenital malformations, and associations are only an indication that further investigation is needed, not that a problem exists. Diphenoxylate's effect on milk of nursing mothers is uncertain, but the atropine component in a diphenoxylate combination product does pass into the milk.

Additional information. Although difenoxin (CAS RN 28782-42-5) is available as a pharmaceutical preparation, body chemistry also produces this substance from a dose of diphenoxylate. By itself, difenoxin is a Schedule I substance illegal to possess under any circumstance (DEA no. 9168), officially classified as having no medical value. When combined with enough atropine sulfate, however, difenoxin is a Schedule IV prescription drug known as Lyspafen and Motofen.

Difenoxin acts much like diphenoxylate and is used to treat diarrhea. Dangers are similar to diphenoxylate's. A two-year experiment gave daily doses of difenoxin and atropine to rats and produced no evidence that the combination causes cancer.

In rat experimentation the difenoxin-atropine combination (Pregnancy Category C) had only a weak impact on fertility, and no birth defects were attributed to the combination after being administered to rats and rabbits at levels that were dozens of times the amount recommended for humans. Pregnant rats, however, did have longer labor and more stillbirths, and a higher percentage of their offspring died as newborns. The difenoxin-atropine combination is not recommended for pregnant women or nursing mothers.

Additional scientific information may be found in:

Favin, F.D. "Chronic High-Dose Lomotil Abuse and Safe Withdrawal." *ASHP Midyear Clinical Meeting* 26 (December 1991): 92D.

Ives, T.J. "Illicit Use of Diphenoxylate Hydrochloride to Prevent Narcotic Withdrawal Symptoms." *Drug Intelligence and Clinical Pharmacy* 14 (1980): 715–16.

Kleinman, M.H., and D. Arnon. "Use of Diphenoxylate Hydrochloride (Lomotil) in the Management of the Minor Withdrawal Syndrome during Methadone Detoxification: Clinical Report." *British Journal of Addiction* 72 (1977): 167–69.

Penfold, D., and G.N. Volans. "Overdose from Lomotil." *British Medical Journal* 2 (1977): 1401–2.

Rumack, B.H., and A.R. Temple. "Lomotil Poisoning." *Pediatrics* 53 (1974): 495–500.

Whitehead, W.E., A. Wald, and N.J. Norton. "Treatment Options for Fecal Incontinence." *Diseases of the Colon and Rectum* 44 (2001): 131–42.

Dipipanone

Pronunciation: dih-PIP-uh-nohn

Chemical Abstracts Service Registry Number: 467-83-4

Formal Names: Diconal, Piperidyl-Methadone, Wellconal

Type: Depressant (opioid class). *See* page 24

Federal Schedule Listing: Schedule I (DEA no. 9622)

USA Availability: Illegal to possess

Pregnancy Category: None

Uses. Actions of this drug are similar to those of **morphine**. Dipipanone has no officially approved medical usage in the United States, but elsewhere it is used as a powerful pain reliever for conditions such as surgery and cancer. Some cancer patients prefer this drug for pain control. The compound can control coughs.

Drawbacks. Persons are supposed to avoid the drug if they suffer from low thyroid activity or enlarged prostate. Dipipanone can make people sleepy, and users are supposed to be cautioned about operating dangerous machinery. Volunteers in one experiment experienced lower alertness after taking dipipanone, but other experiments found the substance to lack sedative action. Study does show that sedation can occur when dipipanone is given together with the antihistamine triprolidine. Dipipanone can cause headache, tremors, nausea, and vomiting, impair vision, interfere with breathing, make urination difficult, lower blood pressure, and reduce production of saliva. Seizures have been reported. Euphoria may occur. A case study notes delusions and hallucinations caused by the drug. Paranoia has occurred occasionally. A case report tells of serious colon difficulty occurring after someone injected three dissolved oral Diconal tablets, a combination product containing dipipanone and the antivomiting drug cyclizine, accompanied by drinking three liters of beer. Even in ordinary medical use, however, dipipanone can cause constipation and is supposed to be used cautiously if a person has bowel obstruction.

Abuse factors. Dipipanone is related to **methadone** and can be substituted for assorted opioids. That property gave dipipanone a role in addiction treatment programs seeking to switch addicts to dipipanone. Tolerance and dependence can occur. Reportedly drug abusers find dipipanone more potent than **heroin**, and in combination with cyclizine, dipipanone reportedly can create a rush of enjoyment that some persons prefer over heroin. In the 1980s some British observers considered dipipanone abuse to be as much a problem as abuse of methadone and **methylphenidate**, with some addicts getting their supplies legally from doctors. Rather little has been heard about the substance since then, however.

Drug interactions. Dipipanone may interact badly with monoamine oxidase inhibitors (MAOIs), which are substances found in some antidepressants and other medication.

Cancer. Potential for causing cancer is unknown.

Pregnancy. Potential for birth defects is unknown. Authorities are uncertain whether the drug passes into a nursing mother's milk, but they believe the level would be so low as to cause no harm to the infant. An infant can be born dependent on the drug if the mother has been using it during the final trimester of pregnancy.

Additional scientific information may be found in:

Bound, D., and S. Greer. "Psychotic Symptoms after Dipipanone." *Lancet* 2 (1978): 480.

Faull, C., et al. "Experience with Dipipanone Elixir in the Management of Cancer Related Pain—Case Study." *Palliative Medicine* 8 (1994): 63–65.

Posner, J., et al. "Effects of an Opiate on Cold-Induced Pain and the CNS in Healthy Volunteers." *Pain* 23 (1985): 73–82.

Stewart, M.J., et al. "Forensic Toxicology in Urban South Africa." *Journal of Toxicology: Clinical Toxicology* 38 (2000): 415–19.

Telekes, A., et al. "Effects of Triprolidine and Dipipanone in the Cold Induced Pain Test, and the Central Nervous System of Healthy Volunteers." *British Journal of Clinical Pharmacology* 24 (1987): 43–50.

Turnbull, A.R., and P. Isaacson. "Ischemic Colitis and Drug Abuse." *British Medical Journal* 2 (1977): 1000.

DMT

Pronunciation: dee-em-tee

Chemical Abstracts Service Registry Number: 61-50-7

Formal Names: Dimethyltryptamine, N,N-Dimethyltryptamine

Informal Names: AMT, Businessman's LSD, Businessman's Special, Business-man's Trip, Cohoba Snuff, Disneyland, Disneyworld, Dmitri, Fantasia, 45 Minute Psychosis, 45 Minute Trip, Instant Psychosis, Psychosis

Type: Hallucinogen. *See* page 25

Federal Schedule Listing: Schedule I (DEA no. 7435)

USA Availability: Illegal to possess

Pregnancy Category: None

Uses. Various plants contain this chemical, and minute quantities are manufactured by body processes in mammals. The substance can also be made in a laboratory and is chemically similar to **bufotenine**. Grasses containing DMT can sicken and kill livestock.

Native peoples of the Amazon use snuffs and drinks containing DMT for religious purposes. Supposedly such drinks can give a person telepathy and other ESP (extrasensory perception) powers, but one researcher failed to achieve such states even though he used the drink 30 times while living among a native population for three years.

In rat experiments the animals acted as if DMT is similar to **LSD**. A human study found DMT to evoke visual and auditory hallucinations so intense that the volunteers lost contact with ordinary reality during the drug experience. The volunteers vacillated back and forth between euphoria and unease. In contrast, a different human study comparing DMT and delta-9-tetrahydrocannabinol (also called THC, the main active ingredient in **marijuana**) found their actions to be equivalent. The finding was exceptional, however; most reports describe DMT as a potent hallucinogen with actions reminiscent of LSD or **mescaline**. Some people are said to become relaxed as DMT's initial actions wear off.

One commonly mentioned DMT effect is awareness of elves, fairies, or some alien intelligence—encounters that users do not necessarily find pleasant. Some users say that time seems to slow. Most scientists seek explanations that do not require acceptance of alternative realities, because throughout the history of science the simplest explanations tend to be correct. For example, time may seem slower if many events crowd simultaneously on someone's consciousness—an explanation that does not require time itself to alter. Likewise, industrious investigators have detected changes in the eye during DMT intoxication, changes that the brain may interpret as light and that a person can "see" as hallucinations.

Drawbacks. While under DMT's influence a person can experience memory trouble, shortened attention span, and altered perception of one's body. Physical effects may include dizziness, nausea, tingling, trembling, weakness, and breathing difficulty, along with higher body temperature, heart rate, and blood pressure. Reportedly a typical human-size dose per body weight is enough to kill a sheep.

Some researchers suspect that excessive natural production of DMT and related substances by a person's body processes may be the cause of schizophrenia and other psychotic conditions. Research along that line has produced mixed results. One study found that DMT levels generally went up and down in psychiatric patients, depending on outbreaks of psychotic behavior and return to normalcy, but timing of the shifts did not always match changes in patients' conditions. In addition, psychologically normal persons with liver disease can have DMT levels about as high as those found in schizophrenic individuals.

Abuse factors. Human experimentation has detected no development of tolerance to DMT's psychological effects. Tolerance to some physical actions (such as higher pulse rate) has been measured, but tolerance to increase of blood pressure has not been seen. Mice form a tolerance to DMT, and rats not only acquire a tolerance to DMT but have also exhibited cross-tolerance with LSD (meaning the drugs can be substituted for each other, in some ways at least). Humans have also shown partial cross-tolerance between those two drugs. Cats and monkeys fail to develop tolerance to various DMT effects (such as changes in appetite, behavior, and coordination) but apparently tolerance can develop to other effects. Some researchers feel that DMT tolerance is an uncertain phenomenon at best.

Drug interactions. Not enough scientific information to report.

Cancer. Not enough scientific information to report.

Pregnancy. Not enough scientific information to report.

Additional scientific information may be found in:

Fish, M.S., and E.C. Horning. "Studies on Hallucinogenic Snuffs." *Journal of Nervous and Mental Disease* 124 (1956): 33–37.

Gillin, J.C., et al. "The Psychedelic Model of Schizophrenia: The Case of N,N-Dimethyltryptamine." *American Journal of Psychiatry* 133 (1976): 203–8.

Riba, J., et al. "Subjective Effects and Tolerability of the South American Psychoactive Beverage Ayahuasca in Healthy Volunteers." *Psychopharmacology* (Berlin) 154 (2001): 85–95.

Rosenberg, D.E., et al. "The Effect of N,N-Dimethyltryptamine in Human Subjects Tolerant to Lysergic Acid Diethylamide." *Psychopharmacologia* 5 (1964): 217–27.

Shulgin, A.T. "Profiles of Psychedelic Drugs—DMT." *Journal of Psychedelic Drugs* 8 (1976): 167–68.

Strassman, R.J. "Human Psychopharmacology of N,N-Dimethyltryptamine." *Behavioural Brain Research* 73 (1996): 121–24.

Strassman, R.J., et al. "Dose-Response Study of N,N-Dimethyltryptamine in Humans. II. Subjective Effects and Preliminary Results of a New Rating Scale." *Archives of General Psychiatry* 51 (1994): 98–108.

Szára, S. "The Comparison of the Psychotic Effect of Tryptamine Derivatives with the Effects of Mescaline and LSD-25 in Self-Experiments." In *Psychotropic Drugs*, ed. S. Garattini and V. Ghetti. New York: Elsevier, 1957. 460–67.

DOB

Pronunciation: dee-oh-bee

Chemical Abstracts Service Registry Number: 53581-53-6

Formal Names: 4-Bromo-2,5-Dimethoxyamphetamine

Informal Names: Bob, Bromo-DMA, Bromo-STP, PBR

Type: Hallucinogen. *See* page 25

Federal Schedule Listing: Schedule I (DEA no. 7391)

USA Availability: Illegal to possess

Pregnancy Category: None

Uses. This drug became available in the 1960s. It can produce hallucinations and affect interpretations of time and space. Some persons who thought they took **LSD** were actually on DOB. Research has found DOB effects to develop more gradually and to be more prolonged than those of LSD.

A chemist who knew he was taking pure DOB reported that a small dose brightened his perception of colors and created a mellow mood. Larger doses created muscle tremors and increased insight into psychological issues. The chemist recommended against attempting to drive a car while intoxicated. In a controlled experimental setting with volunteers interested in using the drug to gain better awareness of themselves, the drug stimulated thoughts, feelings, and physical senses. People became more articulate, saw new meaning in ordinary experiences, and became more inclined to self-examination. In contrast to **MDA** experiences, the **DOB** volunteers showed less lethargy and were more interested in what was going on around them. No hallucinations occurred.

Drawbacks. In canines DOB can elevate body temperature and blood pressure. In humans DOB's physical effects can include nausea, diarrhea, muscle spasms, blood vessel spasms, sensations of tingling and burning, impaired sense of touch, convulsions, and seizures. The drug may be safe from a technical pharmaceutical standpoint because there is a huge difference between the size of a therapeutic dose and a lethal one, but the drug is so potent that small doses are known to kill. Effects may last for hours and suddenly intensify and become fatal. Characteristics of overdose can resemble those of amphetamine, including fear and physical aggression. The medical literature includes a DOB case somewhat resembling ergotism (see **ergot**), resulting in the patient's lower legs being amputated.

Abuse factors. Not enough scientific information to report.

Drug interactions. **Alcohol** may increase the strength of a DOB dose.

Cancer. Not enough scientific information to report.

Pregnancy. Not enough scientific information to report.

Additional scientific information may be found in:

Buhrich, N., G. Morris, and G. Cook. "Bromo-DMA: The Australasian Hallucinogen?" *Australian and New Zealand Journal of Psychiatry* 17 (1983): 275–79.

Davis, W.M. "LSD or DOB?" *American Journal of Psychiatry* 139 (1982): 1649.

Delliou, D. "4-Bromo-2,5-Dimethoxyamphetamine: Psychoactivity, Toxic Effects and Analytical Methods." *Forensic Science International* 21 (1983): 259–67.

Shulgin, A.T., T. Sargent, and C. Naranjo. "4-Bromo-2,5-Dimethoxyphenylisopropylamine, a New Centrally Active Amphetamine Analog." *Pharmacology* 5 (1971): 103–7.

Toennes, S.W., et al. "Aufklärung eines unklaren neurologischen Syndroms durch toxikologische Untersuchungen [Explanation of an Unclear Neurological Syndrome by Toxicologic Investigation]." *Deutsche Medizinische Wochenschrift* 125 (2000): 900–902. (Abstract in English).

DOM

Pronunciation: dee-oh-em

Chemical Abstracts Service Registry Number: 15588-95-1

Formal Names: 4-Methyl-2,5-Dimethoxyamphetamine

Informal Names: Serenity, Stop the Police, STP, Super Terrific Psychedelic, Too Stupid to Puke, Tranquility

Type: Hallucinogen. *See* page 25

Federal Schedule Listing: Schedule I (DEA no. 7395)

USA Availability: Illegal to possess

Pregnancy Category: None

Uses. This substance was a classic of the 1960s drug scene, where it was likened to **LSD** and nicknamed STP for "Serenity, Tranquility, and Peace" and apparently performed as advertised. Because of the nickname initials some persons have confused the drug with a motor oil additive called STP, but they are different substances.

DOM is a powerful drug, 50 to 100 times stronger than **mescaline**, to which DOM is chemically related. Rats respond to DOM and mescaline in similar ways. Chemically DOM is not only related to mescaline but also to amphetamine, and an experiment using low dosages of DOM found that the drug had a typical stimulant effect of improving performance on simple learning tasks.

Psychological and hallucinogenic effects depend on size of dose. As the size increases, so do intensity and longevity of effects. Many reports of alleged DOM experiences exist, but typically we do not know if the illicit substance really was DOM. One person who did ingest the real thing described hallucinations, brightened mood, more awareness of colors, more enjoyment of music and sex, and various insights into personal issues facilitated by the drug. Volunteers who received DOM in a formal experiment also experienced improved spirits and insights, but the amount of DOM was not enough to produce hallucinations. Results from another experiment showed increased awareness of emotion and thoughts, leading researchers to conclude that the substance might be useful in psychotherapy. In still another experiment psychological effects included disturbed perceptions of time and space, a sensation of voices being distant, echoing sound, seeing sound as light, seeing ordinary movement as stroboscopic jerkiness, seeing surfaces moving sinuously, and feeling like one was no longer located in one's body.

Drawbacks. An experiment documented physical sensations that included warmth, tingling, dizziness, nausea, tremors, rapid heartbeat, impaired movement, coughing, sweating, and lack of hunger. Insomnia has also been reported. In rats DOM can raise body temperature and lower appetite.

Supposedly effects from a single dose can last for three days, but in a group of 25 volunteers who took substantial doses, only 2 persons experienced effects lasting past the day of the experiment, and none had any effects on the second day afterward. Some users who expect the drug to act like LSD have not realized that DOM effects take longer to develop, and after waiting the amount of time they would wait for LSD actions to begin, those persons have taken more DOM in a mistaken belief that the original amount was not enough. The result can be an overdose emergency. Achieving such an overdose apparently takes dedication; one estimate puts DOM's safety index at 10,000 (meaning a person would have to take 10,000 times the amount of a standard effective dose in order to be poisoned). Some investigators wonder if previous use of psychoactive drugs makes people more sensitive to DOM, thereby making overdose easier.

Abuse factors. Tolerance can develop.

Drug interactions. Not enough scientific information to report.

Cancer. Not enough scientific information to report.

Pregnancy. Not enough scientific information to report.

Additional scientific information may be found in:

Hollister, L.E., M.F. Macnicol, and H.K. Gillespie. "An Hallucinogenic Amphetamine Analog (DOM) in Man." *Psychopharmacologia* 14 (1969): 62–73.

Ropero-Miller, J.D., and B.A. Goldberger. "Recreational Drugs: Current Trends in the 90s." *Clinics in Laboratory Medicine* 18 (1998): 727–46.

Shulgin, A.T., T. Sargent, and C. Naranjo. "4-Bromo-2,5-Dimethoxyphenylisopropylamine, a New Centrally Active Amphetamine Analog." *Pharmacology* 5 (1971): 103–7.

Snyder, S.H., L.A. Faillace, and H. Weingartner. "DOM (STP), a New Hallucinogenic Drug, and DOET: Effects in Normal Subjects." *American Journal of Psychiatry* 125 (1968): 357–64.

Snyder, S.H., L. Faillace, and L. Hollister. "2,5-Dimethoxy-4-Methyl-Amphetamine (STP): A New Hallucinogenic Drug." *Science* 158 (1967): 669–70.

Dronabinol

See also **Marijuana**

Pronunciation: droh-NAB-i-nol
Chemical Abstracts Service Registry Number: 1972-08-3
Formal Names: Delta-9-Tetrahydrocannabinol, Marinol, THC
Type: Hallucinogen. *See* page 25
Federal Schedule Listing: Schedule III (DEA no. 7369)
USA Availability: Prescription
Pregnancy Category: C

Uses. This is a pure form of THC, the main active ingredient found in the Schedule I substance **marijuana**. Dronabinol can be obtained from marijuana or manufactured synthetically. Compared to infrequent marijuana users, frequent marijuana users are better at identifying whether they have received dronabinol or a placebo.

Dronabinol is used to reduce nausea in persons undergoing cancer chemotherapy and to stimulate appetite in AIDS (acquired immunodeficiency syndrome) patients. Alzheimer's patients who received experimental dronabinol showed improved appetites and reduction of behavior associated with the disease. Research indicates that the drug may widen airways, a help to persons suffering from breathing difficulty. Experimental success has also been achieved in treating spasticity, reducing not only that affliction but its associated rigidity and pain. Research has also examined whether dronabinol may work as a cough medicine. Human testing shows that oral dosage of dronabinol's active ingredient THC can help reduce pain.

Drawbacks. Dronabinol can redden eyes and accelerate or slow heartbeat. Sometimes users feel faint upon suddenly standing up. Many of marijuana's actions are experienced with dronabinol: euphoria, hallucinations, more acuteness in physical senses, altered time perception, memory trouble, confusion, and drowsiness. Not everyone finds marijuana actions to be pleasant, and some nausea patients find those effects so unpleasant that they would rather forgo the dronabinol and endure the nausea. Some other effects associated with marijuana have not been observed with medical use of dronabinol, such as trouble with thinking skills and lack of ambition.

Abuse factors. Tolerance occurs to some of the drug's actions but not to appetite stimulation. Dependence is reported, with withdrawal symptoms including sleeping difficulty, peevishness, fidgeting, perspiration, runny nose, appetite loss, and loose bowel movements. In one study withdrawal symptoms lasted three days and gradually cleared up over that time. Addiction is uncommon. No one in a five-month study, including persons who had previously abused other drugs, began abusing dronabinol; nor did any of these persons exhibit changes of personality or changes of ability to function in society. An effort to discover evidence of illicit use in San Francisco found none. Apparently persons interested in recreational effects of dronabinol prefer marijuana.

Drug interactions. Animal experimentation has found that dronabinol substantially increases the pain relieving qualities of **codeine, heroin, hydromorphone, meperidine, methadone, morphine,** and **oxymorphone.** The antinausea drug prochlorperazine appears to reduce the unwanted marijuana actions of dronabinol.

Cancer. Dronabinol's potential for causing cancer is unknown. The Ames test, a standard laboratory procedure for detecting cancer-causing potential, revealed none.

Pregnancy. No birth defects have been attributed to dronabinol in mice and rat experiments, although more pregnancy failures occurred. THC passes from a pregnant animal into the fetus. Pregnant women are advised to be cautious with the drug. It passes into milk of nursing mothers, and levels in milk are higher than in the mothers' bloodstream.

Additional scientific information may be found in:

Beal, J.E., et al. "Long-Term Efficacy and Safety of Dronabinol for Acquired Immuno-deficiency Syndrome–Associated Anorexia." *Journal of Pain and Symptom Management* 14 (1997): 7–14.

Calhoun, S.R., G.P. Galloway, and D.E. Smith. "Abuse Potential of Dronabinol (Marinol)." *Journal of Psychoactive Drugs* 30 (1998): 187–96.

Devine, J.W., L.A. Mahr, and C.R. Rieck. "Effectiveness of Delta-9-Tetrahydrocannabinol in Chemotherapy-Induced Nausea and Vomiting." *Journal of the Iowa Pharmacy Association* 54 (1999): 22–24, 47–50.

Gonzalez-Rosales, F., and D. Walsh. "Intractable Nausea and Vomiting Due to Gastrointestinal Mucosal Metastases Relieved by Tetrahydrocannabinol (Dronabinol)." *Journal of Pain and Symptom Management* 14 (1997): 311–14.

Haney, M., et al. "Abstinence Symptoms Following Oral THC Administration to Humans." *Psychopharmacology* 141 (1999): 385–94.

Kirk, J.M., and H. de Wit. "Responses to Oral Delta-9-Tetrahydrocannabinol in Frequent and Infrequent Marijuana Users." *Pharmacology, Biochemistry, and Behavior* 63 (1999): 137–42.

Struwe, M., et al. "Effect of Dronabinol on Nutritional Status in HIV Infection." *Annals of Pharmacotherapy* 27 (1993): 827–31.

Wright, P.L., et al. "Reproductive and Teratologic Studies with DELTA-9-Tetrahydrocannabinol and Crude Marijuana Extract." *Toxicology and Applied Pharmacology* 38 (1976): 223–35.

Ephedrine

See also **Ma Huang**

Pronunciation: e-FED-rin (also pronounced EF-uh-dreen)

Chemical Abstracts Service Registry Number: 299-42-3. (Hydrochloride form 50-98-6; sulfate form 134-72-5)

Formal Names: Broncholate Syrup, Elsinore, Kie Syrup, Letigen, Marax, Pretz-D, Primatene, Rynatuss

Informal Names: Chinese Speed, Herbal Ecstasy, Herbal XTC

Type: Stimulant (amphetamine class). *See* page 12

Federal Schedule Listing: Unlisted

USA Availability: Varies by state and by product formulation

Pregnancy Category: C

Uses. Although natural products containing the drug have a long history, ephedrine was not isolated from **ma huang** until the 1880s. Ephedrine is found in other plants as well. It can be refined from plants or synthesized in a laboratory. Despite ma huang's familiar use as a medicinal herb, Western medicine did not accept ephedrine until the 1920s. Ephedrine has found usage in standard medicine, alternative medicine, and recreation. Responding to a survey, 14 companies reported they sold the equivalent of 425 million individual doses in 1995, 976 million in 1997, and 3 billion in 1999.

Some early uses have since become outmoded, such as against leprosy and whooping cough. Weight loss experiments have found ephedrine, alone or in combination with **caffeine** or aspirin, to be more effective than placebos and also more effective than dexfenfluramine (see **fenfluramine**). A study found ephedrine useful in helping heavy smokers to reduce the number of cigarettes they consume. Standard medicine has also exploited ephedrine's urinary retention effect to help incontinent persons. The drug has been employed against asthma, runny noses, narcolepsy, painful menstruation, and depression.

In alternative medicine ephedrine is marketed for losing weight, increasing muscle mass, facilitating intellectual concentration, and promoting vigor. A scientific study found that ephedrine in combination with caffeine (but not by itself) significantly improves endurance in physical exercise. Many sports organizations ban use of ephedrine by athletes.

Although not a true amphetamine, ephedrine has qualities reminiscent of that stimulant class and has been commonly used to manufacture illicit **meth-**

cathinone and **methamphetamine**. Indeed, ephedrine's chemical relationship to amphetamine and methamphetamine is so close that urine tests can misidentify ephedrine as those drugs. In an experiment where people received a substance without knowing what it was, ephedrine produced the same physical and mental effects as **phenmetrazine**, **methylphenidate**, **dextroamphetamine**, and methamphetamine. Ephedrine's legal status was in flux as this book was written: Depending on the federal or state jurisdiction, ephedrine might be Schedule IV or a freely available unscheduled substance; commerce as a medical drug might be legal, but commerce as a raw chemical might be a crime.

Drawbacks. Amphetamine was designed in a laboratory to provide a substitute for ephedrine because of the latter's drawbacks. A double dose of ephedrine can be poisonous, in comparison to other drugs with the same therapeutic effects but that require 10 or 20 times the regular dose to become severely toxic. For that reason many physicians prefer to avoid prescribing ephedrine.

Ephedrine can cause skin rash, nausea, diarrhea, constipation, hepatitis, rise in body temperature, jitteriness, insomnia, hyperactivity, irregular heartbeat, high blood pressure, heart attack, stroke, seizures, kidney stones, visual and auditory hallucinations, and paranoid psychosis. Ephedrine can worsen muscle tics; animal experimentation shows the drug causing brain damage that can lead to the tics seen in Parkinson's disease. During strong physical exertion, such as bodybuilding, ephedrine may increase danger of heart attack. Suspicion exists that persons who stop taking ephedrine may be more sensitive to it if they start using the drug again.

Many reports of adverse events come from cases in which a person was using ephedrine diet supplements commonly found in health food stores. Perhaps people regard such products as inherently "healthy" and fail to realize that an ephedrine food supplement can produce a drug overdose or be hazardous if used moderately but for too long.

The U.S. Food and Drug Administration (FDA) became particularly alarmed at the prevalence of medical problems developed by young healthy users, and regulatory efforts were increasing when this book was written. Some scientists say the FDA's concerns are unfounded and that many physical problems after ephedrine ingestion derive from a person's prior medical history or massive overdose. Nonetheless, the FDA believes that ephedrine may harm people who already have the following conditions: prostate trouble, psychological afflictions (including depression and nervousness), high blood pressure, diabetes, glaucoma, and ailments of thyroid, kidney, or heart.

Alcohol is an ingredient in some ephedrine inhalers and can influence readings in breathalyzer tests for drunk driving. That problem can be avoided by a 15-minute wait between using the inhaler and administering a test.

Abuse factors. Historically ephedrine has seldom been abused, but in the 1990s it was cited as growing in popularity among youths, as a recreational stimulant with euphoric and aphrodisiac effects. Such characteristics have allowed illicit dealers to market ephedrine falsely as **cocaine**, methamphetamine, and **MDMA**. Some cocaine users find ephedrine less satisfying but still a satisfactory substitute. Reports of ephedrine addiction exist.

Drug interactions. Caffeine boosts ephedrine's power and can transform a normal dose into a dangerous one. Aspirin and yohimbine (from **yohimbe**) may also strengthen some ephedrine effects. Dangerous interactions can occur with monoamine oxidase inhibitors (MAOIs, typically antidepressants). Less serious adverse effects may occur if ephedrine is taken with the antiasthma medicine theophylline.

Cancer. The FDA has noted research indicating that substances like ephedrine may promote lung cancer, especially among tobacco smokers.

Pregnancy. Safety for use during pregnancy is unestablished. The drug is known to raise fetal heart rate, and fetal blood levels can reach about 70% of the pregnant woman's blood level of ephedrine. The drug is transferred to breast milk in sufficient quantity to affect nursing infants, making them grouchy and interfering with their sleep. Chicken experiments with ephedrine produce defects in embryos, but such testing is considered inconclusive regarding human impact. Rabbit experiments find a mix of ephedrine, theophylline, and **phenobarbital** to cause birth defects similar to those observed in the child of a woman who took that drug combination while pregnant. The same drug combination is suspected in another birth defect case. Although a study of 373 human pregnancies found no malformations attributable to ephedrine even when used in the first trimester, the drug is associated with a small increase in likelihood of birth defects and is not recommended for use during pregnancy.

Additional information. Many nonprescription remedies for common colds include pseudoephedrine (CAS RN 345-78-8), which is related to ephedrine and has similar effects, both desired and undesired. Depending on actions being measured, pseudoephedrine may have from 25% to 50% of ephedrine's strength. Pseudoephedrine can be used to make methamphetamine and methcathinone.

Pseudoephedrine is believed to promote a dangerous bowel disease called ischemic colitis, particularly in women around the time they go into menopause. A case report indicates that taking pseudoephedrine with serotonin reuptake inhibitor antidepressants may create a medical emergency called "serotonin syndrome." Typical signs of that condition are hyperactivity, confusion, nervousness, vomiting, fast heartbeat, excessive body temperature, shivering, tremors, weakness, or losing consciousness. Caution is advised about using pseudoephedrine shortly after receiving vaccinations, which temporarily increase body temperature. Nonetheless, in the 1980s research on more than 100,000 individuals using prescription pseudoephedrine found no hospitalizations caused by the drug.

Influence on fetal development is uncertain, although pseudoephedrine is suspected of causing birth defects when used in the first trimester. The drug is known to accelerate fetal heartbeat but has no particular effect on fetal blood flow, nor does the substance seem to hinder passing nutrients and gases between woman and fetus. Although excreted into human milk, the amount of excretion is so slight as to be considered safe for infants of nursing mothers.

Additional scientific information may be found in:

"Adverse Events Associated with Ephedrine-Containing Products—Texas, December 1993–September 1995." *Morbidity and Mortality Weekly Report* 45 (1996): 689–93.

Astrup, A., et al. "The Effect and Safety of an Ephedrine/Caffeine Compound Compared to Ephedrine, Caffeine and Placebo in Obese Subjects on an Energy Restricted Diet. A Double Blind Trial." *International Journal of Obesity and Related Metabolic Disorders* 16 (1992): 269–77.

"Dietary Supplements Containing Ephedrine Alkaloids; Proposed Rule." *Federal Register* 62 (1997): 30677–724.

Gruber, A.J., and H.G. Pope, Jr. "Ephedrine Abuse among 36 Female Weightlifters." *American Journal on Addictions* 7 (1998): 256–61.

James, L.P., et al. "Sympathomimetic Drug Use in Adolescents Presenting to a Pediatric Emergency Department with Chest Pain." *Journal of Toxicology. Clinical Toxicology* 36 (1998): 321–28.

Pipe, A., and C. Ayotte. "Nutritional Supplements and Doping." *Clinical Journal of Sport Medicine* 12 (2002): 245–49.

Whitehouse, A.M., and J.M. Duncan. "Ephedrine Psychosis Rediscovered." *British Journal of Psychiatry* 150 (1987): 258–61.

Ergot

Pronunciation: UR-guht

Chemical Abstracts Service Registry Number: 12126-57-7

Formal Names: *Claviceps purpurea*

Informal Names: Cockspur Rye, Hornseed, Mother of Rye, Muttercorn, Smut Rye, Spur Kernels, Spurred Rye

Type: Hallucinogen. *See* page 25

Federal Schedule Listing: Unlisted

USA Availability: Nonprescription natural product

Pregnancy Category: None

Uses. The history of ergot is composed of madness and disfiguring disease but might still be an obscure footnote to medicine except for the discovery of a related chemical in the 1930s called **LSD**. That link brought modern attention to a normally inconspicuous natural product. Ergot comes from a rather fishy-smelling fungus growing on improperly stored grain (typically rye). In cool and damp conditions ergot is also found on various grains and grasses in the field. This happens around the world; in the 1990s Iowa's barley crop suffered infection. Ergot chemicals are also found in **morning glory** seeds. Although ergot is typically an unwanted contamination in grain, sometimes the fungus is deliberately cultivated to be harvested for pharmaceutical purposes.

Ergot is a traditional treatment to reduce menstrual blood flow and bleeding after childbirth. The substance promotes contractions of the uterus, and the raw product has been used for centuries as an aid to birthing. Unskilled administration, however, can rupture the uterus. In more recent times ergonovine (CAS RN 129-51-1) has been isolated from ergot as the active chemical for promoting childbearing. Chemicals from ergot can induce abortions in cows and sheep, but reports conflict on whether ergot has this effect on humans. One authority notes that such attempted use can kill the pregnant woman. Ergot preparations are still used as a fallback if no other drug provides sufficient aid in childbirth, but they are generally avoided in modern obstetrics.

Ergotamine, a substance derived from ergot, is used to treat migraine headache. Raw ergot is not used for that purpose because the unprocessed natural product would have too many unwanted effects, making the headache cure worse than the disease. Ergot chemicals have also been used to treat menopause and for experimental treatment of patients suffering from Parkinson's disease and from mental deterioration associated with old age, including Alzheimer's disease. After volunteers took an ergot drug called co-dergocrine they were stimulated and did better than normal on tests of thinking, decisions, and physical movement. That finding is not surprising, given that LSD is related to ergot and can act as a powerful stimulant.

Drawbacks. Entire communities have been devastated when residents ate food contaminated with ergot. Such outbreaks of ergotism come in two varieties, convulsive and gangrenous. Both can occur simultaneously. The gangrenous kind is characterized by weeks of severe burning pain in appendages, sometimes called St. Anthony's Fire or Holy Fire. The convulsive kind can involve dizziness, ringing in the ears, tingling fingers, hallucinations, vomiting, convulsions, delirium, and a sensation that vermin are crawling underneath the skin. Ergotism incidents occurred in Ethiopia in the 1970s, in India during the 1950s, in Russia during the 1920s, and in the United States during the 1800s. Some authorities argue that convulsions and hallucinations caused by ergot were responsible for the Salem witchcraft accusations in colonial America during the 1600s. Such instances are good examples of why herbal medicine authorities recommend avoiding the natural product.

Ergot constricts blood vessels in fingers and toes, enough that repeated use can cause gangrene. Extreme human cases can kill substantial portions of entire limbs; the same result was seen in cows that grazed in an ergot-contaminated pasture and in cattle that ate contaminated feed. Less serious unwanted effects can include nausea, vomiting, chest pain, itching, weak legs, and numb fingers. Extended dosage can cause difficulty in movement, impair vision by damaging blood vessels in the eye, and produce inability to use words.

Ergotamine can cause heart trouble and gangrenous ergotism. Rat tests show that a wide variety of health problems are caused by chronic consumption of ergocryptine, an ergot chemical.

Abuse factors. Not enough scientific information to report about tolerance, dependence, withdrawal, or addiction. Deliberate consumption of the natural product is probably rare.

Drug interactions. Ergot problems can be exacerbated by **caffeine**, by tobacco cigarettes, by the HIV/AIDS drug ritonavir, and possibly by the antidepressant fluoxetine (Prozac). A case report relates instances of bad reactions occurring when people used ergot products along with "beta blockers," a type of drug that is typically prescribed for heart problems.

Cancer. In 1990 a World Health Organization study reported that no information was available on ergot's potential for causing cancer. Research published in 1976, however, said that ergotamine and two other ergot chemicals did not cause cell mutations in mice and hamsters (mutations can indicate potential for cancer).

Pregnancy. Using ergot during pregnancy and nursing is considered hazardous. Ergot chemicals consumed by a pregnant cow can pass into the fetus and also appear in the cow's milk. In pigs ergot can interfere with reproduction and milk supply. Ergotamine is known to cause human fetal stress, is known to cause birth defects in animals, and is suspected of causing birth defects in humans. Pregnant women who took drugs in unsuccessful suicide attempts were the subjects of a study that tentatively concluded that ergotamine did not cause congenital malformations, but the researchers felt they needed more data to be sure. Other investigators have noted reports of ergotamine birth defects consistent with reduced blood flow (a known action of ergot preparations), but those reports have not been scientifically confirmed. Clinical observations have noted that when nursing mothers use ergotamine in the first week after birth, their infants show normal milk consumption and normal weight gain during that week. Ergot passes into human milk, however, and instances have been noted of infants poisoned from ergot in the milk.

Bromocriptine and cabergoline, drugs related to ergot, have been used in circumstances when milk production needs to be suppressed in women who have recently given birth. Cabergoline has been used experimentally to treat pituitary cancer and Parkinson's disease, and in certain circumstances the drug should increase female fertility, but scientists are unsure about its potential for causing birth defects. Cabergoline experiments with rabbits and mice did not produce malformations. A study of pregnant women who used cabergoline found several instances of birth defects, but no more than would be expected if the drug had not been used. Congenital malformations among offspring were noted in another set of pregnant women who used the drug, but researchers reported no conclusion on the drug's role.

Additional scientific information may be found in:

Hofmann, A. "Historical View on Ergot Alkaloids." *Pharmacology* 16 (1978, Suppl. 1): 1–11.

Merhoff, G.C., and J.M. Porter. "Ergot Intoxication: Historical Review and Description of Unusual Clinical Manifestations." *Annals of Surgery* 180 (1974): 773–79.

Moir, J.C. "Ergot: From 'St. Anthony's Fire' to the Isolation of Its Active Principle, Ergometrine (Ergonovine)." *American Journal of Obstetrics and Gynecology* 120 (1974): 291–96.

Van Dongen, P., and A. De Groot. "History of Ergot Alkaloids from Ergotism to Ergometrine." *European Journal of Obstetrics and Gynecology and Reproductive Biology* 60 (1995): 109–16.

Woolf, A. "Witchcraft or Mycotoxin? The Salem Witch Trials." *Journal of Toxicology. Clinical Toxicology* 38 (2000): 457–60.

Estazolam

Pronunciation: ess-TA-zoh-lam

Chemical Abstracts Service Registry Number: 29975-16-4

Formal Names: ProSom

Type: Depressant (benzodiazepine class). *See* page 21

Federal Schedule Listing: Schedule IV (DEA no. 2756)

USA Availability: Prescription

Pregnancy Category: X

Uses. Estazolam's main medical uses are for relaxing muscles, fighting convulsions, and inducing sleep. The compound can also reduce anxiety in insomniacs but is not intended for long-term use against insomnia. Estazolam has been used successfully to treat auditory hallucinations and to improve the general mental state of schizophrenics. The drug is considered more potent than **diazepam**. Insomnia studies show estazolam to be about 15 times stronger than **flurazepam**.

Drawbacks. Estazolam may, at inappropriate times, make people lightheaded or sleepy and interfere with movement. Constipation and dry mouth are common. Even at high doses the drug's hindrance of respiration is of no concern in persons who breathe normally but might be troublesome for persons who have impaired breathing—although experimental results have been reassuring even for that population. A rebound effect can occur when people stop taking the drug for insomnia, meaning that sleep disturbance temporarily becomes worse than it was before treatment. In one study the most common adverse effect was feeling tired the day after using the drug. Other volunteers have experienced lower mental acuity and pulse rate 10 hours after taking the drug, even after getting a good night's sleep.

Abuse factors. Withdrawal symptoms are usually minor if a person takes estazolam long enough to produce dependence, but unusual reports exist of delirium and dangerous seizures during withdrawal.

Drug interactions. Estazolam actions can be boosted by **alcohol**, barbiturates, opiates, antihistamines, and monoamine oxidase inhibitors (MAOIs—found in some antidepressants). Cigarette smoking can shorten the time that an estazolam dose lasts.

Cancer. Long-term experiments with rats and mice found no sign that estazolam causes cancer. Potential for causing human cancer is unknown.

Pregnancy. A rat experiment produced no change in fertility. Estazolam is known to cause human birth defects, and pregnant women are never supposed to take the drug. Analysis of milk from nursing rats shows that estazolam and its breakdown products can pass into milk.

Additional scientific information may be found in:

Astrup, C., and L. Vatten. "Effect of the Benzodiazepine Derivative Estazolam in Schizophrenia." *Biological Psychiatry* 19 (1984): 85–88.

Cohn, J.B. "Hypnotic Efficacy of Estazolam Compared with Flurazepam in Outpatients with Insomnia." *Journal of Clinical Pharmacology* 31 (1991): 747–50.

"Estazolam—A New Benzodiazepine Hypnotic." *Medical Letter on Drugs and Therapeutics* 33 (1991): 91–92.

Lingjaerde, O. "Effect of the Benzodiazepine Derivative Estazolam in Patients with Auditory Hallucinations. A Multicentre Double-Blind, Cross-Over Study." *Acta Psychiatrica Scandinavica* 65 (1982): 339–54.

Pierce, M.W., V.S. Shu, and L.J. Groves. "Safety of Estazolam. The United States Clinical Experience." *American Journal of Medicine* 88, no. 3A (1990): 12S–17S.

Rosen, R.C., et al. "Psychophysiological Insomnia: Combined Effects of Pharmacotherapy and Relaxation-Based Treatments." *Sleep Medicine* 1 (2000): 279–88.

Vogel, G.W., and D. Morris. "The Effects of Estazolam on Sleep, Performance, and Memory: Long-term Sleep Laboratory Study of Elderly Insomniacs." *Journal of Clinical Pharmacology* 32 (1992): 647–51.

Ethchlorvynol

Pronunciation: eth-KLOR-vih-nahl
Chemical Abstracts Service Registry Number: 113-18-8
Formal Names: Arvynol, ECV, Ethylchlorovinyl, Placidyl, Serensil
Informal Names: Green Weenies
Type: Depressant. *See* page 19
Federal Schedule Listing: Schedule IV (DEA no. 2540)
USA Availability: Prescription
Pregnancy Category: C

Uses. Insomnia is the main medical condition treated by this drug, although it has also been used as a tranquilizer. The compound has been used to assist pain relief, on the theory that its calming and sleep-inducing qualities can allow pain relievers to work better. Although ethchlorvynol is considered safe for adults under medical supervision, ordinarily medical personnel are not supposed to dose children with ethchlorvynol, as adequate testing of impact on juveniles has not been done. Normally the drug is not supposed to be used for more than one week, as longer dosage increases risk of adverse effects.

The substance was introduced in the 1950s and is considered old-fashioned. It has mostly been superseded by newer pharmaceuticals that are more effective and that have fewer adverse effects.

Drawbacks. Because the drug makes people sleepy, they should avoid running dangerous machinery (such as motor vehicles) while under the influence. Symptoms of ethchlorvynol intoxication are similar to those of **alcohol** intoxication. The drug can cause nausea and vomiting, dizziness, and fainting. Confusion, stammering, intense headache, and general loss of vigor have also been reported. Intravenous abuse of the drug has caused vomiting, low blood pressure and body temperature, liver damage, fluid buildup in the lungs, and coma.

Persons suffering from porphyria should avoid ethchlorvynol. Porphyria is a body chemistry disease that can cause sudden violent outbursts, and the disease can be promoted by ethchlorvynol. The substance should also be avoided by people who experience "paradoxical reactions" to barbiturates or alcohol. A paradoxical reaction is an effect opposite from the expected one—for example, barbiturates causing hyperactivity rather than mellowness. In an unusual accident the drug squirted into someone's eyes and seriously injured the corneas. One capsule format of an ethchlorvynol preparation called Placidyl includes FD&C Yellow No. 5 (tartrazine), which can cause asthma attacks in some people.

Abuse factors. A case report indicates that tolerance may develop, but the indication was complicated by influence from the patient's thyroid disease. Another case report tells of the opposite effect, with a person becoming so sensitive to the drug that a trivial dose put him into a coma for a week. Experts generally feel, however, that tolerance is a more typical development. Taking the drug long enough to produce dependence can also produce slurred speech, amnesia, discoordination, tremors, eyesight difficulty, and facial numbness. The drug has a withdrawal syndrome that may not start until days after dosage suddenly stops. Withdrawal may include the dependence symptoms just noted, plus excitability, convulsions, delirium, hallucinations, nervousness, and loss of normal emotional reactions. Delirium tremens can occur. Standard treatment involves temporary reinstatement of the drug followed by tapering off doses, but **phenobarbital** has enough cross-tolerance to substitute for this purpose. Typically such detoxification is delicate enough to require hospitalization. In 1981 U.S. Supreme Court Justice William Rehnquist was reported to be so dependent upon medically prescribed ethchlorvynol that his mind was clouded while undergoing withdrawal in a hospital. A case report tells of someone who had months of hallucinations requiring weeks of hospitalization while trying to cope with ethchlorvynol withdrawal complicated by alcohol use. Alcohol abusers may find ethchlorvynol attractive. Medical authorities have noted close similarities between symptoms of dependence and withdrawal evoked by alcohol and ethchlorvynol.

Drug interactions. Individuals are not supposed to use ethchlorvynol along with other depressants (including alcohol and barbiturates) or with monoamine oxidase inhibitors (MAOIs, included in some antidepressants and other medication). Delirium has occurred in persons who take ethchlorvynol along with the tricyclic antidepressant amitriptyline hydrochloride, and caution is advised about taking other tricyclic antidepressants along with ethchlorvynol. Ethchlorvynol may interact with medications given to prevent blood clots. In animals injected with THC, the main active component of **marijuana**, ethchlorvynol becomes more potent than usual.

Cancer. Rat experiments using many times the recommended human dose of ethchlorvynol have yielded no evidence that the substance causes cancer. In contrast, mice experiments indicate (but have not confirmed) a cancer-causing potential. In the body the drug converts into other chemicals; results from laboratory testing have yielded mixed results concerning their cancer-causing potential.

Pregnancy. The drug is associated with fetal and newborn death in rat experiments. In one experiment using the drug on pregnant rats, offspring appeared normal but behaved abnormally and showed body chemistry aberrations. Effects on human pregnancy are uncertain. The substance passes into a human fetus, and in dogs the fetal blood level reaches the same strength as the maternal level. A baby born to a woman using the drug showed withdrawal symptoms; in an infant these may include abnormal reflexes, nervousness, and peevishness. Standard advice is to avoid ethchlorvynol during pregnancy. Although the drug's presence in milk of nursing mothers is unclear, the potential hazard of dosing infants through the milk makes nursing inadvisable.

Additional scientific information may be found in:

Flemenbaum, A., and B. Gunby. "Ethchlorvynol (Placidyl) Abuse and Withdrawal (Review of Clinical Picture and Report of 2 Cases)." *Diseases of the Nervous System* 32 (1971): 188–92.

Garetz, F.D. "Ethchlorvynol (Placidyl). Addiction Hazard." *Minnesota Medicine* 52 (1969): 1131–33.

Heston, L.L., and D. Hastings. "Psychosis with Withdrawal from Ethchlorvynol." *American Journal of Psychiatry* 137 (1980): 249–50.

Kripke, D.F., P. Lavie, and J. Hernandez. "Polygraphic Evaluation of Ethchlorvynol (14 Days)." *Psychopharmacology* (Berlin) 56 (1978): 221–23.

Kurt, T.L., G. Reed, and R.J. Anderson. "Pulmonary Edema after Intravenous Ethchlorvynol (Placidyl)." *Veterinary and Human Toxicology* 24 (1982, Suppl.): 76–78.

Marshall, E. "Rehnquist's Drug Dependence Poses Dilemma." *Science* 215 (1982): 379–80.

Yell, R.P. "Ethchlorvynol Overdose." *American Journal of Emergency Medicine* 8 (1990): 246–50.

Ether

Pronunciation: EE-thur

Chemical Abstracts Service Registry Number: 60-29-7

Formal Names: Diethyl Ether, Diethyl Oxide, Ethoxyethane, Ethyl Ether, Ethyl Oxide, Sulfuric Ether

Informal Names: Anesthesia Ether, Sweet Vitriol

Type: Inhalant. *See* page 26

Federal Schedule Listing: Unlisted

USA Availability: Some sales of the chemical are restricted because it can be used for manufacturing controlled substances

Uses. Although the substance has been available for hundreds of years it was not used as a drug until the nineteenth century began. The compound relaxes muscles and increases blood sugar levels. For decades it was a standard anesthetic but has been superseded by chemicals that work faster, that are better tolerated by patients, and that are less of a fire hazard. Nonetheless, knowledgeable medical personnel can use ether safely without complicated equipment, and the drug remains common where high-tech medical facilities are not common or nonexistent. In liquid form ether is used medically to clean skin surfaces before putting on adhesive tape and is used to help take off adhesive tape.

The gas format is used recreationally (sometimes along with chloroform), but drinking liquid ether is a more common recreational usage. Effects of drinking are similar to those produced by **alcohol** but appear faster and last briefly. People feel stimulated and confused, may experience euphoria and hallucinations, may have difficulty walking, and sometimes pass out. Ether drinking is associated with Ireland, where the custom was adopted in response to temperance movement restrictions on alcohol's availability in the 1800s. Ether drinking has been known in other European countries also, as well as the United States. In America during the 1800s ether was drunk on occasions ranging from a professional medical society meeting to weddings and quilting bees. Such a range indicates wide social acceptance of the practice. The substance was considered less harmful than alcohol. While using ether, nineteenth-century writer and physician Oliver Wendell Holmes made notes about spiritual insight that he felt was opening to him with the drug's help, but afterward he found the notes to be gibberish.

Drawbacks. Lighter doses of the gas stimulate breathing, but larger doses depress it. The gas irritates airways. At higher doses pulse rate and blood pressure decline. A serious unwanted effect can be a fatal convulsion. Using ether as a beverage can cause headache, increase salivation, irritate the passageway from mouth to stomach (resulting in vomiting), and produce heavy flatulence. In liquid form the substance can irritate skin and be absorbed through it.

Ether is highly flammable, and various regulations govern medical usage to reduce chances of ignition. These rules even control types of clothing worn by caregivers and types of linen used on carts, lest a static electricity spark create an explosion. Ether vapor is heavier than air and can accumulate in depressions such as the area of a pillow around a patient's head, making ignition all the more catastrophic. Stories are told of ether drinkers being killed when lighting a tobacco pipe or while indulging too close to an open flame. Even releasing ether fumes from the mouth toward a lit fireplace was considered a hazard to avoid, lest ether ignition flash back and down a person's throat.

Abuse factors. Some accounts describe ether usage as potentially addictive.

Drug interactions. Not enough scientific information to report.

Cancer. Laboratory tests indicate ether may have potential for causing cancer, but whether the substance produces the disease in animals is unknown.

Pregnancy. The drug has caused congenital malformations and fetal death in experiments on chicken embryos, but impact on humans is unclear. Women with industrial exposure are somewhat more likely to suffer spontaneous abortion. Ether passes from a pregnant woman into the fetus, but neither chronic exposure nor acute medical exposure is known to cause birth defects. Nursing infants seem unharmed by milk from women using ether.

Additional information. "Petroleum ether" and the drug ether are different substances.

Additional scientific information may be found in:

Connell, K.H. "Ether Drinking in Ulster." *Quarterly Journal of Studies on Alcohol* 26 (1965): 629–53.
Nagle, D.R. "Anesthetic Addiction and Drunkenness: A Contemporary and Historical Survey." *International Journal of the Addictions* 3 (1968): 25–39.
Strickland, R.A. "Ether Drinking in Ireland." *Mayo Clinic Proceedings* 71 (1996): 1015.

Ethylestrenol

Pronunciation: eth-ill-EHS-treh-nol

Chemical Abstracts Service Registry Number: 965-90-2

Formal Names: Duraboral, Maxibolin, Orabolin, Orgabolin

Type: Anabolic steroid. *See* page 24

Federal Schedule Listing: Schedule III (DEA control no. 4000)

USA Availability: Prescription

Uses. Researchers have given the substance to children who needed improvement in appetite. In places where the drug is illegal for agricultural use, some stockmen occasionally use it illegally to promote cattle growth.

Ethylestrenol has been used to help normalize blood disorders, including low white blood cell levels caused by leukopenia and conditions involving unwanted blood clotting. Experiments indicate that heart attack patients may gain particular benefit from blood actions of the drug. It has also worked as an experimental treatment for hemophilia. The drug can reduce purpura (purple blotches caused by blood leaking just below the skin). Ethylestrenol has been used experimentally to treat frostbite, and case reports note success in using ethylestrenol to help treat a painful ulcerative skin disease called livedo vasculitis and another called atrophie blanche, but experiments with a similar affliction had mixed results. Persons suffering from rheumatoid arthritis and from Raynaud's disease, an ailment involving poor blood circulation in fingers and toes, have improved while taking ethylestrenol. The drug has also been used to treat Behcet's syndrome, another disease involving problems in blood circulation. Mice experiments using ethylestrenol show limited success in treating symptoms of the skin disease lupus erythematosus and also Sjögren's syndrome, an immune system disease that includes destruction of the salivary glands and sweat glands.

Drawbacks. Among anabolic steroids ethylestrenol is considered to have few masculinizing effects, and it also helps maintain normal functioning of female organs. Nonetheless, in women the drug can cause acne, increase facial hair, and produce hoarseness that can transform into permanent deepening of the voice. The substance can bring on premature sexual development in boys and girls. In sexually mature females ethylestrenol can disrupt or even halt menstrual periods. Men can become less fertile. The substance promotes fluid and salt retention, which can aggravate assorted medical conditions. The drug is not recommended for men suffering from breast or prostate cancer. The substance can worsen porphyria, a disease that can make people violent and sensitive to light. Ethylestrenol has been used to help short youths grow taller but if used incorrectly may instead terminate bone growth, preventing young users from attaining the full adult stature that they would otherwise have achieved. Effective usage to promote height requires careful medical supervision.

Abuse factors. Some bodybuilders use ethylestrenol in hopes of promoting muscle mass even though the substance is banned by international athletic organizations.

Drug interactions. Rats that receive ethylestrenol are better able to survive massive exposure to **meprobamate** or **nicotine** and high exposure to the insecticides paraoxon and parathion. Ethylestrenol also makes rats act less affected by **LSD**. Ethylestrenol can counteract anesthesia actions of barbiturates, diminish ulcers caused by the pain reliever indomethacin, and reduce consequences of vitamin D overdose.

Cancer. Not enough scientific information to report.

Pregnancy. Pregnant women and nursing mothers are supposed to avoid ethylestrenol. In rat experiments the drug masculinized female fetuses.

Additional scientific information may be found in:

Chakrabarti, R., and G.R. Fearnley. "Phenformin Plus Ethylestrenol in Survivors of Myocardial Infarction: Three-Year Pilot Study." *Lancet* 2 (1972): 556–59.

Hecht, A. "Anabolic Steroids: Pumping Trouble." *FDA Consumer* 18 (September 1984): 12–15.

Kawashima, K., et al. "Virilizing Activities of Various Steroids in Female Rat Fetuses." *Endocrinologia Japonica* 24 (1977): 77–81.

Kerrebijn, K.F., and A. Delver. "Ethylestrenol (Orgabolin): Effects on Asthmatic Children during Corticosteroid Treatment." *Scandinavian Journal of Respiratory Diseases* 68 (1969, Suppl.): 70–77.

Murchison, L. "Uses and Abuses of Anabolic Steroids." *Prescribers' Journal* 26 (1986): 129–35.

Van Puymbroeck, M., et al. "17alpha-ethyl-5beta-estrane-3alpha, 17beta-diol, a Biological Marker for the Abuse of Norethandrolone and Ethylestrenol in Slaughter Cattle." *Journal of Chromotography. B, Biomedical Sciences and Applications* 728 (1999): 217–32.

Etorphine

Pronunciation: et-OR-feen

Chemical Abstracts Service Registry Number: 14521-96-1. (Hydrochloride form 13764-49-3)

Formal Names: Immobilon, M99

Informal Names: Elephant Juice

Type: Depressant (opiate class). *See* page 22

Federal Schedule Listing: Schedule I (DEA no. 9056). Hydrochloride form Schedule II (DEA no. 9059)

USA Availability: Illegal to possess except in hydrochloride form, which is prescription

Uses. This pain-relieving drug is derived from **thebaine**. In jurisdictions where etorphine is legal, it is used as a veterinary sedative. The substance is powerful. Depending on dosage method and animal species receiving the drug, its strength is estimated as anywhere from 10 times to 80,000 times that of **morphine**, so a person administering the drug must be skilled in order to avoid a serious overdose. The related Schedule II controlled substance dihydroetorphine is also powerful—10 to 10,000 times stronger than morphine. Etorphine acts quickly. Veterinarians and naturalists use etorphine darts to knock down wild elephants and grizzly bears. Zoos utilize the drug on white rhinoceros, giraffes, and other animals when medical necessity requires them to be unconscious.

Human tests show that etorphine can relieve intense pain without causing unconsciousness. Tests using dihydroetorphine alone and in combination with acupuncture have found the drug to be safe and effective for easing labor pain in childbirth. The substance has relieved pain in cancer patients. Experimenters suspect that as well as being a more powerful pain reliever than morphine, dihydroetorphine may also be less likely to create dependence in a patient.

Opiates and other depressants normally interfere with physical performance. Administered in a particular way, however, etorphine reliably produces a "paradoxical" effect (opposite to an expected effect) of increasing athletic performance by stimulating physical activity while reducing pain. Racehorses have been doped with the drug to make them run faster. Many lovers of the sport disapprove of the practice not only for its illegality but because the horse is harmed. Perhaps the most notorious incident occurred in the late 1980s when Rocket Racer won the Perth Cup by eight lengths and continued running. The horse would not stop despite the jockey's efforts; after nearly another lap around the track, the horse collapsed and died. Reportedly some human track competitors have used the same drug, accelerated their pace as a race progressed, and had difficulty stopping after crossing the finish line.

Drawbacks. In animal experiments dihydroetorphine interferes with the immune system, interference that may make infections more likely. Etorphine can send blood pressure up or down, reduce body temperature, and impair heartbeat and breathing. Impaired breathing is also an unwanted effect observed with dihydroetorphine, along with constipation, nausea, vomiting, dizziness, and drowsiness.

Although etorphine is a standard veterinary medicine, knowledgeable users treat it with great respect and keep an antidote on hand because accidental injection can be fatal. The drug may be absorbed though the skin, and supplies of etorphine are generally dyed red so users can readily tell if they have touched it (such as a smear across a shirt or hand). Swift administration of an antidote can prevent death.

The quantity needed to kill a person is so minute that its presence in a body can be difficult or even impossible to detect. Harmless chemicals added to a dose can make etorphine even harder to discover through laboratory tests. The drug has also attracted military attention as a possible chemical warfare agent.

Abuse factors. When humans in an experiment received etorphine they experienced euphoria and described the drug as feeling like morphine. Researchers who administered etorphine in that experiment concluded that the drug is likely to be abused. Misuse has been noted in China. Other investigators reached the same conclusion about dihydroetorphine from the way rats responded to it. The U.S. Drug Enforcement Administration has ruled that dihydroetorphine's abuse potential is similar to **heroin**'s. The government of Hong Kong has noted dihydroetorphine's lower price and less stringent control make it appealing to heroin addicts. Lawsuits against the tobacco industry unearthed documentation indicating one company considered the possibility that competitors might lace cigarettes with etorphine to add an addictive need that could not be satisfied by other brands, thereby coercing consumer loyalty to a particular product.

A mice study found no dependence at all after dihydroetorphine had been administered for six days, but rat and mice research demonstrates that dihydroetorphine eventually produces enough dependence to cause withdrawal symptoms. Investigators have noted that rats act as if dihydroetorphine is a satisfactory substitute for heroin. Etorphine can prevent withdrawal symptoms in morphine addicts, an action demonstrating cross-tolerance between the two drugs, but an etorphine dose holds off withdrawal symptoms for a shorter time than morphine would. In rhesus monkey experiments etorphine and dihydroetorphine are both cross-tolerant with morphine. In those same experiments, when dihydroetorphine dosage was suddenly stopped, few withdrawal signs appeared. Withdrawal symptom research on mice indicates that dihydroetorphine may do more than substitute for morphine: A dihydroetorphine dose may actually make morphine withdrawal symptoms go away, so further doses of either drug become unnecessary. Such a result would be inconsistent with what is known about opiate dependence, but discovery of new facts can change scientific understandings. Some researchers believe that etorphine and dihydroetorphine have potential for treating opiate addiction. Dihydroetorphine has been used for that purpose in China but seems to produce even stronger dependence among heroin addicts than **methadone**. So perhaps animal experiment findings that indicate low dependence potential in dihydroetorphine cannot be extrapolated to humans.

Drug interactions. Giving etorphine and morphine together increases pain relief in mice, while the etorphine does not seem to increase the strength of opiate dependence in the combination. Researchers speculate that the improved pain control might be great enough to allow much smaller doses of morphine in humans than would otherwise be needed, which in turn would greatly decrease the amount of dependence otherwise created by normal-size morphine doses.

Cancer. Not enough scientific information to report.

Pregnancy. Not enough scientific information to report.

Additional scientific information may be found in:

Firn, S. "Accidental Poisoning by an Animal Immobilizing Agent." *Lancet* 2 (1973): 95–96.

"Immobilon: Curiously Strong." *Lancet* 2 (1977): 178.

Jasinski, D.R., J.D. Griffith, and C.B. Carr. "Etorphine in Man. 1. Subjective Effects and Suppression of Morphine Abstinence." *Clinical Pharmacology and Therapeutics* 17 (1975): 267–72.

Marcoux, G.S. "Etorphine: A New Opiate of Abuse?" *Canadian Journal of Psychiatry* 41 (1996): 261.

"Schedule II Control of Dihydroetorphine under the Controlled Substances Act (CSA)." *Federal Register* 65 (2000): 69442–43.

Fenfluramine

Pronunciation: fen-FLOO-ra-meen

Chemical Abstracts Service Registry Number: 458-24-2. (Hydrochloride form 404-82-0)

Formal Names: Miniphage, Ponderal, Ponderax, Pondimin, Ponflural, Redux

Type: Stimulant (anorectic class). *See* page 15

Federal Schedule Listing: Schedule IV (DEA no. 1670). In 2002 federal authorities were planning to make the substance unscheduled.

USA Availability: Prescription

Pregnancy Category: C

Uses. For convenience this drug is here classified as a stimulant simply because other anorectics controlled by the U.S. Drug Enforcement Administration are stimulants. Chemistry operates independently of classification schemes, however, and fenfluramine does not act like typical stimulants even though it is related to amphetamine. Fenfluramine can sedate users and has only modest influence on body temperature and blood pressure. Yet it also has characteristics of powerful stimulants: euphoria, hallucinations, paranoia. High doses can pep up a person rather than sedate. Fenfluramine can alter time perceptions and snap moods from one extreme to another. Some scientists classify it as a hallucinogen. Occasionally it can act as an aphrodisiac in females. Fenfluramine also lowers cholesterol levels.

In humans fenfluramine has been found effective for diminishing panic attacks but has had mixed success when used to treat obsessive behavior. Experimental use against schizophrenia has been unsuccessful, with patients worsening under the drug regimen. Indeed, reports asked whether the drug might be inducing psychotic reactions. A four-week study found fenfluramine useful in improving the conduct of mentally retarded children suffering from attention deficit hyperactivity disorder (ADHD). A longer study (11 months) found the drug provided only limited help to autistic children, and a still longer study (27 months) found such long-term administration impractical due to unwanted effects and due to changes in the autistic children's lives. A scientific review of such studies concluded that the drug's potential nonetheless merited further trials.

Fenfluramine is a drug of many effects, but medically its primary use has been for weight loss. Studies consistently indicate the drug's effectiveness for that purpose. One study found it comparable to **dextroamphetamine** in producing weight loss.

Drawbacks. Fenfluramine tends to dry out the mouth, a condition promoting tooth decay. Other unwanted actions can include headache, peevish feelings, dizziness, tiredness, nausea, vomiting, diarrhea, and frequent urination. Experience indicates that persons need to be weaned off the drug; cold turkey cessation can cause depression or even a medical emergency called "serotonin syndrome." That syndrome may include hyperactivity, confusion, nervousness, vomiting, too-rapid heartbeat, excessive body temperature, shivering, tremors, weakness, or passing out.

Abuse factors. Experimental animals have shown little interest in receiving fenfluramine doses, a classic sign of small addiction potential. Human amphetamine addicts have found fenfluramine to feel like a placebo.

Drug interactions. If the compound is taken along with migraine headache remedies or antidepressants (particularly monoamine oxidase inhibitors—MAOIs) serotonin syndrome can arise.

Researchers discovered that fenfluramine could be administered in combination with **phentermine**, an anorectic that works in a different way. The combination became known as fen-phen (or phen-fen). Rat experiments showed that fen-phen reduces food intake far more than either drug can do alone, and experience confirmed the same kind of multiplier effect in humans. Such impact allows persons to take lower doses than would be necessary with either drug alone, thereby minimizing any undesired actions of the drugs. Phentermine counteracts fenfluramine's common sedative quality, allowing users to function more normally.

Weight control is one of the most challenging conditions encountered by medical practitioners, and fen-phen became tremendously popular. One study found that almost 90% of 88 obesity patients taking fenfluramine or the closely related drug dexfenfluramine were also taking phentermine and that almost 33% of the 88 patients lacked obesity levels for which these or other anti-obesity drugs were an appropriate treatment.

Suddenly, after many years of wide use without much report of alarming adverse effects, in 1997 accounts began associating fenfluramine with rapidly developing fatal heart valve disorders. The U.S. Food and Drug Administration asked the manufacturer to withdraw fenfluramine and dexfenfluramine from the market. In that litigious era the manufacturer instantly and voluntarily complied. Hot debate then erupted in medical circles about whether heart disease was caused by fenfluramine, phentermine, or the two drugs in combination. Studies purported to confirm that the drugs alone or in combination really did create heart valve affliction. Other research purported to find no evidence of the drugs' involvement. Highly knowledgeable and distinguished medical authorities took differing stances on the question and raged at one another in scientific journals. An issue also arose of whether fen-phen caused fatal pulmonary hypertension (high pressure in blood circulation to lungs), with researchers reminding fellow scientists that fenfluramine works in ways similar to the anorectic drug aminorex, which had been linked to pulmonary hypertension in the 1960s and was thereafter withdrawn from the market. Particular concern was expressed about fenfluramine's impact on pulmonary hypertension and edema among users living or traveling in high altitudes. Phentermine is a monoamine oxidase inhibitor, and despite a lack of reports about acute adverse interaction with fenfluramine, some researchers noted that a more chronic interaction could cause the kind of heart and pulmonary damage that was appearing. Researchers began reporting organic brain damage from fenfluramine and dexfenfluramine in animal experiments. Investigators now noticed many instances of psychiatric disturbance among persons taking fenfluramine and noted that the disorders implied organic brain damage. The drug was also linked to human angina pectoris (a frightening sensation of pain and suffocation typically caused by insufficient oxygen supply to the heart) and to a case of a gangrenous condition resulting in amputation of fingers. As time passed, evidence appeared that the heart valve and pulmonary hypertension disorders could stabilize and even improve after patients stopped taking fen-phen. Scientific debate continues about fenfluramine's role in heart ailments and pulmonary hypertension.

Despite the beating that fen-phen took from the news media and from many scientists, researchers remain curious about whether the drug combination still has a role in medicine. Even though fenfluramine can cause depression, interest arose in possible psychotherapeutic uses. As the twenty-first century began, experimenters reported that fen-phen can ease withdrawal from **cocaine**. Rat experiments find that fen-phen reduces **alcohol** intake and eliminates alcohol withdrawal symptoms, findings that may be relevant to treatment of alcoholism. Indeed in 1995 one medical practitioner reported success in treating alcohol and cocaine addicts with fen-phen, sometimes substituting **pemoline** for phentermine.

Cancer. Not enough scientific information to report.

Pregnancy. Experimenters who gave fenfluramine to pregnant mice found no measurable effect on fetal development and no effect on offspring's ability to perform in learning tests. For primates evidence exists that the drug passes into the fetus and reaches high levels there. The combination fen-phen has not seemed to harm human fetal development.

Additional information. Dexfenfluramine (CAS RN 3239-44-9) is a stereoisomer of fenfluramine, meaning the two molecules have the same chemical formula and the same atomic bonds, but the molecules look different (as a person's left and right hands look different even though both have the same components). Studies comparing the two drugs find little or no difference in effect, although dexfenfluramine was introduced with the hope that it had fewer unwanted actions than fenfluramine when used for weight loss. A report praising dexfenfluramine characterized its weight loss capability as equaling that produced by the antidepressant fluoxetine (Prozac) or by a combination of **ephedrine** and **caffeine**. Diarrhea is noted as a dexfenfluramine effect, and concern arose that the drug can aggravate glaucoma. Depending on laboratory manipulations of circumstances, it can promote or diminish panic attacks.

Additional scientific information may be found in:

Davis, R., and D. Faulds. "Dexfenfluramine. An Updated Review of Its Therapeutic Use in the Management of Obesity." *Drugs* 52 (1996): 696–724.

Griffith, J.D., J.G. Nutt, and D.R. Jasinski. "Comparison of Fenfluramine and Amphetamine in Man." *Clinical Pharmacology and Therapeutics* 18 (1975): 563–70.

Gross, S.B. "Appetite Suppressants and Cardiac Valvulopathy. Current Clinical Perspectives." *Advance for Nurse Practitioners* 7 (1999): 36–40.

McCann, U.D., V. Eligulashvili, and G.A. Ricaurte. "Adverse Neuropsychiatric Events Associated with Dexfenfluramine and Fenfluramine." *Progress in Neuropsychopharmacology and Biological Psychiatry* 22 (1998): 1087–102.

McCann, U.D., et al. "Brain Serotonin Neurotoxicity and Primary Pulmonary Hypertension from Fenfluramine and Dexfenfluramine: Systematic Review of the Evidence." *Journal of the American Medical Association* 278 (1997): 666–72.

Schiller, N.B. "Fen/Phen and Valvular Heart Disease: If It Sounds Too Bad to Be True, Perhaps It Isn't." *Journal of the American College of Cardiology* 34 (1999): 1159–62.

Vivero, L.E., P.O. Anderson, and R.F. Clark. "A Close Look at Fenfluramine and Dexfenfluramine." *Journal of Emergency Medicine* 16 (1998): 197–205.

Wellman, P.J, and T.J. Maher. "Synergistic Interactions between Fenfluramine and Phentermine." *International Journal of Obesity and Related Metabolic Disorders* 23 (1999): 723–32.

Fentanyl

Pronunciation: FEN-ta-nill

Chemical Abstracts Service Registry Number: 437-38-7. (Citrate form 990-73-8)

Formal Names: Actiq, Alfenta, Alfentanil, Duragesic, Durogesic, Innovar, Sublimaze, Sufenta, Sufentanil

Informal Names: Apache, Bear, China, China Girl, China Town, China White, Dance Fever, Fen, Friend, Goodfellas, Great Bear, He Man, Jackpot, King Ivory, Murder, Murder 8, Persian White, Poison, Synthetic Heroin, Tango & Cash, TNT

Type: Depressant (opioid class). *See* page 24

Federal Schedule Listing: Schedule II (DEA no. 9801)

USA Availability: Prescription

Pregnancy Category: C

Uses. Developed in Europe during the 1950s, this drug became available for medical use in the United States during the 1960s. It is also used in veterinary medicine, especially with cats. Depending on means of administration (injection, oral) fentanyl can be 10 times stronger than **morphine**, and fentanyl citrate can be 8 to 100 times stronger. One report claims fentanyl is 40 times stronger than **heroin**.

Relieving cancer pain is a standard use for fentanyl. With cancer, the drug is normally given only when a patient is dying and unable to experience enough pain control from other opioids. Fentanyl does not necessarily reduce the amount of pain per se but can make people less aware of discomfort. The substance also has sedative actions and suppresses coughs. The drug has been used to help treat tetanus. Fentanyl can alter a person's spirits, making someone euphoric or provoking an opposite feeling of sadness and discontent. One dosage format is the fentanyl patch, allowing the drug to be absorbed through the skin.

Drawbacks. Patches are potent enough in themselves, but a case report tells of one drug abuser who decided to heat a patch and inhale the vapor; he instantly lost consciousness, but prompt attention by skilled medical personnel saved his life.

Fentanyl may cause serious and even fatal breathing difficulty, and this problem can still arise after the drug's action has apparently lifted. Risk of that unwanted effect is heightened among "opioid naive" patients who have not developed tolerance to pain relief from other opioids; so because of the breathing hazard those opioid-naive patients often do not receive fentanyl. Nonetheless, it is sometimes used for childbirth, surgery, and dentistry and for persons suffering from lower back ache and pain in bones and joints. Physicians even give fentanyl to infants.

The drug can promote sleepiness and slow a person's pulse rate, alertness, and physical motions. Such effects interfere with ability to operate automobiles or machinery. Other unwanted actions include itching, constipation, urine retention, nausea and vomiting, increased blood pressure, and fainting upon standing up. Cases of muscle rigidity have been reported. Laboratory tests suggest fentanyl might worsen a body chemistry disease called porphyria.

Fentanyl can provoke seizures in persons prone to such affliction. A drastic treatment for seizures is surgical removal of a brain lobe where seizures originate, and instrument readings during the operation guide surgeons on how much of the brain to remove. Fentanyl is a standard surgical anesthetic, and one study found that the drug can temporarily create seizures in healthy portions of the brain, thereby misleading surgeons about how much they should remove.

Like many other drugs, fentanyl has stronger effects on older persons, and dosage should be adjusted accordingly.

Abuse factors. Tolerance and dependence can occur, with typical opioid withdrawal symptoms. Just three days of medical dosing can produce enough dependence to cause uncomfortable withdrawal upon sudden stoppage of the drug, an exceptionally short time compared to most opioids. Animal experiments indicate that **buprenorphine** can alleviate fentanyl withdrawal.

Drug interactions. Normally people should avoid fentanyl if they have taken monamine oxidase inhibitors (MAOIs—found in some antidepressants and other medicine) in the past two weeks, as MAOIs can greatly increase opioid actions. For the same reason, using fentanyl with other depressants (including **alcohol**) can be risky. **Midazolam** hydrochloride and fentanyl appear to boost each other's actions. The HIV/AIDS medicine ritonavir makes a fentanyl dose last longer.

Cancer. Whether fentanyl causes cancer is unknown, although laboratory tests with one version of the drug yielded no indication of cancer-causing potential.

Pregnancy. Rats receiving fentanyl have lower fertility rates and bring fewer pregnancies to term, compared to rats not receiving the drug, and those effects occurred at smaller doses than humans typically receive. When fentanyl citrate has been given to pregnant rats, birth defects in their offspring have not been attributed to the drug. Whether fentanyl causes congenital malformations in humans is unknown. An infant can be born with dependence if the mother has been using fentanyl. The drug passes into a nursing mother's milk but not in amounts deemed harmful to an infant.

Additional information. Alfentanil (Schedule II, CAS Registry No. 71195-58-9) is a derivative of fentanyl used for pain control and anesthesia. Effects last only a few minutes. Depending on dosage form, pain relief is 1 to 10 times stronger than morphine. When given to a pregnant woman alfentanil apparently passes into the fetus. The drug can produce muscle rigidity in infants.

Sufentanil (Schedule II, CAS Registry No. 56030-54-7, citrate form 60561-17-3) is a derivative of fentanyl used for pain control and anesthesia. It is 50 to 100 times stronger than morphine and is used to knock out wild animals. The drug takes effect faster than fentanyl but lasts a shorter time. Sufentanil can lower heart rate and blood pressure, create muscle rigidity, and cause typical unwanted opioid effects such as itching and vomiting. At normal doses sufentanil can halt breathing, so medical personnel stand by to provide respiration assistance when they administer the drug. Laboratory and animal experiments indicate no potential for causing cancer. Tests with rats and rabbits did not produce birth defects. Researchers examining the results when sufentanil is used in childbirth found no harm to mother or infant. Sufentanil is assumed to pass into the milk of nursing mothers, but the amount is assumed harmless to the infant.

Other fentanyl derivatives exist. They are used illicitly to experience heroin sensations and can be 1,000 times stronger than heroin.

Fentanyl has the same molecular formula as the Schedule I substance acetyl-alpha-methylfentanyl (DEA no. 9815), but the two drugs are different substances.

Additional scientific information may be found in:

Baylon, G.J. "Comparative Abuse Liability of Intravenously Administered Remifentanil and Fentanyl." *Journal of Clinical Psychopharmacology* 20 (2000): 597–606.

Henderson, G.L. "Designer Drugs: Past History and Future Prospects." *Journal of Forensic Sciences* 33 (1988): 569–75.

Patt, R.B., and L.A. Hogan. "Comment: Transdermal Fentanyl." *Annals of Pharmacotherapy* 27 (1993): 795–96.

Schneider, U., et al. "Effects of Fentanyl and Low Doses of Alcohol on Neuropsychological Performance in Healthy Subjects." *Neuropsychobiology* 39 (1999): 38–43.

Zacny, J.P., et al. "Subjective and Behavioral Responses to Intravenous Fentanyl in Healthy Volunteers." *Psychopharmacology* (Berlin) 107 (1992): 319–26.

Flunitrazepam

Pronunciation: flyoo-neye-TRAYZ-eh-pam

Chemical Abstracts Service Registry Number: 1622-62-4

Formal Names: Rohypnol

Informal Names: Candy, Circles, Darkene, Date Rape Drug, Drop Drug, Dulcitas, Forget Me Drug, Forget Pills, La Rocha, La Roche, Lunch Money Drug, Mexican Valium, Mind Erasers, Pappas, Pastas, Peanuts, Pingus, Potatoes, Remember All, Reynol, Reynolds, Rib, Roaches, Roachies, Roach-2, Roapies, Robinol, Robutal, Rochas, Rochas Dos, Roche, Roche Dos, Roches, Rochies, Rohibinol, Roofenol, Roofies, Ropanol, Ropers, Ropes, Rophies, Rophs, Rophy, Ropies, Roples, Ro-Shay, Row-Shay, R05-4200, R-25, R-2, Rubies, Ruffies, Ruffles, Trip & Fall, Whiteys, Wolfies

Type: Depressant (benzodiazepine class). *See* page 21

Federal Schedule Listing: Schedule IV (DEA no. 2763), but Schedule I in many state schedules

USA Availability: Prescription where legal

Uses. This quick-acting and long-lasting drug is widely used around the world for legitimate medical purposes. Flunitrazepam is prescribed to treat insomnia and anxiety, to relax muscles, to stop convulsions, and to calm people. In the 1990s it was Western Europe's most commonly prescribed calming and sleep-inducing medicine. The drug is administered to treat **alcohol** withdrawal syndrome, and experimental use in treating depression has found flunitrazepam promising. Some unauthorized use of the drug is believed to be for self-medication of depression and low self-esteem. The drug has specialized usefulness in surgery as a medication given prior to administration of anesthesia, and its tendency to reduce pressure inside the eyeball can avert the rise caused by the anesthetic succinylcholine (important if patients are at risk for glaucoma). In hospice care where doses can be higher and more frequent than normal, flunitrazepam has reduced nausea and vomiting from cancer chemotherapy.

Actions are similar to those of **diazepam**, but flunitrazepam is 7 to 10 times stronger. Nonetheless, compared to other benzodiazepine class drugs an overdose of flunitrazepam does not seem more poisonous, nor does flunitrazepam appear more prone to cause medical crises.

Drawbacks. The drug may cause euphoria, raise self-esteem, and give a sense of power in users while at the same time decreasing fear. Such effects may promote violence in a person who is already prone to such conduct, particularly when the substance is combined with alcohol.

Users are sometimes unable to remember what happened while they were under flunitrazepam's influence. Immediate effects aside, researchers have documented that people still experience trouble when doing laboratory memory tests 10 hours after taking a medical dose of the drug, a dose that may be much lighter than some abusers take. Many other benzodiazepine class drugs cause memory trouble as well, although their effect is less publicized than flunitrazepam's.

Flunitrazepam can slow reaction times, reduce ability to pay attention to tasks, and leave people too woozy and discoordinated to drive a car safely. Difficulty in driving has been demonstrated in simulations and in an instrumented automobile actually driven for several miles the day after drivers took a nighttime dose. In experiments (including a test of potential drug effects on shift workers) people took various sleep aids at bedtime; flunitrazepam harmed persons' ability to move their limbs the next day. Such effects appear to be dose-related; an experiment using much smaller doses found little or no impact on performance the next day. Large doses can cause breathing trouble. Injection can kill skin around the needle site.

Abuse factors. Abuse of the drug has become a concern among public health authorities in several countries. Under provisions of international treaties the federal government lists flunitrazepam as a Schedule IV controlled substance but has forbidden sale of this pharmaceutical in the United States. State governments have begun reclassifying the substance as Schedule I, certifying it as having no medical value and allowing anyone possessing it to be prosecuted under state law.

In the 1990s law enforcement agencies declared flunitrazepam to be a date rape drug, allowing men to commit sexual assault against unresisting victims who have foggy or even no memory of the circumstances. In this regard the drug is little different from alcohol, though faster acting. In a survey of 53 women who willingly used flunitrazepam, 10% said they were afterward assaulted physically or sexually. When 66 other "flunitrazepam users" described the tablet, many descriptions were of some other drug even though the people believed they had taken flunitrazepam. Untoward events may be real, but the identity of an involved drug may be less certain than law enforcement officials say. The U.S. Drug Enforcement Administration (DEA) says detection of flunitrazepam is nearly impossible in rape cases because urine samples must be analyzed within 72 hours of ingesting flunitrazepam, making the drug's prevalence as a tool in sexual assault impossible to demonstrate. Nonetheless, the DEA describes the problem's extent as serious. A student of the topic found that from 1994 to 1998 a nationwide total of "at least" 26 sexual assaults "potentially involved" the drug. One laboratory conducted a two-year study of 1,179 urine specimens from sexual assault victims in 49 states, specimens selected because of suspicion that some drug was involved—and thereby more likely to have positive results than if samples were chosen randomly from sex crime cases. The lab found 6 positive for flunitrazepam (0.5%), 97 (8%) positive for a benzodiazepine class substance (a category including many drugs other than flunitrazepam), 451 positive for alcohol, and 468 negative for any drug of abuse that was searched for. A two-year study of 2,003 urine samples from sexual assault victims believed to have ingested a drug found less than 2% containing flunitrazepam or **GHB**. The same study reported that as of 1999 utilization of those two drugs seemed to be waning. Flunitrazepam's legal manufacturer has offered to provide free and definitive analysis of samples submitted by medical and law enforcement personnel. Researchers at the University of Miami report that detection of flunitrazepam in urine samples is easy and that, in contrast to ambiguous results from sex crime investigations, flunitrazepam had been confirmed in "up to" 10% of drunk driving cases in 1995 and 1996 in Miami-Dade County, Florida, but plummeted after the drug became Schedule I under state law in 1997.

Despite hype about flunitrazepam, a review article published in 1997 noted absence of evidence that the substance's actions differ from those of other drugs in the benzodiazepine class. Flunitrazepam is simply a very strong benzodiazepine, and its potency may have much to do with stories told about it. To produce similar drug effects, a small amount of flunitrazepam may be about equal to a large amount of some other benzodiazepine.

Tolerance can occur. A person's body can develop dependence with flunitrazepam, resulting in a withdrawal syndrome if dosage stops. Withdrawal symptoms are similar to those with other benzodiazepine class substances. Severe cases can include delirium, hallucinations, and seizures. When researchers cut off the drug supply to dependent monkeys they became agitated and peevish, had tremors and poor control of muscles, and sometimes vomited and ran a fever. Although flunitrazepam is much stronger than diazepam, a canine experiment found those two drugs roughly equivalent in ability to produce dependence. Flunitrazepam reduced the **morphine** withdrawal syndrome in mice; if the same effect carries over to humans flunitrazepam might appeal to opiate addicts who have an unreliable supply of opiates. Surveys show flunitrazepam to be a favorite among opiate abusers, although among other people the substance seems no more attractive than other benzodiazepines.

Drug interactions. Alcohol and flunitrazepam boost each other's actions. Some illicit drug users find flunitrazepam to be a pleasing addition to a dose of inferior **heroin**, and some find that flunitrazepam eases harsh effects from **cocaine**. However, using multiple illicit drugs, particularly if the combination tends to make the body produce opposite actions simultaneously, is an invitation to problems. **Buprenorphine** disrupts the body's ability to break down flunitrazepam.

Cancer. Laboratory testing of the drug itself and of urine from rats and humans who have received doses indicates that flunitrazepam can induce gene mutations, a possible sign of cancer-causing potential.

Pregnancy. In pregnant women the drug passes into amniotic fluid and the fetal blood supply, although fetal levels are lower than maternal levels. Excessive muscular motions have been observed in a fetus after the drug is administered to a pregnant woman. When given to infants the drug lowers their blood pressure (an effect noted in adults as well). Although the drug passes into breast milk, levels are considered too low to affect a nursing infant if a mother does not take the drug regularly.

Additional scientific information may be found in:

Anglin, D., K.L. Spears, and H.R. Hutson. "Flunitrazepam and Its Involvement in Date or Acquaintance Rape." *Academic Emergency Medicine* 4 (1997): 323–26.

Calhoun, S.R., et al. "Abuse of Flunitrazepam (Rohypnol) and Other Benzodiazepines in Austin and South Texas." *Journal of Psychoactive Drugs* 28 (1996): 183–89.

Daderman, A.M., and L. Lidberg. "Flunitrazepam (Rohypnol) Abuse in Combination with Alcohol Causes Premeditated, Grievous Violence in Male Juvenile Offenders." *Journal of the American Academy of Psychiatry and the Law* 27 (1999): 83–99.

"Flunitrazepam Misuse and Abuse in South Africa." *South African Medical Journal* 89 (1999): 1155.

Mattila, M.A., and H.M. Larni. "Flunitrazepam: A Review of Its Pharmacological Properties and Therapeutic Use." *Drugs* 20 (1980): 353–74.

Ott, H., et al. "Anterograde and Retrograde Amnesia after Lormetazepam and Flunitrazepam." *Psychopharmacology Series* 6 (1988): 180–93.

Waltzman, M.L. "Flunitrazepam: A Review of 'Roofies.' " *Pediatric Emergency Care* 15 (1999): 59–60.

Woods, J.H., and G. Winger. "Abuse Liability of Flunitrazepam." *Journal of Clinical Psychopharmacology* 17 (1997, Suppl. 2): S1–S57.

Fluoxymesterone

Pronunciation: floo-ok-see-MESS-ter-ohn

Chemical Abstracts Service Registry Number: 76-43-7

Formal Names: Androfluorene, Android-F, Halotestin, Ora-Testryl, Stenox

Type: Anabolic steroid. *See* page 24

Federal Schedule Listing: Schedule III (DEA no. 4000)

USA Availability: Prescription

Pregnancy Category: X

Uses. This compound became available in the 1950s. Standard medical uses in males include treatment for delayed puberty and underdeveloped male organs. Experiments demonstrate that fluoxymesterone can improve the growth, weight, and social interactions of boys having slow physical maturation. Compared to some other anabolic steroids, this drug has less tendency to promote masculine body signs (facial hair, deeper voice) in girls, and fluoxymesterone has been used to nurture increased height in girls. The drug can be administered to treat female sexual dysfunction.

In women the drug is used to fight breast cancer by interfering with hormones that encourage the disease. Research has found fluoxymesterone effective in reducing a cancer called myeloma and for counteracting anemia caused by myeloma. Mixed results have occurred when using the drug for correcting anemia associated with kidney failure. The substance has been a treatment for osteoporosis, a condition in which bones become susceptible to easy breakage, and for hereditary angioedema—an affliction that may involve throat swelling that interferes with breathing.

Although anabolic steroids have potential for preventing young users from achieving expected adult height, with fluoxymesterone that outcome does not occur among females suffering from Turner's syndrome (the expected adult height in persons with this condition, however, is already short). Several studies tracking boys using the drug under close medical supervision found adult height to be normal.

A research team studied effects on normal males who received doses three times a day for a three-month period. Little impact could be detected, although a few unwanted effects such as headaches occurred. Perhaps the most notable reported change was a 30% drop in triglyceride levels; excessive triglycerides are associated with heart attack and stroke.

Drawbacks. Another study using normal men measured a drop in their **testosterone** levels, an unsurprising finding as fluoxymesterone is supposed to replace testosterone. Extended usage may interfere with male sexual function and fertility. General unwanted actions have included acne, itching, dizziness, nausea, vomiting, yellowish tinge to body color (an indication of jaundice), constipation, and frequent urination. Fluid retention can cause swelling. The drug may interfere with blood clotting and may reduce the amount of insulin needed by diabetics. The compound also can be harmful to a person who suffers from porphyria, an affliction that can involve violence and sensitivity to light. Fluoxymesterone can pass into a sexual partner, enough to affect that person. Because of that, barrier contraceptives are recommended for sexually active fluoxymesterone patients and their partners.

The substance is banned from athletic competitions. Scientists have not confirmed that the substance helps sport abilities, but nonetheless some bodybuilders use it. Supposedly the drug can increase strength without increasing weight, an important factor in some classes of sporting competition. Reportedly the substance promotes aggressiveness, enhancing its appeal to athletes who must physically attack opponents. Some athletic users describe the drug as unpleasant. Athletic abuse of fluoxymesterone is not necessarily limited to human competitions; concern exists that the substance may be given to racehorses.

Abuse factors. Not enough scientific information to report about tolerance, dependence, withdrawal, or addiction.

Drug interactions. In female breast cancer patients receiving levothyroxine to boost thyroid gland activity, fluoxymesterone can interact and elevate thyroid activity too much. Experiments have administered fluoxymesterone in combination with other drugs to alter the mood of older persons exhibiting nervousness, irritation, and suspiciousness toward caregivers. One study reported no change; another reported substantial change; the difference may have involved what drugs were used in addition to fluoxymesterone, along with differing dosages.

Cancer. Laboratory tests have provided uncertain guidance on whether fluoxymesterone causes cancer. A case report mentions that two men developed prostate cancer after receiving the drug to treat impotence; cause and effect were not asserted, but the coincidence was considered important enough to merit caution. Men with prostate cancer should avoid the drug. A case report mentions liver cancer developing in a patient undergoing fluoxymesterone therapy for over four years, but again cause and effect were not claimed. A survey examined all reported deaths from hepatic angiosarcoma, a type of liver cancer, in the United States from 1964 to 1974; from the total of 168 cases, 1 was associated with taking fluoxymesterone. Once again, however, "association" is not "cause."

Pregnancy. In humans the compound may harm fetal development of female sexual organs, introducing male characteristics. The drug is not recommended for pregnant women, but the substance has been used to control milk production. Fluoxymesterone passes into milk, and nursing mothers should avoid the drug.

Additional scientific information may be found in:

Dhillon, V.S., et al. "In Vitro and in Vivo Genotoxicity of Hormonal Drugs. VI. Fluoxymesterone." *Mutation Research* 342 (1995): 103–11.

Kirkland, R.T., and G.W. Clayton. "Growth Increments with Low Dose Intermittent Growth Hormone and Fluoxymesterone in First Year of Therapy in Hypopituitarism." *Pediatrics* 63 (1979): 386–88.

Lenko, H.L., J. Maenpaa, and J. Perheentupa. "Acceleration of Delayed Growth with Fluoxymesterone." *Acta Paediatrica Scandinavica* 71 (1982): 929–36.

Novak, E., et al. "Pharmacologic Evaluation of Fluoxymesterone in Normal Men." *Current Therapeutic Research: Clinical and Experimental* 16 (1974): 251–260.

Strickland, A.L. "Long-Term Results of Treatment with Low-Dose Fluoxymesterone in Constitutional Delay of Growth and Puberty and in Genetic Short Stature." *Pediatrics* 91 (1993): 716–20.

Flurazepam

Pronunciation: flur-AZ-eh-pam

Chemical Abstracts Service Registry Number: 17617-23-1. (Hydrochloride form 1172-18-5)

Formal Names: Dalmane, Paxane

Type: Depressant (benzodiazepine class). *See* page 21

Federal Schedule Listing: Schedule IV (DEA no. 2767)

USA Availability: Prescription

Pregnancy Category: X

Uses. Flurazepam has become one of the most common benzodiazepine class compounds in medical use around the globe. One reason for its popularity is flurazepam's high therapeutic index, meaning the dose needed for medical action is much smaller than a fatal dose, making accidental poisoning unlikely. Caregivers mainly use this long-acting drug to help people sleep, and it has been used experimentally to reduce sleepwalking.

Drawbacks. Flurazepam often leaves people groggy the next day, impairing their mental abilities (including memory and accuracy of perceptions). Such problems can decrease after weeks or months of using the drug, but in one experiment users never achieved normal performance while taking flurazepam. Researchers find that volunteers may be unaware of the trouble they are having. In contrast to those typical findings, experiments using healthy college students found no effect on performance the day after taking a nighttime dose of the drug.

Laboratory tests of users demonstrate impairment in reaction time, eye-hand coordination, making decisions, and maintaining attention. All those skills are relevant to operating an automobile. Twelve hours after taking a nighttime dose of flurazepam, volunteers drove a test vehicle. Researchers conducting the experiment concluded that such drivers were much more likely to have a road accident than controls who received a placebo. Bolder experimenters had drivers take a car into actual traffic the day after ingesting flurazepam, and drivers had trouble keeping the car aligned in the proper lane. An experiment using a driving simulator also showed people to have trouble driving the morning after using flurazepam.

Users tend to be more accident prone in general, not just behind the steering wheel of a car. A case report tells of a person's muscular discoordination clearing up when he stopped taking flurazepam, and experimental work has documented the drug's tendency to interfere with movement. In elderly persons that unsteadiness is associated with falls causing broken hips, and caution is advised in prescribing flurazepam to older people. One factor with flurazepam problems experienced by the elderly is that, compared to younger persons, the elderly maintain higher levels of the drug in their bodies from a given dose.

Researchers find that the substance can help people shift their sleep schedules from night to daytime, while promoting good-quality rest, yet the drug still has hangover effects that degrade ability to function after awakening.

The drug can worsen verbal communication, causing voices to become indistinct and grammar to become garbled. Studies measuring sleep-time breathing find that the drug can exacerbate respiration problems; in some experiments researchers concluded that the change has no practical effect on health, but medical literature notes an instance in which the drug's influence on breathing did cause trouble for a sleeping person. In a mice experiment flurazepam lowered body temperature. In humans long-term use of the drug is suspected of causing hallucinations and confusion, and a case report exists of a single dose creating those symptoms along with euphoria. Investigators in the 1970s found mild euphoria to be a routine effect of flurazepam. Headache, low blood pressure, eyesight trouble, nausea, vomiting, and constipation can occur. A case report relates that a woman's interest in sexual activity increased when she stopped taking flurazepam and **diazepam**. Flurazepam is believed to interfere with women's ability to achieve a sexual orgasm.

Abuse factors. Tests with normal persons find that flurazepam has equal or less appeal compared to placebo. Medical authorities examining the drug in the 1970s concluded that it probably had little potential for abuse. Despite the drug's apparent low appeal, it can create a physical dependence with a person's body. Withdrawal symptoms can include peevishness, fidgeting, anxiety, sweating, tremors, high blood pressure, and intolerance to light and sounds. One longtime user of flurazepam and diazepam developed such a strong dependence with them that a severe withdrawal syndrome occurred when she suddenly halted dosage: cramps, stomach discomfort, nervous unease, sleep difficulty, and nightmares. Milder versions of such symptoms are reported if the original level of dependence is lighter. Symptoms can be avoided if flurazepam usage is tapered off rather than stopped suddenly. Volunteers who received flurazepam in a long-term experiment consistently detected the difference between the drug and a placebo, an ability causing investigators to conclude that users of flurazepam do not develop tolerance to the drug (tolerance is a classic indicator of addictive potential). This conclusion is not accepted by all experts, however, and some believe tolerance does occur.

Drug interactions. A catalepsy effect from **marijuana** may become stronger in mice if they also receive flurazepam, but the reason is unclear. **Alcohol** and flurazepam boost some of each other's effects. Experimenters find that **caffeine** can lessen flurazepam's adverse next-day effects on performance. The heartburn medicine cimetidine lengthens the time that flurazepam's metabolite desalkylflurazepam stays in the body. In a monkey experiment, that metabolite produced performance deficiencies reminiscent of those seen in humans with flurazepam and also lowered inhibitions.

Cancer. No indication of a cancer-causing potential has emerged.

Pregnancy. Experiments with rats and rabbits produced no birth defects. Researchers tracking assorted birth defects examined medical records of 50 to 99 women who took flurazepam during pregnancy and found no malformations in offspring. Nonetheless, birth defects are considered a serious risk from the drug, and pregnant women are advised to avoid it. Newborns from mothers using the drug may have "floppy infant syndrome" involving sedation, inferior muscle tone, breathing trouble, and poor feeding.

Additional scientific information may be found in:

Council on Drugs. "Evaluation of a New Hypnotic Agent—Flurazepam Hydrochloride (Dalmane)." *Journal of the American Medical Association* 218 (1971): 246.

De Wit, H., E.H. Uhlenhuth, and C.E. Johanson. "Lack of Preference for Flurazepam in Normal Volunteers." *Pharmacology, Biochemistry, and Behavior* 21 (1984): 865–69.

"Flurazepam (Dalmane)." *Medical Letter on Drugs and Therapeutics* 17 (1975): 29–30.

Judd, L.L., E. Ellinwood, and L.A. McAdams. "Cognitive Performance and Mood in Patients with Chronic Insomnia during 14-Day Use of Flurazepam and Midazolam." *Journal of Clinical Psychopharmacology* 10 (1990, Suppl.): S56–S67.

Juhl, R.P., V.M. Daugherty, and P.D. Kroboth. "Incidence of Next-Day Anterograde Amnesia Caused by Flurazepam Hydrochloride and Triazolam." *Clinical Pharmacy* 3 (1984): 622–25.

Mendelson, W.B., et al. "A Clinical Study of Flurazepam." *Sleep* 5 (1982): 350–60.

Wesnes, K., and D.M. Warburton. "A Comparison of Temazepam and Flurazepam in Terms of Sleep Quality and Residual Changes in Performance." *Neuropsychobiology* 11 (1984): 255–59.

Younus, M., and M.J. Labellarte. "Insomnia in Children: When Are Hypnotics Indicated?" *Paediatric Drugs* 4 (2002): 391–403.

Freon

Pronunciation: FREE-on

Chemical Abstracts Service Registry Number: 11126-05-9

Type: Inhalant. *See* page 26

Federal Schedule Listing: Unlisted

USA Availability: Generally unrestricted

Pregnancy Category: None

Uses. Freon is most familiar as a component of refrigeration and air-conditioning systems. The compound is commonly used to clean metal, and other industrial uses exist as well. In past times freon was routinely used in pressurized aerosol spray cans, but that usage ended after scientists discovered that freon contributes to the destruction of the Earth's ozone layer. Some persons have experienced hallucinations from inhaling freon vapor. A medical case report mentions that heavy polydrug abusers have used freon to experience flashbacks of those experiences. Various chemical formulations of freon exist, some of which may have hallucinogenic effect, and some of which may not.

Drawbacks. Freon may produce lung spasms. The substance has caused high blood pressure, perhaps as a consequence of kidney damage resulting from the substance. Users have described acccelerated heartbeat. Inhalation has also brought on a cardiac emergency called ventricular fibrillation, which is fatal without immediate medical intervention. Even if the person survives, most individuals do not receive sufficient help in time to prevent lasting brain injury from lack of oxygen. In one case a 15-year-old freon user not only experienced the heart emergency but suffered lung and muscle damage as well. Using enough freon in a closed space can be fatal due to oxygen starvation. Inhalers have also reported injuries ranging from lacerations to a broken neck when they lost consciousness and collapsed while sniffing freon; such harm may not be attributable to the substance itself but can be a consequence of using it.

Pressurized freon gas can be cold enough to cause frostbite. Case reports note cold damage to fingers, along with drooling caused by frostbite injury to lips, tongue, and inside of the mouth. One report described "notable deformation" of someone's face; in another case, plastic surgery was necessary to reconstruct the damaged face of one recreational user.

Injection of freon is possible but seems to occur as industrial accidents to fingers rather than as an effort to obtain psychological effects. Upon injection, the gas, which has been under pressure in a container, is free to expand inside the body, producing uncomfortable results. Case reports indicate that victims fully recover.

Injury has also occurred from exposure to liquid freon, which is extremely cold and can cause severe frostbite. In one case, portions of a stomach died from freezing, causing holes that had to be surgically repaired. As with injections, injuries from liquid freon seem to be industrial accidents rather than results of recreational use.

Abuse factors. Not enough scientific information to report about tolerance, dependence, withdrawal, or addiction.

Drug interactions. Not enough scientific information to report.

Cancer. Not enough scientific information to report.

Pregnancy. Not enough scientific information to report.

Additional scientific information may be found in:

"Aerosols for Colds." *Medical Letter on Drugs and Therapeutics* 15 (1973): 86–88.

Brady, W.J., Jr., et al. "Freon Inhalational Abuse Presenting with Ventricular Fibrillation." *American Journal of Emergency Medicine* 12 (1994): 533–36.

Goldsmith, R.J. "Death by Freon." *Journal of Clinical Psychiatry* 50 (1989): 36–37.

Lee, T., et al. "Oral Frostbite Secondary to Freon Propellant Abuse." *Journal of Toxicology. Clinical Toxicology* 34 (1996): 562.

Maxwell, J.C. "Deaths Related to the Inhalation of Volatile Substances in Texas: 1988–1998." *American Journal of Drug and Alcohol Abuse* 27 (2001): 689–97.

Wegener, E.E., K.R. Barraza, and S.K. Das. "Severe Frostbite Caused by Freon Gas." *Southern Medical Journal* 84 (1991): 1143–46.

Gasoline

Pronunciation: gas-uhl-EEN (also pronounced GAS-uhl-een)

Chemical Abstracts Service Registry Number: 8006-61-9. (Benzine form 86290-81-5)

Formal Names: Petrol, White Gasoline

Type: Inhalant. *See* page 26

Federal Schedule Listing: Unlisted

USA Availability: Generally unrestricted

Pregnancy Category: None

Uses. Inhaling gasoline fumes can produce effects that researchers liken to those of **mescaline**: euphoria, hallucinations, and distortions of sensory perception including sensations of revolving and floating. Some users experience feelings of increased power and reduced fear, effects that may encourage mischief from users who are already social outcasts.

Drawbacks. Sniffers have complained of tasting gasoline for days afterward. Other unwanted effects may include fear, lonely feelings, sleepiness, weakness, headache, poor appetite, nausea, too much salivation, breathing difficulty, dizziness, lightheadedness, ringing in the ears, and amnesia. Conflicting evidence exists about possible inhalation harm to kidneys in male rats and in humans, although the human risk is considered low to nonexistent. Case reports tell of muscle injury from inhaling gasoline. Nerve damage can arise, causing trouble in walking and other movements. Manic behavior and seizures are reported. As with most other inhalant abuse, sudden death can occur.

The human body reacts to gasoline vapor in the same way regardless of a person's motive for inhaling it, and researchers have expressed concern about health hazards faced by automobile filling station attendants who receive long-term low-level exposure to gasoline fumes.

Fumes from other types of fuels can have similar actions. In a training exercise JP-5 aviation fuel vapor leaked into the cockpit of a T-34C turboprop aircraft. One pilot gradually lost control proficiency, becoming euphoric and mirthful even though he was told an emergency had been declared. The other pilot was nauseated but managed to land the craft. Both had trouble walking, were weary, and had problems completing familiar written reports. The next day the pilot who had been more severely affected had allergic symptoms (sneezing, nasal discharge, eyes watering and itching) and poor appetite.

Sniffing leaded gasoline is uncommon in the United States, as federal regulations halted motor fuel sales of that substance (although the product was still available in Mexico and Canada in the 1990s). In addition to injury from gasoline the product can cause lead poisoning. Leaded gasoline damage to thinking ability has been documented: attention, learning, and memory. Recreational users of leaded gasoline may also suffer organic brain damage leading to tremors, difficulty in moving arms and legs, personality change, psychosis, sleepiness, and dementia. Recovery may occur, but fatal outcome is possible. One study of persons hospitalized for chronic leaded gasoline sniffing in Australia noted a 40% death rate, but that was the death rate for persons so sick that they required hospital care, not for chronic leaded gasoline users as a whole. Persons with industrial exposure to leaded gasoline fumes have exhibited psychotic behavior, occasionally followed by death. Gasoline sold as a motor fuel may contain **toluene** or various other chemicals that are hazardous to breathe and that may account for some unwanted effects attributed to gasoline.

Injection of liquid gasoline for recreational purposes is disastrous; in Nazi Germany gasoline injection was an experimental method of execution. A case report about a drug abuser who survived gasoline injection noted nerve damage that reduced motion capability in the arm and hand. Drinking gasoline can also have serious medical consequences; one case report listed kidney and respiratory failure along with damage to liver and blood, accompanied by seizures.

Injury may occur by combining dangerous activity with impaired judgment during intoxication. Unconscious persons may let a gasoline container spill its flammable contents all over them. Recreational users have suffered major burns from ignition of vapor and liquid. Open flame is unnecessary; a static electricity spark can set off the gasoline. Inhaled gases can spread into other parts of the body besides the lungs, and fire from ignited gasoline vapor can instantly reach into the body's interior with devastating consequences. One scientific journal article is entitled "Death Due to 'Harakiri' or Gasoline Fumes?"

Abuse factors. Gasoline gets little attention as a substance of abuse in the United States, but researchers in India studied nine teenage and younger persons who declared gasoline to be their top choice among recreational substances. These users were all from lower social and economic backgrounds, and their fathers tended to be alcoholics. Authorities have described the practice as more popular in rural American communities than in big cities. A study of the habit among Navajo teenagers found them doing poorly in school and prone to trouble with police, factors probably having nothing to do with effects of the chemical but that indicate that gasoline misuse appeals to social misfits. Research in Australia and Canada has also linked the practice to individuals experiencing personal and social discontent. The practice seems more prevalent among males than among females. Gasoline sniffing is often a social occasion rather than a solitary practice, suggesting that the custom has elements of promoting group identity and solidarity.

Development of dependence with gasoline is indicated by a withdrawal syndrome: dry mouth, watery eyes, sleeping difficulty, peevishness, problems in moving arms and legs.

Drug Interactions. Not enough scientific information to report.

Cancer. Some types of DNA damage indicate cancer-causing potential, and evidence of DNA damage has been detected in persons with workplace exposure to gasoline fumes. A large study examining medical records of 19,000 automobile service station attendants through a 20-year period found higher-than-normal rates of cancer in the nose, throat, lungs, and kidneys. Gasoline vapor is suspected of causing acute myeloid leukemia. Gasoline fumes cause cancer in animal experiments.

Pregnancy. Infants born to women who were recreational gasoline inhalers during pregnancy may exhibit improper muscle tension, head deformities, mental retardation, and other deficiencies, leading some researchers to suspect that gasoline causes birth defects.

Additional scientific information may be found in:

Beckmann, G., and G. Hauck. "Tod durch 'Harakiri' oder Benzindampfe? [Death due to 'Harakiri' or Gasoline Fumes?]" *Archiv für Kriminologie* 154 (1974): 77–82.

Edminster, S.C., and M.J. Bayer. "Recreational Gasoline Sniffing: Acute Gasoline Intoxication and Latent Organolead Poisoning. Case Reports and Literature Review." *Journal of Emergency Medicine* 3 (1985): 365–70.

Maruff, P., et al. "Neurological and Cognitive Abnormalities Associated with Chronic Petrol Sniffing." *Brain* 121 (1998): 1903–17.

Nurcombe, B., et al. "A Hunger for Stimuli: The Psychosocial Background of Petrol Inhalation." *British Journal of Medical Psychology* 43 (1970): 367–74.

Poklis, A., and C.D. Burkett. "Gasoline Sniffing: A Review." *Clinical Toxicology* 11 (1977): 35–41.

Seshia, S.S., et al. "The Neurological Manifestations of Chronic Inhalation of Leaded Gasoline." *Developmental Medicine and Child Neurology* 20 (1978): 323–34.

Tolan, E.J., and F.A. Lingl. " 'Model Psychosis' Produced by Inhalation of Gasoline Fumes." *American Journal of Psychiatry* 120 (1964): 757–761.

Valpey, R., et al. "Acute and Chronic Progressive Encephalopathy Due to Gasoline Sniffing." *Neurology* 28 (1978): 507–10.

GHB

Pronunciation: jee-eightch-bee

Chemical Abstracts Service Registry Number: 591-81-1. (Sodium salt form 502-85-2)

Formal Names: 4-Hydroxybutanoic Acid, Gamma Hydroxybutyrate, Gamma-Hydroxybutyric Acid, Sodium Oxybate, Sodium Oxybutyrate

Informal Names: Blue Verve, Cherry Menth, Cherry Meth, Easy Lay, Everclear, EZ Lay, Fantasy, G, Gamma Oh, GBH, Georgia Home Boy, Ghana Marijuana, Gib, Goop, Great Hormones at Bedtime, Grievous Bodily Harm, G-Riffick, Growth Hormone Booster, Jib, Jib Gamma, Lemons, Liquid E, Liquid Ecstasy, Liquid X, Max (combination with amphetamines), Mickey Finn Special, Natural Sleep-500, Nature's Quaalude, Organic Quaalude, Oxy-Sleep, Poor Man's Heroin, Salty Water, Soap, Scoop, Somatomax, Somsanit, Vita-G, Water, Wolfies, Zonked

Type: Depressant. *See* page 19

Federal Schedule Listing: Schedule I (DEA no. 2010)

USA Availability: Illegal to possess

Pregnancy Category: None

Uses. Although GHB is commercially manufactured, it is also produced within the bodies of mammals where it may promote hibernation and help the brain to withstand deficient oxygen supply. The substance was once widely available as a nutritional supplement in health food stores. People consumed it in hopes that the product would promote fat reduction and muscle development. Human experiments confirm that the drug can increase the body's levels of human growth hormone while the substance is circulating in the bloodstream, but the studies did not last long enough to show whether this GHB effect built muscles or reduced fat. The hope for muscle development has been tested in experiments with rats and dogs, but without success; the drug failed to increase the animals' growth hormone levels.

Where this drug is legal, its main medical use is for anesthesia and for treating drug abuse patients. It has been used experimentally to study epilepsy, to reduce damage from exposure to nuclear radiation, and to treat fibromyalgia (a rheumatic disease causing weariness, muscle pain, and stiff joints). Some efforts to help schizophrenics with the substance have been successful; some have not. Experiments with hamsters indicate the drug may have potential for reducing damage from bleeding. Animal experiments also suggest the drug may have potential in treating heart attack. Although GHB is a depressant that has been used successfully to treat insomnia, it has also been used to treat narcolepsy, a condition in which people have difficulty staying awake.

According to law enforcement authorities, rapists have exploited GHB's sedative effect to make victims pliable. From 1996 to 1999 a total of 22 such reports reached the U.S. Drug Enforcement Administration. From 1996 to 1999 a group of 2,003 urine samples were compiled from victims across the United States in sexual assault cases where drugs were a suspected weapon used by the assailant. Analysis found GHB or **flunitrazepam** in fewer than 2%, and the number of instances declined in each passing year. At about the same time, a 26-month study collected 1,179 samples from sexual assault cases nationwide in which a drug was suspected of playing a role and found 4% to be positive for GHB.

Persons wanting GHB sometimes obtain GBL instead (gamma butyrolactone, nicknamed Blue Nitro Vitality or Firewater). The body converts a dose of GBL into GHB, so their effects are about the same. Products containing GBL can be poisonous, a fact that some drug abusers learn in dramatic ways.

Recreational users take GHB for euphoria and hallucinations, to increase sociability, to promote interest in sexual activity, and to lower inhibitions. One drug misuser who used GBL likened its effects to **alcohol**. GBL is also marketed as a mood elevator, a quality that some GHB users ascribe to that substance as well. Researchers using various scientific measurements have confirmed that GHB promotes mental calmness but may simultaneously make a person feel discontented.

Drawbacks. Tests using medical-size doses (which may be smaller than ones taken by illicit users) reveal no impairment of mental or physical abilities; the researchers concluded that GHB does not hurt job performance or ability to drive a car. Nevertheless, GHB is suspected of causing an automobile driver to pass out, and the drug's sleep-inducing properties make it inadvisable to use while operating dangerous machinery. Supposedly the drug causes amnesia about events that occur while a person is intoxicated with the substance, although experiments using medical-size doses find no effect on short-term memory. A large-enough dose can slow heart rate and interfere with a person's ability to move and make a person vomit and fall asleep. Breathing difficulty can occur. Seizures have been reported, but some authorities believe those reports have misidentified various muscle contractions as seizures. In monkeys the drug lowers body temperature. In rats that effect depends on a dose's size, with small amounts raising body temperature and large amounts lowering it. An odd overdose effect has been observed in persons who temporarily stop breathing yet become violent despite that impairment. The drug reduces control of urination and defecation. Although GHB can cause blood to appear in urine, no damage to body organs has been observed. People can take medical doses for years without showing any psychotic symptoms.

Abuse factors. Experiments with monkeys show little abuse potential in the drug, but some medical personnel who treat drug abusers consider the potential to be high. GHB abusers, however, tend to have bad relationships with other drugs as well, so using such a population to evaluate GHB's particular abuse potential is treacherous.

GHB has been used successfully to reduce or even eliminate withdrawal symptoms in alcohol addicts. One alcohol withdrawal study found GHB as effective as **diazepam**, a standard drug given to aid alcohol withdrawal; in addition, GHB worked faster than diazepam at alleviating sadness, restlessness, and anxiety among patients. GHB has also reduced craving for alcohol on a long-term basis. One group of researchers administering GHB for this purpose observed no troublesome unwanted effects, and barely 1% of patients began abusing GHB—a disturbing percentage in a general population but a very low rate for a drug addict population. Tightly controlled dispensing conditions, however, may be the reason for that low rate; abuse might be heavier among persons with ready access to the drug. GHB is cross-tolerant enough with **heroin** and **methadone** to diminish their withdrawal symptoms. Animal experiments have found modest cross-tolerance with **morphine**, **dextroamphetamine**, and **LSD**.

In studies measuring GHB's usefulness for treating narcolepsy, no tolerance was observed even though some patients had been taking the drug for up to nine years. Dispute exists about whether tolerance develops in nonmedical usage. GHB dependence can emerge after taking large doses for a long time. Diazepam can ease GHB withdrawal symptoms. Tremors, uneasiness, difficulty with sleep, visual and auditory hallucinations, high blood pressure, faster heartbeat, sweating, nausea, and vomiting can be part of the withdrawal syndrome. Symptoms may last for over two weeks. GHB withdrawal can include psychosis so severe that people have to be restrained, but how much of that reaction is caused by the drug and how much is caused by the individual's underlying personality may be unclear. Dosage affects severity of withdrawal, with heavy users having the most trouble.

Drug interactions. The HIV (human immunodeficiency virus) drugs saquinavir and ritonavir can have serious and potentially fatal interactions with GHB. Simultaneous use of alcohol or other depressants with GHB increases risk of overdose. The drug has a high sodium content, which might be a problem for persons needing to limit their intake of sodium.

Cancer. Tests on rats and mice indicate GHB does not cause cancer.

Pregnancy. Whether the drug causes birth defects is unknown. It passes into the fetus if a pregnant woman takes a dose and can reduce fetal respiration. When the substance was still a legal medical drug, GHB was used as an aid to childbirth.

Additional scientific information may be found in:

"Adverse Events Associated with Ingestion of Gamma-butyrolactone—Minnesota, New Mexico, and Texas, 1998–1999." *MMWR. Morbidity and Mortality Weekly Report.* 48 (1999): 137–40.

Bernasconi, R., et al. "Gamma-hydroxybutyric Acid: An Endogenous Neuromodulator with Abuse Potential?" *Trends in Pharmacological Sciences* 20 (1999): 135–41.

Dyer, J.E. "Gamma-hydroxybutyrate: A Health-Food Product Producing Coma and Seizurelike Activity." *American Journal of Emergency Medicine* 9 (1991): 321–24.

Ferrara, S.D., et al. "Effects of Single Dose of Gamma-hydroxybutyric Acid and Lorazepam on Psychomotor Performance and Subjective Feelings in Healthy Volunteers." *European Journal of Clinical Pharmacology* 54 (1999): 821–27.

Galloway, G.P., et al. "Gamma-hydroxybutyrate: An Emerging Drug of Abuse That Causes Physical Dependence." *Addiction* 92 (1997): 89–96.

Hernandez, M., et al. "GHB-Induced Delirium: A Case Report and Review of the Literature on Gamma Hydroxybutyric Acid." *American Journal of Drug and Alcohol Abuse* 24 (1998): 179–83.

Li, J., S.A. Stokes, and A. Woeckener. "A Tale of Novel Intoxication: A Review of the Effects of Gamma-hydroxybutyric Acid with Recommendations for Management." *Annals of Emergency Medicine* 31 (1998): 729–36.

Glutethimide

Pronunciation: gloo-TETH-ih-meyed

Chemical Abstracts Service Registry Number: 77-21-4

Formal Names: Doriden, Elrodorm, Noxyron

Informal Names: CB, CD, Ciba, D, Glue, Goofballs, Goofers. *With **codeine***: Doors & 4s, Dors & 4s, 4 Doors, G & C, Hits, Loads, Packets, Pancakes & Syrup, Sets, Setups, 3s & 8s

Type: Depressant. *See* page 19

Federal Schedule Listing: Schedule II (DEA no. 2550)

USA Availability: Prescription

Pregnancy Category: C

Uses. The substance became available in the 1950s as an alternative to barbiturates. As a medicine this drug is mainly used to calm people and make them sleepy. It has also been used to help prevent jaundice in newborns and to reduce muscle tremors in adults. Glutethimide intoxication has been likened to that from **alcohol** or barbiturates.

Drawbacks. Glutethimide can have a rebound effect, meaning that if a person is taking the drug to combat anxiety or insomnia and stops taking it, those conditions can temporarily become worse than before. One study found that after several months the drug's ability to induce sleep deteriorates so badly that users have more trouble falling asleep than insomniacs who don't use any sleep-inducing drug.

A test of the drug's influence on mental ability found little effect, but tobacco smokers seemed to be affected more than nonsmokers. A test of skills related to automobile driving found little influence from glutethimide. The drug produced inconsistent results in another experiment measuring alertness, reaction time, and decision making. Those tests, however, involve normal doses during relatively brief time spans. Generally people are advised to become aware of how the drug affects them before attempting to run dangerous machinery. Long-term heavy abuse can reduce mental skills in ways that resemble organic brain damage. Animal experiments suggest that the substance may worsen porphyria, a body chemistry disorder that can make a person violent. The drug can aggravate urinary tract blockage and should be used cautiously by persons with enlarged prostate. Eyesight difficulty and dry mouth are among typical unwanted effects.

A severe overdose can produce what looks like skin burns, and muscle spasms or even convulsions may occur. Case reports note that long-term use of glutethimide can decrease a person's calcium levels; one report tells of bones softening in a person who took the drug routinely for 10 years, and another report notes seizures occurring due to low calcium. The drug can also reduce a body's supply of vitamin D. After a dozen years of daily glutethimide ingestion, one person had lost so much muscle control that speech was difficult, unassisted walking was impossible, and control of urination and bowel movements was no longer possible. Similar case reports exist. Others, however, mention persons who took the drug for years without noticeable ill effect.

Abuse factors. Some illicit drug users take glutethimide with **codeine**. The combination supposedly produces a euphoria and stupor like **heroin**'s. Users of the combination report increased sociability and feelings of intellectual insight in discussions that were actually about nothing. The drug mix can seriously impair breathing, and deaths are verified. Some of these deaths involve dosages of each drug that were theoretically safe, outcomes implying that glutethimide and codeine may boost each other's actions. Users of the combination have experienced typical unwanted actions of both drugs in addition to headaches, grouchiness, tremors, cramps, and trouble sleeping.

Glutethimide tolerance and dependence can develop. Withdrawal has symptoms similar to those seen with barbiturates. Seizures are noted in case reports. Among persons taking medical doses of glutethimide for months, a withdrawal syndrome can include hallucinations, fever, delirium, and convulsions. Case reports tell of withdrawal experiences that included catatonia. For addiction treatment, **phenobarbital** can be substituted for glutethimide, and a person can then be gradually weaned off the phenobarbital.

Drug interactions. The drug reduces effectiveness of warfarin, a medicine that fights heart attack and stroke by reducing blood clotting. Glutethimide is also supposed to be avoided if someone is taking the anti-blood-clotting substance coumarin. A U.S. Army aerospace test found that using alcohol with glutethimide did not harm breathing. That finding has rather narrow significance for most persons, but a more generally relevant finding came from an experiment showing that glutethimide raised blood alcohol levels of persons who had been drinking. Alcohol and glutethimide may be a mix to avoid. Antihistamines should be used cautiously with glutethimide. Animal experimentation shows that injection of **marijuana**'s main active component THC (tetrahydrocannabinol) increases the potency of glutethimide, thereby increasing risk of overdose.

Cancer. Not enough scientific information to report.

Pregnancy. Glutethimide is related to thalidomide, perhaps the most notorious pharmaceutical cause of human birth defects. In experimentation with rats and rabbits glutethimide did not produce physically apparent birth defects. The death rate among rabbit offspring was 6%, however, compared to a 2% rate among offspring with no fetal drug exposure—a rate three times higher for the glutethimide group than for the nondrug group. One experiment found the death rate of rats with prenatal glutethimide exposure to be three times that of rats with no drug exposure. Surviving rats with fetal exposure to glutethimide exhibit abnormal behavior, but their own offspring behave normally. Pregnant women have routinely received glutethimide for insomnia, nausea, and vomiting. Humans with sufficient fetal exposure may be born dependent on the drug. It has been used to ease labor. Nursing mothers who take the drug may have enough glutethimide in their milk to make their infants sleepy.

Additional scientific information may be found in:

Bender, F.H., J.V. Cooper, and R. Dreyfus. "Fatalities Associated with an Acute Over-dose of Glutethimide (Doriden) and Codeine." *Veterinary and Human Toxicology* 30 (1988): 332–33.

DiGiacomo, J.N., and C.L. King. "Codeine and Glutethimide Addiction." *International Journal of the Addictions* 5 (1970): 279–85.

Haas, D.C., and A. Marasigan. "Neurological Effects of Glutethimide." *Journal of Neurology, Neurosurgery, and Psychiatry* 31 (1968): 561–64

Jones, A.H., and J.F. Mayberry. "Chronic Glutethimide Abuse." *British Journal of Clinical Practice* 40 (1986): 213.

Kovacs, T. "[Acute Toxicological Cases during a Ten-Year Period in Our Clinic]." *Orvosi Hetilap* [*Hungarian Medical Journal*] 143 (2002): 71–76. Abstract in English.

Mould, G.P., S.H. Curry, and T.B. Binns. "Interaction of Glutethimide and Phenobarbital with Ethanol in Man." *Journal of Pharmacy and Pharmacology* 24 (1972): 894–99.

Reveri, M., S.P. Pyati, and R.S. Pildes. "Neonatal Withdrawal Symptoms Associated with Glutethimide (Doriden) Addiction in the Mother during Pregnancy." *Clinical Pediatrics* 16 (1977): 424–25.

Shamoian, C.A. "Codeine and Glutethimide; Euphoretic, Addicting Combination." *New York State Journal of Medicine* 75 (1975): 97–99.

Halazepam

Pronunciation: hal-AZ-eh-pam

Chemical Abstracts Service Registry Number: 23092-17-3

Formal Names: Paxipam

Type: Depressant (benzodiazepine class). *See* page 21

Federal Schedule Listing: Schedule IV (DEA no. 2762)

USA Availability: Prescription

Pregnancy Category: D

Uses. Halazepam's main medical usage is for reducing anxiety. Because the drug promotes drowsiness, it is sometimes prescribed to be taken at bedtime, aiding both sleep and calmness. One experiment found the compound to be more effective than **clorazepate** dipotassium in helping anxiety. Another study found that halazepam can diminish anxiety significantly on the very first day of administration. Halazepam is also used to treat symptoms of **alcohol** withdrawal and has had some experimental success in alleviating schizophrenic psychoses. Physicians have observed that halazepam can reduce stress and depression and can improve epilepsy. An experiment found that halazepam did not increase belligerence, unlike some benzodiazepine class drugs. Canine studies show that in the body the drug converts into nordiazepam and **oxazepam**, which are also metabolites of **diazepam**.

Drawbacks. The compound can reduce saliva output. With stronger dosages elderly persons sometimes experience difficulty in manual dexterity and other muscle control; during an experiment several elderly individuals fell. In certain kinds of tests mice exhibit memory trouble after the drug is given.

Abuse factors. In an experiment some alcoholics had difficulty distinguishing halazepam from placebo, an outcome suggesting that the drug has low potential for abuse (as abusers of alcohol and other drugs should be particularly susceptible). Nonetheless, a person's body can develop physical dependence with halazepam, which is a traditional sign of addictive potential. One group of researchers found withdrawal symptoms to be so mild, however, that a placebo could control them.

Drug interactions. The heartburn medicine cimetidine is suspected of interfering with halazepam's effects.

Cancer. No cancer developed in rats and mice at daily dosage levels 5 to 50 times the maximum human dose.

Pregnancy. Experiments with rats and rabbits have produced no evidence that the drug causes birth defects.

Additional scientific information may be found in:

Fann, W.E., W.M. Pitts, and J.C. Wheless. "Pharmacology, Efficacy, and Adverse Effects of Halazepam, a New Benzodiazepine." *Pharmacotherapy* 2 (1982): 72–79.

Fann, W.E., B.W. Richman, and W.M. Pitts. "Halazepam in the Treatment of Recurrent Anxiety Attacks in Chronically Anxious Outpatients: A Double Blind Placebo Controlled Study." *Current Therapeutic Research: Clinical and Experimental* 32 (1982): 906–10.

Griffiths, R.R., and B. Wolf. "Relative Abuse Liability of Different Benzodiazepines in Drug Abusers." *Journal of Clinical Psychopharmacology* 10 (1990): 237–43.

"Halazepam (Paxipam)—Another Benzodiazepine." *Medical Letter on Drugs and Therapeutics* 24 (1982): 50.

Jaffe, J.H., et al. "Abuse Potential of Halazepam and of Diazepam in Patients Recently Treated for Acute Alcohol Withdrawal." *Clinical Pharmacology and Therapeutics* 34 (1983): 623–30.

Pecknold, J.C., et al. "Controlled Comparative Study of Halazepam in Anxiety." *Current Therapeutic Research: Clinical and Experimental* 32 (1982): 895–905.

Heroin

Pronunciation: HAIR-oh-in (also pronounced HEAR-oh-in)

Chemical Abstracts Service Registry Number: 561-27-3

Formal Names: Acetomorphine, Diacetylmorphine, Diamorphine

Informal Names: Agua de Chango, AIP, Al Capone, Alquitran, Alquitranat, Amsterdam Marble, Antifreeze, Aries, Aunt Hazel, Bad Seed, Ball, Ballot, Bart Simpson, Beast, Big H, Big Harry, Birdie Powder, Black Pearl, Black Stuff, Black Tar, Blanca, Blanco, Blows, Blue Bag, Blunt, Bomb, Bombido, Bombita, Bombs Away, Bonita, Boy, Bozo, Brain Damage, Brea, Brick Gum, Broja, Brown, Brown Crystal, Brown Marijuana, Brown Rhine, Brown Sugar, Brown Tape, Bundle, Butu, Caballo, Caca, Calbo, Canade, Cap, Capital H, Carga, Carne, Chapopote, Charley, Chatarra, Cheese, Chicle, Chieva, China Cat, China White, Chinese Red, Chip, Chiva, Climax, Cocofan, Coffee, Cotics, Courage Pills, Crank, Crap, Crop, Crown Crap, Cura, Cut-Deck, Dava, Dead on Arrival, Deck (quantity), Deuce, Diesel, Dirt, DOA, Dog Food, Dogie, Doogie, Dooje, Doojee, Dooley, Dope, Dreck, Dr. Feelgood, Dugie, Duji, Dujie, Dust, Dyno, Dyno-Pure, Eighth, Estuffa, Ferry Dust, Flea Powder, Foil, Foo Foo Stuff, Foolish Powder, Fry Daddy (with crack), Furra, Galloping Horse, Gallup, Gamot, Garbage, Gato, George, Georgia Smack, Girl, Glacines, Glass, Gold, Golden Girl, Golpe, Goma, Good, Good & Plenty, Good H, Good Horse, Goofball (combination with **cocaine**), Gravy, H, H & C (with cocaine), H-Bomb (with **MDMA**), Hache, H Caps, Hairy, Hard, Hard Candy, Hard Stuff, Harry, Hazel, Heaven, Heaven Dust, Helen, Hell Dust, Henry, Hera, Hero, Heroina, Herone, Hero of the Underworld, Hessle, Him, Hombre, Hong-Yen, Horse, Horsebite, Hot Dope, HRN, Indian Pink, Iroini, Isda, Jee Gee, Jee Jee, Jerry Springer, Jive, Jive Doo Jee, Joharito, Jojee, Jones, Joy, Joy Flakes, Joy Powder, Junco, Junk, Kabayo, Karachi (with **methaqualone** and **phenobarbital**), Kompot, La Buena, LBJ, Lemonade, Little Bomb, Load (quantity), Malaysian Pink, Manteca, Matsakow, Mayo, Mexican, Mexican Brown, Mexican Horse, Mexican Mud, Mojo, Monkey Water, Moonrock (with crack cocaine), Morotgara, Mortal Combat, Mud, Murder 1 (with cocaine), Murotugora, Muzzle, Nanoo, New Jack Swing (with **morphine**), Nice & Easy, Noise, Nose, Nose Drops, Number 8, Number 4, Number 3, Nurse, Ogoy, Oil, Old Steve, Orange Line, Pack, Pangonadalot, Parachute (alone or with crack), P-Dope, Peg, Penang Pink, Perfect High, Perica, Perico, Persian, Persian Brown, P-Funk, Piedra, Poison, Polvo, Poppy, Powder, Predator, Preza, Primo (with cocaine), Pulborn, Punk Rocker (with assorted other substances), Pure, Quill, Racehorse Charlie, Ragweed, Rambo, Rane, Raw

Fusion, Raw Hide, Ready Rock, Red, Red Chicken, Red Eagle, Red Rock, Red Rock Opium (with barbital, **caffeine**, and strychnine), Red Rum (with barbital, caffeine, and strychnine), Red Stuff (with barbital, caffeine, and strychnine), Reindeer Dust, Rhine, Rufus, Sack, Salt, Scag, Scat, Scate, Schmeek, SCOT, Scott, Scramble, Second to None, Shit, Shmeck, Shoot, Shoot-Up, Silk, Skag, Skid, Skunk, Sleeper, Slime, Smack, Smoke (with crack cocaine), Smoking Gun (with cocaine), Snow, Snowball (with cocaine), Speedball (with cocaine or **methylphenidate**), Spider Blue, Spike, Spoon (quantity), Stuff, Sugar, Sweet Dreams, Sweet Jesus, Sweet Stuff, Tar, Taste, Tecata, Thanie, Thing, Thunder, Tigre, Tigre Blanco, Tigre del Norte, Tits, TNT, Tongs, Tootsie Roll, Vidrio, Whack (with **PCP**), White, White Boy, White Girl, White Junk, White Lady, White Nurse, White Stuff, Whiz Bang (with cocaine), Wicked, Wings, Witch, Witch Hazel, Z (quantity), Zoquete

Type: Depressant (opiate class). *See* page 22

Federal Schedule Listing: Schedule I (DEA no. 9200)

USA Availability: Illegal to possess

Pregnancy Category: None

Uses. For most of the twentieth century drug addiction and heroin were synonymous in the United States; all substance abuse was assumed to lead to heroin. Only in the 1980s did heroin become displaced as the devil drug, supplanted in public fear and disapproval by **cocaine**. Being a Schedule I substance, heroin has no officially approved medical use in the United States.

Heroin is produced from **morphine**, and body chemistry converts a heroin dose back into morphine. Most users cannot detect a difference between those two substances. Depending on means of administration and the effect being measured, heroin is 1.5 to 8.0 times stronger than morphine and is used medically to suppress coughs and relieve pain in children and adults. One study of pain relief found heroin comparable to **hydromorphone**, a standard medication administered to fight severe pain. Physicians have judged heroin to be a safe anesthetic for use during childbirth, with no apparent ill effect on mother or child. The drug is also used to treat porphyria, a body chemistry disorder making people sensitive to light and occasionally making them violent. Heroin users of both genders have reported increased sexual activity upon starting the compound, with decline in that activity as usage continues. That sequence would be consistent with the drug at first reducing psychological anxiety, an effect gradually evolving into indifference about the world. As noted below, heroin has hormonal actions that reduce male sexual activity.

Extrapolating from severity of withdrawal symptoms, any particular size heroin dose taken by intravenous injection is five times stronger than one taken by inhaling heated vapor ("chasing the dragon"). Other measurements show a dose to be four times more potent when taken intravenously instead of by inhaling powder.

Sometimes intravenous injection of heroin produces a rush of feeling likened to a total body sexual orgasm. Heroin may allow some nonmedical users to experience euphoria, but more typically an intoxicating dose increases psychic distance between the user and the world, making reality seem unimportant. Used in that way the drug is an escape—not into happiness but into emptiness. Someone intoxicated by a dose of heroin does not care what happens any more. Lesser doses simply reduce tension, taking the edge off life's stresses. People using lesser doses of heroin in that way may function more productively, or they may experience trouble because they feel confident enough to get into situations they would otherwise avoid.

Drawbacks. Classic unwanted heroin actions are nausea, vomiting, and constipation. Many other afflictions attributed to the drug actually come from adulterants in illicit supplies or from dosage techniques—such as addicts sharing the same hypodermic needle with one another, a custom promoting diseases ranging from hepatitis to AIDS (acquired immunodeficiency syndrome). Researchers find, however, that injectors of a heroin variety called "black tar" have an increased risk for botulism infection at the injection site, no matter how hygienic their equipment and technique. Injectors of any type heroin are more prone to all sorts of infections, and some researchers suspect that heroin impairs the immune system. Inhaling heated heroin vapor can rapidly produce enough brain damage to cripple a person, although case reports indicate that partial recovery is possible. Inhaling either the vapor or powder can also cause breathing trouble, and injection can cause swift fluid buildup in the lungs. A study found reduced bone density in chronic male heroin users, making broken bones more likely, and researchers suspected the problem resulted from lower **testosterone** levels caused by heroin (a heroin action that is also known to reduce male sex drive). Apparently the bone density and testosterone problems can correct themselves if heroin use stops. Although stroke is an uncommonly reported outcome of heroin use, autopsy examinations of 100 heroin addict brains indicate that 5% to 10% of injectors suffer small strokes that may not cause the person to seek medical treatment but that may thereafter affect the person's behavior. One experiment with heroin addicts found still another unwanted effect: Most of them see colors somewhat differently than nonusers do.

Abuse factors. All the above hazards are real, but experience also shows that addicts can take maintenance doses (enough to hold off withdrawal symptoms but not enough to get high) for years with no apparent ill effect. The behavior of people on a maintenance dose can be indistinguishable from someone using no drug at all; while on a maintenance dose of heroin ordinary middle-class persons can function well in all aspects of life at work and at home.[1] Such factors are highly influenced by the legal setting of heroin use. When federal legislation outlawed the drug in the early twentieth century, the kinds of persons who took the drug changed, as did the common reasons for using the drug.

Achieving heroin addiction is normally a lengthy process; people do not become addicts instantly with a single dose. Indeed, persons can use heroin intermittently for years and not develop dependence, let alone develop a compulsion to take the drug. Someone with a fulfilling life is unlikely to become addicted even if heroin is used occasionally. In contrast, people with nothing to live for may find heroin to be the best part of their lives, a discovery leading to addiction.

Breaking heroin addiction depends on the reason someone takes the drug. Severe withdrawal symptoms mimic influenza, but someone willing to put up with them for a couple of days can emerge with no more dependence on the drug. Physical dependence with heroin is a relatively trivial part of addiction. Few addicts take the substance simply to avoid the withdrawal syndrome. Instead, they take the drug to cope with assorted frustrations in life. If those frustrations are resolved, the heroin addiction will resolve. If those difficulties remain, heroin may remain the best way the addict knows to cope with them, and addiction will persist.[2] Both heroin and tobacco can reduce stress, and if heroin users cut back on that drug, they often increase their cigarette consumption.

Although heroin is traditionally considered the final step in illicit drug use, with previous substances leading from one to another until the climax of heroin is reached, scientific research does not support that scenario. Experienced drug users have typically used assorted substances over the years, but the "gateway" hypothesis in which one substance leads to another has been refuted time and again. Nor is heroin necessarily the final stopping place for addicts. For example, research demonstrates that some heroin users move on to amphetamines as their main drug.

Drug interactions. Some persons use heroin and amphetamines together or heroin and cocaine together, a potentially fatal practice called speedballing, in order to get a variety of simultaneous drug sensations. Analysis of fatalities attributed to heroin suggests that **alcohol** increases risk of death.

Cancer. Whether heroin can cause cancer is unknown. One study found that cells of heroin addicts show chromosome damage that might promote cancer, but the damage becomes less over a period of months if addicts switch from heroin to **methadone**. Other research has found that intravenous heroin users are more likely to get cancer than the general population, but factors other than heroin may be involved.

Pregnancy. Although heroin usage apparently damages chromosomes, the damage may be from breakdown products rather than heroin itself. A study of several dozen infants found that those from heroin-using mothers had six or seven times the amount of chromosome damage found in infants from mothers who did not use the drug. This damage did not translate into congenital malformations, however. Researchers have examined children born to women who abused heroin during pregnancy and found no indication that the drug causes birth defects. Infants may be smaller than normal upon birth, but heroin's role is uncertain because the women tend to abuse additional drugs and engage in other conduct harmful to fetal development. Infants born to such mothers may have dependence with heroin and undergo withdrawal symptoms. Sudden infant death syndrome is more common in babies with fetal exposure to heroin than in babies without any illicit drug exposure, but researchers are uncertain whether the drug is a more important factor than overall home environment. Physical and mental development of children whose mothers used heroin during pregnancy is slightly slower than normal, an observation supported by findings in rat experiments. Examination of school-age boys who had fetal exposure to heroin finds them to be much like other children despite lower scores on various physical and psychological tests; one group of researchers noted that prenatal exposure to alcohol has much more impact than heroin, and another investigator noted that girls' test scores were normal.

Among pregnant Australian women in drug treatment programs who use both heroin and methadone, infant mortality is higher than among women who only use methadone, but researchers believe the difference is not due to heroin but due to multiproblem lifestyles in which heroin is just one of many problems. This theme was also brought out by a study in Israel comparing children of parents who abused heroin and children of parents who did not, while at the same time comparing home environments. The investigators discovered that assorted problems suffered by children of heroin users had much more to do with general conditions at home than with any chemical influence of the drug on fetal development, a conclusion supported by still more Israeli research and consistent with findings by the U.S. National Institute on Drug Abuse and other researchers.

Breast-feeding by heroin-using mothers is considered safe for their infants. Passage of heroin into the milk is doubtful, and levels of heroin's breakdown products (such as morphine) are low enough to avoid hazard.

Additional scientific information may be found in:

Cygan, J., M. Trunsky, and T. Corbridge. "Inhaled Heroin-Induced Status Asthmaticus: Five Cases and a Review of the Literature." *Chest* 117 (2000): 272–75.

"Diamorphine." In *Therapeutic Drugs*, ed. C. Dollery. 2d ed. New York: Churchill Livingstone, 1999. D70–D75.

Ornoy, A., et al. "The Developmental Outcome of Children Born to Heroin-Dependent Mothers, Raised at Home or Adopted." *Child Abuse and Neglect* 20 (1996): 385–96.

Sawynok, J. "The Therapeutic Use of Heroin: A Review of the Pharmacological Literature." *Canadian Journal of Physiology and Pharmacology* 64 (1986): 1–6.

Schneider, J.W., and S.L. Hans. "Effects of Prenatal Exposure to Opioids on Focused Attention in Toddlers during Free Play." *Journal of Developmental and Behavioral Pediatrics* 17 (1996): 240–47.

Sneader, W. "The Discovery of Heroin." *Lancet* 352 (November 21, 1998): 1697–99.

Zuckerman, G.B., et al. "Neurologic Complications Following Intranasal Administration of Heroin in an Adolescent." *Annals of Pharmacotherapy* 30 (1996): 778–81.

Notes

1. P. Biernacki, *Pathways from Heroin Addiction: Recovery without Treatment*. Health, Society, and Policy series, ed. S. Ruzek and I.K. Zola (Philadelphia: Temple University Press, 1986), 6, 36, 55; T.S. Blair, "The Relation of Drug Addiction to Industry," *Journal of Industrial Hygiene* 1 (October 1919): 288; Blum, "Student Characteristics and Major Drugs," in R.H. Blum, et al., *Students and Drugs: College and High School Observations*, The Jossey-Bass Behavioral Science Series and the Jossey-Bass Series in Higher Education (published jointly) (San Francisco: Jossey-Bass, 1969), 77–78; I. Chein, et al., *The Road to H: Narcotics, Delinquency, and Social Policy* (New York: Basic Books, 1964), 358; T.D. Crothers, *Morphinism and Narcomanias from Other Drugs* (Philadelphia: W.B. Saunders and Company, 1902), 31 (Not all of the Crothers book has withstood later scientific advances); W.R. Cuskey, A.W. Klein, and W. Krasner, *Drug-Trip Abroad: American Drug Refugees in Amsterdam and London* (Philadelphia: University of Pennsylvania Press, 1972), 94–96; W.C. Cutting, "Morphine Addiction for 62 Years," *Stanford Medical Bulletin* 1 (August 1942): 39–41; T. Duster, *The Legislation of Morality: Law, Drugs, and Moral*

Judgment (New York: The Free Press, 1970), 9, 117–28, 241; C.W. Earle, "The Opium Habit: A Statistical and Clinical Lecture," *Chicago Medical Review* 2 (1880): 445; L.S. Goodman and A. Gilman, *The Pharmacological Basis of Therapeutics*, 2nd ed. (New York: The Macmillan Company, 1955), 242–44; N. Hentoff, *A Doctor Among the Addicts* (Chicago: Rand McNally, 1968), 43–44; L. Hutchins, et al., "A Two-Year Follow-Up of a Cohort of Opiate Users from a Provincial Town," *British Journal of Addiction* 66 (1971): 129–40; Jaffe, "Drug Addiction and Drug Abuse," in Goodman and Gilman, *Pharmacological* 7th ed. (1985), 542, 547; Jaffe and Martin, "Opioid Analgesics and Antagonists," in Goodman and Gilman, *Pharmacological* 7th ed. (1985), 498; L. Johnston, *Drugs and American Youth* (Ann Arbor, MI: Institute for Social Research, University of Michigan, 1973), 193, 218; J. Kaplan, *The Hardest Drug: Heroin and Public Policy*, Studies in Crime and Justice (Chicago: University of Chicago Press, 1983), 136; R. King, *The Drug Hang-Up: America's Fifty Year Folly* (New York: W.W. Norton & Company, 1972), 18, 76; L. Kolb, *Drug Addiction: A Medical Problem* (Springfield, IL: Charles C. Thomas, 1962), 10–11, 46, 57–58, 64, 104–5, 114; Mellinger et al., "Drug Use, Academic Performance, and Career Indecision: Longitudinal Data in Search of a Model," in D.B. Kandel, ed., *Longitudinal Research on Drug Use: Empirical Findings and Methodological Issues* (Washington, DC: Hemisphere Publishing Corporation, 1978), 167–69, 172–73; H.W. Morgan, *Drugs in America: A Social History, 1800–1980* (Syracuse, NY: Syracuse University Press, 1981), 31; H.W. Morgan, *Yesterday's Addicts: American Society and Drug Abuse 1865–1920* (Norman: University of Oklahoma Press, 1981), 8; E.J. Morhous, "Drug Addiction in Upper Economic Levels: A Study of 142 Cases," *West Virginia Medical Journal* 49 (July 1953): 189; J.A. O'Donnell, *Narcotics Addicts in Kentucky*, U.S. Public Health Service Publication No. 1881 (National Institute of Mental Health, 1969) [SuDocs FS2.22:N16/3], 56, 60, 79–80, 94–98, 204, 211, 214, 217, 223–33, 241; S. Peele, with A. Brodsky, *Love and Addiction* (New York: Taplinger Publishing Company, 1975), 35; J.J. Platt and C. Labate, *Heroin Addiction: Theory, Research, Treatment*, Wiley Series on Personality Processes, A Wiley Interscience Publication (New York: John Wiley & Sons, 1976), 171; H.G. Pope, Jr., M. Ionescu-Pioggia, and J.D. Cole, "Drug Use and Life-Style among College Undergraduates: Nine Years Later," *Archives of General Psychiatry* 38 (1981): 588–91; C. Raymond, "Researchers Say Debate over Drug War and Legalization Is Tied to Americans' Cultural and Religious Values," *Chronicle of Higher Education* 36 (March 7, 1990): A6–A7, A10–A11 (Craig Reinarman comments); "Report of Committee on the Acquirement of Drug Habits," *Proceedings of the American Pharmaceutical Association* 51 (1903): 473; J. Rublowsky, *The Stoned Age: A History of Drugs in America*, Capricorn Books (New York: G.P. Putnam's Sons, 1974), 138, 191; E.M. Schur, *Narcotic Addiction in Britain and America: The Impact of Public Policy* (Bloomington: Indiana University Press, 1962), 28, 151; G.V. Stimson, *Heroin and Behaviour: Diversity among Addicts Attending London Clinics* (New York: John Wiley & Sons, 1973), 149, 178; G.M. Smith, C.W. Semke, and H.K. Beecher, "Objective Evidence of Mental Effects of Heroin, Morphine and Placebo in Normal Subjects," *Journal of Pharmacology and Experimental Therapeutics* 136 (1962): 53, 58; A.S. Trebach, *The Great Drug War and Radical Proposals That Could Make America Safe Again* (New York: Macmillan Publishing Company, 1987), 345; U.S. Congress, House, Select Committee on Crime, Hearings, *The Improvement and Reform of Law Enforcement and Criminal Justice in the United States* (91 Cong., 1 sess., 1969) [SuDocs Y4.C86/3:L41], 287, 291 (Stephen Waldron statement); U.S. Congress, Senate, Committee on the Judiciary, Subcommittee on Improvements in the Federal Criminal Code, Hearings, *Illicit Narcotics Traffic* (84 Cong., 1 sess., 1955) [SuDocs Y4.J89/2:N16/1–10], 1326, 1339 (Hubert S. Howe testimony); A. Weil, *The Natural Mind: An Investigation of Drugs and the Higher Consciousness*, Rev. ed. (Boston: Houghton Mifflin Company, 1986), 55, 57–58; White House Conference on Narcotic and Drug Abuse, *Proceedings* (1962) [SuDocs Y3.W58/5:2P94/962], 305; N.E. Zinberg, *Drug, Set, and Setting: The Basis for Controlled*

Intoxicant Use (New Haven: Yale University Press, 1984): 157, 162; N.E. Zinberg and R.C. Jacobson, "The Natural History of 'Chipping,' " *American Journal of Psychiatry* 133 (1976): 38; N.E. Zinberg and D.C. Lewis, "Narcotic Usage: I. A Spectrum of a Difficult Medical Problem," *New England Journal of Medicine* 270 (1964): 989, 992.

2. J.B. Bakalar and L. Grinspoon, *Drug Control in a Free Society* (Cambridge: Cambridge University Press, 1984), 47, 58, 135, 144; D.J. Bellis, *Heroin and Politicians: The Failure of Public Policy to Control Addiction in America* (Westport, CT: Greenwood Press, 1981), 25, 134, 210, 223; Biernacki, *Pathways*, 27, 43–44, 52, 95, 97, 99, 124–25, 161, 179, 226–28, 231; P.H. Blachly, *Seduction: A Conceptual Model in the Drug Dependencies and Other Contagious Ills* (Springfield, IL: Charles C. Thomas, 1970), 30, 37–38, 43, 80; J.S. Blackwell, "Drifting, Controlling and Overcoming: Opiate Users Who Avoid Becoming Chronically Dependent," *Journal of Drug Issues* 13 (1983): 219–35; P.G. Bourne, "Issues in Addiction," in P.G. Bourne, ed., *Addiction* (New York: Academic Press, 1974), 11; J.M. Boyle and A.F. Brunswick, "What Happened in Harlem? Analysis of a Decline in Heroin Use Among a Generation Unit of Urban Black Youth," *Journal of Drug Issues* 10 (1980): 109; E.M. Brecher, and the Editors of Consumer Reports, *Licit and Illicit Drugs: The Consumers Union Report on Narcotics, Stimulants, Depressants, Inhalants, Hallucinogens, and Marijuana—Including Caffeine, Nicotine, and Alcohol* (Boston: Little, Brown and Company, 1972), 39; Chein et al., *Road*, 6, 14, 22–23, 159, 364; I. Chein and E. Rosenfeld, "Juvenile Narcotics Use," *Law and Contemporary Problems* 22 (1957): 54; Childress, "Extinction of Conditioned Responses in Abstinent Cocaine or Opioid Users," in L.S. Harris, ed., *Problems of Drug Dependence, 1986: Proceedings of the 48th Annual Scientific Meeting, The Committee on Problems of Drug Dependence, Inc.* (National Institute on Drug Abuse, Research Monograph Series, No. 76, 1987) [SuDocs HE20.8216/5:986], 189–95; Cuskey and Edington, "Drug Abuse as Self-Destructive Behavior," in A.R. Roberts, ed. and comp., *Self-Destructive Behavior* (Springfield, IL: Charles C. Thomas, 1975), 138–39; Duster, *Legislation*, 209–11; Falk, "The Place of Adjunctive Behavior in Drug Abuse Research," in T. Thompson and C.E. Johanson, eds., *Behavioral Pharmacology of Human Drug Dependence* (National Institute on Drug Abuse, Research Monograph no. 37, 1981) [SuDocs HE20.8216:37], 276; D.B. Graeven and K.A. Graeven, "Treated and Untreated Addicts: Factors Associated with Participation in Treatment and Cessation of Heroin Use," *Journal of Drug Issues* 13 (1983): 207–18; R.E. Hinson and S. Siegel, "Nonpharmacological Bases of Drug Tolerance and Dependence," *Journal of Psychosomatic Research* 26 (1982): 496–502; L.G. Hunt and C.D. Chambers, *The Heroin Epidemics: A Study of Heroin Use in the United States 1965–75*, Sociomedical Science Series (New York: Spectrum Publications, 1976), 117; R. Jacobson and N.E. Zinberg, *The Social Basis of Drug Abuse Prevention*, Special Studies Series, no. 5 (Washington, DC: The Drug Abuse Council, 1975), 8, 14–15, 48, 50, 53, 60; B.D. Johnson, et al., *Taking Care of Business: The Economics of Crime by Heroin Abusers* (Lexington, MA: D.C. Heath and Company, 1985), 2; H.F. Judson, *Heroin Addiction in Britain: What Americans Can Learn from the English Experience* (New York: Harcourt Brace Jovanovich, 1973), 78, 80, 143–44; Kandel, "Convergences in Prospective Longitudinal Surveys of Drug Use in Normal Populations," in Kandel, *Longitudinal*, 15–16; Kaplan, *Hardest*, 10, 33–34, 36–38, 43–46; King, *Drug*, 234, 261; Kolb, *Drug*, 83–84, 127; I.D. Leader-Elliott, "Heroin in Australia: The Costs and Consequences of Prohibition," *Journal of Drug Issues* 16 (1986): 136; D.B. Louria, *Overcoming Drugs: A Program for Action* (New York: McGraw-Hill Book Company, 1971), 84; E.A. Nadelmann, "Drug Prohibition in the United States: Costs, Consequences, and Alternatives," *Science* 245 (1989): 944; Peele, *Love*, 19, 59–60, 64–65, 67, 87; Platt and Labate, *Heroin*, 102, 107, 159–61, 193; D.H. Powell, "A Pilot Study of Occasional Heroin Users," *Archives of General Psychiatry* 28 (1973): 586–94; V.H. Raveis and D.B. Kandel, "Changes in Drug Behavior from the Middle to the Late Twenties:

Initiation, Persistence, and Cessation of Use," *American Journal of Public Health* 77 (1987): 607–11; R.M. Restak, *The Mind* (New York: Bantam Books, 1988), 118; Robins, "The Interaction of Setting and Predisposition in Explaining Novel Behavior: Drug Initiations Before, In, and After Vietnam," in Kandel, *Longitudinal*, 181; L.N. Robins, *The Vietnam Drug Abuser Returns*, Final Report (Special Action Office for Drug Abuse Prevention, 1974) [SuDocs PrEx20.9:A/2], 31–32; L.N. Robins, D.H. Davis, and D.N. Nurco, "How Permanent Was Vietnam Drug Addiction?" *American Journal of Public Health* 64 (Suppl. 1974): 38–43; L.N. Robins and J.E. Helzer, "Drug Use Among Vietnam Veterans: Three Years Later," *Medical World News* 16 (October 27, 1975): 44–45, 49; L.N. Robins, J.E. Helzer, and D.H. Davis, "Narcotic Use in Southeast Asia and Afterward: An Interview Study of 898 Vietnam Returnees," *Archives of General Psychiatry* 32 (1975): 959; Rublowsky, *Stoned*, 128; C.R. Sanders, "Doper's Wonderland: Functional Drug Use by Military Personnel in Vietnam," *Journal of Drug Issues* 3 (Winter 1973): 71–72; Scher, "The Impact of the Drug Abuser on the Work Organization," in J.M. Scher, ed., *Drug Abuse in Industry: Growing Corporate Dilemma* (Springfield, IL: Charles C. Thomas, 1973), 11; R.C. Schroeder, *The Politics of Drugs: An American Dilemma*, 2d ed. (Washington, DC: Congressional Quarterly Press, 1980), 72–73, 76, 82; H.B. Spear and M.M. Glatt, "The Influence of Canadian Addicts on Heroin Addiction in the United Kingdom," *British Journal of Addiction* 66 (1971): 141–49; J. Stewart, H. de Wit, and R. Eikelboom, "Role of Unconditioned and Conditioned Drug Effects in the Self-Administration of Opiates and Stimulants," *Psychological Review* 91 (1984): 251–68; T. Szasz, *Ceremonial Chemistry: The Ritual Persecution of Drugs, Addicts, and Pushers*, Rev. ed. (Holmes Beach, FL: Learning Publications, 1985), 82–83; Trebach, *Great*, 110; A.S. Trebach, *The Heroin Solution* (New Haven: Yale University Press, 1982), 203; Trebach, "The Potential Impact of 'Legal' Heroin in America," in A.S. Trebach, ed., *Drugs, Crime, and Politics* (New York: Praeger Publishers, 1978), 167–68; U.S. Congress, House, Select Committee on Crime, *Improvement*, 287, 290 (Stephen Waldron statement); Weil, *Natural*, 108; D.M. Wilner, et al., "Heroin Use and Street Gangs," *Journal of Criminal Law, Criminology, and Police Science* 48 (1957): 401; C. Winick, "Epidemiology of Narcotics Use," in D.M. Wilner and G.G. Kassebaum, eds., *Narcotics*, University of California Medical Extension Series—Los Angeles (New York: McGraw-Hill Book Company, 1965), 8–9; N.E. Zinberg, "G.I.'s and O.J.'s in Vietnam," *New York Times Magazine*, Dec. 5, 1971, pp. 122–23; Zinberg, "Non-Addictive Opiate Use," in J.C. Weissman and R.L. DuPont, eds., *Criminal Justice and Drugs: The Unresolved Connection*, Multi-Disciplinary Studies in the Law (Port Washington, NY: Kennikat Press, 1982), 5–11, 15; N.E. Zinberg, W.M. Harding, and R. Apsler, "What is Drug Abuse?" *Journal of Drug Issues* 8 (1978): 13, 28.

Hydrocodone

Pronunciation: high-droh-KOH-done

Chemical Abstracts Service Registry Number: 125-29-1. (Bitartrate form 34195-34-1)

Formal Names: Anexsia, Dicodid, Dihydrocodeinone, Duratuss HD Elixir, Histussin D, Hycodan, Hycomine, Hycotuss, Hydrocet, Lorcet, Lortab, Norco, Tussend, Tussionex, Tylox, Vicodin (tablets, ES tablets, HP tablets, and Tuss expectorant), Vicoprofen, Zydone

Informal Names: Tuss

Type: Depressant (opiate class). *See* page 22

Federal Schedule Listing: Schedule II if dispensed by itself (DEA no. 9193); Schedule III if dispensed as part of a combination product

USA Availability: Prescription

Pregnancy Category: C

Uses. Physicians use this drug to suppress coughs and relieve pain. Commercial formulations of the substance routinely combine it with other drugs so a patient obtains multiple therapeutic effects. The combinations can also worsen effects from overdose. Hydrocodone is derived from **thebaine**, and body chemistry apparently converts some of a hydrocodone dose into **hydromorphone**. Hydrocodone's effects are likened to those of **codeine**, but depending on circumstances of dosage, hydrocodone is two to eight times stronger. Taking into account the differences in potency, hydrocodone produces more sedation than codeine.

Drawbacks. Unwanted effects can include hiccups, muscle spasms, dizziness, nausea, vomiting, constipation, and impairment of breathing. The drug can dull mental and physical alertness, so users should avoid operating dangerous machinery. Some pharmaceutical formats of hydrocodone combine that drug with the pain reliever acetaminophen, and excessive usage of that combination can cause deafness.

Abuse factors. Hydrocodone can produce euphoria, and the compound's potential for abuse is rated similar to codeine's. A medical experiment testing both those drugs found that 18 doses were not enough to produce tolerance. Urine from a person using codeine can test positive for hydrocodone. Drug abuse treatment programs seeking to switch **heroin** addicts to some other opiate have successfully used hydrocodone instead of **methadone**.

Drug interactions. Tricyclic antidepressants and monoamine oxidase inhibitors (MAOIs, found in some antidepressants and other medication) may boost hydrocodone effects, and vice versa. When taken with other narcotics, hydrocodone may boost their actions. Taking the substance with anticholinergics, which are drugs affecting the parasympathetic nervous system that controls much of the abdomen, can cause intestinal blockage.

Cancer. Hydrocodone's potential for causing cancer is unknown.

Pregnancy. Hydrocodone's potential for causing birth defects is unknown, although malformations occurred when pregnant rabbits received hydrocodone bitartrate along with the pain reliever ibuprofen at doses strong enough to be poisonous. Malformations did not occur when the same combination was given at poisonous levels to rats. Hydrocodone by itself produced birth defects in hamsters at 700 times the normal human dose. A study of human pregnancy outcomes found no indication that hydrocodone causes birth defects or miscarriage, but nonetheless the drug should be avoided during pregnancy unless the woman's condition unquestionably requires treatment by the substance. Infants born to women who have been using hydrocodone can have dependence with the drug. Whether hydrocodone passes into a nursing mother's milk is unknown.

Additional scientific information may be found in:

Friedman, R.A., et al. "Profound Hearing Loss Associated with Hydrocodone/Acetaminophen Abuse." *American Journal of Otology* 21 (2000): 188–91.

Hopkinson, J.H. "Hydrocodone—A Unique Challenge for an Established Drug: Comparison of Repeated Oral Doses of Hydrocodone (10 Mg) and Codeine (60 Mg) in the Treatment of Postpartum Pain." *Current Therapeutic Research: Clinical and Experimental* 24 (1978): 503–16.

Schick, B., et al. "Preliminary Analysis of First Trimester Exposure to Oxycodone and Hydrocodone." *Reproductive Toxicology* 10 (1996): 162.

Vandam, L.D. "Drug Therapy: Analgetic Drugs—The Mild Analgetics." *New England Journal of Medicine* 286 (1972): 20–23.

Vivian, D. "Three Deaths Due to Hydrocodone in a Resin-Complex Cough Medicine." *Drug Intelligence and Clinical Pharmacy* 13 (1979): 445–46.

Hydromorphone

Pronunciation: high-droh-MOR-fohn

Chemical Abstracts Service Registry Number: 466-99-9. (Hydrochloride form 71-68-1)

Formal Names: Dilaudid, Hydrostat IR, Palladone

Informal Names: Big D, D, Delantz, Delats, Delaud, Delida, Dillies, Drugstore Heroin, Hospital Heroin, Little D, Lords, Pills

Type: Depressant (opiate class). *See* page 22

Federal Schedule Listing: Schedule II (DEA no. 9150)

USA Availability: Prescription

Pregnancy Category: C

Uses. This pain reliever and cough suppressant was first produced in the 1920s. It is made from **morphine**. For pain relief hydromorphone is 2 to 10 times stronger than morphine (depending on why and how the drugs are administered), but hydromorphone effects do not last as long as morphine's. Hydromorphone is recommended to reduce particularly severe pain, such as that encountered in cancer, kidney stone attack, heart attack, sickle-cell anemia crisis, burns, or surgery. One study of seriously ill persons and another study of surgery patients found hydromorphone to be as effective as morphine in pain relief. No difference emerged from surveys asking patients whether morphine or hydromorphone was the more effective pain reliever. In one study patients preferred hydromorphone to **meperidine** for reducing pain, although medical personnel observed no superiority of one over the other. In another study medical personnel judged hydromorphone as better than meperidine for pain control, and in still another study hydromorphone's effects lasted longer than meperidine's.

Drawbacks. Unwanted effects can include itching, nausea, vomiting, constipation, urination difficulty, sedation, sleepiness, dizziness, poor appetite, low blood pressure, muscle spasms, impairment of breathing, reduced mental clarity, and impaired male sexual function. Users should avoid running dangerous machinery such as an automobile until they know the drug is not impeding skills necessary for such tasks. One study involving abdominal surgery patients found that hydromorphone impaired thinking and reasoning more than morphine did, but the same study found that patients' spirits rose more with hydromorphone.

Generally the drug should be avoided by persons suffering from asthma, urinary retention, enlarged prostate, deficient adrenal or thyroid glands, gall-bladder trouble, or epilepsy.

Abuse factors. Dependence can develop after hydromorphone has been taken regularly for several weeks. Although tolerance is unusual for medical effects of drugs, tolerance has been observed when hydromorphone is used for pain relief, with patients needing more of the drug for the same amount of relief.

Heroin addicts find hydromorphone to be a satisfactory substitute. Through cross-tolerance hydromorphone can reduce opiate withdrawal symptoms, and the drug has been used as an experimental medication in programs trying to switch opiate addicts to **methadone** or **buprenorphine**.

Drug interactions. Normally hydromorphone should not be taken along with antihistamines or various tranquilizers and antidepressants, including monoamine oxidase inhibitors (MAOIs, found in some antidepressants and in other medicine). Taking hydromorphone and **cocaine** together can increase each drug's effects.

Cancer. Hydromorphone does not seem to cause cancer.

Pregnancy. In general the drug fails to produce birth defects, but some did appear when pregnant hamsters received 600 times the normal human dose. The potential for malformations is unknown among infants from pregnant women who use the drug in a medical context. Infants can be born with dependence if the mother has used hydromorphone during pregnancy. The drug is used to ease childbirth. Whether the substance passes into a nursing mother's milk is unknown but is considered safe for the infant.

Additional information. The cough syrup form of Dilaudid may contain tartrazine (FD&C Yellow No. 5) to which some persons are allergic, particularly if they are allergic to aspirin.

Additional scientific information may be found in:

Hill, J.L., and J.P. Zacny. "Comparing the Subjective, Psychomotor, and Physiological Effects of Intravenous Hydromorphone and Morphine in Healthy Volunteers." *Psychopharmacology* 152 (2000): 31–39.

"Hydromorphone HCl." In *Therapeutic Drugs*, ed. C. Dollery. 2d ed. New York: Churchill Livingstone, 1999. H69–H71.

McBride, D.C., et al. "Dilaudid Use: Trends and Characteristics of Users." *Chemical Dependencies* 4 (1980): 85–100.

Walker, D.J., and J.P. Zacny. "Subjective, Psychomotor, and Physiological Effects of Cumulative Doses of Opioid Mu Agonists in Healthy Volunteers." *Journal of Pharmacology and Experimental Therapeutics* 289 (1999): 1454–64.

Ibogaine

Pronunciation: i-BOH-gah-in

Chemical Abstracts Service Registry Number: 83-74-9

Formal Names: Endabuse, *Tabernanthe iboga*

Informal Names: Bitter Grass, Iboga, Leaf of God

Type: Hallucinogen. *See* page 25

Federal Schedule Listing: Schedule I (DEA no. 7260)

USA Availability: Illegal to possess

Pregnancy Category: None

Uses. This drug comes from roots of an equatorial African rainforest shrub called *Tabernanthe iboga*. Traditionally the natural product has been used in low doses as a mild stimulant, rather like **coca** or **areca nut**, to fight hunger, thirst, and weariness and also to improve confidence. The natural product's active ingredient ibogaine was found in 1901. Its stimulant qualities gave it a potential role in Western medicine as a means of treating nervous exhaustion and generally helping sick persons recover from worn-down states. The drug was also viewed as a treatment for influenza and for illness caused by microscopic animals called Trypanosmatina protozoa. None of those applications received wide use. Ibogaine is, however, used as an aphrodisiac and has also seen illicit duty as a performance-enhancing substance in athletics.

In strong dosages ibogaine has been a component of African religious life. In that context the substance is used in its natural product format for meditation and to facilitate divine communication. Users may see rainbows around objects, lose barriers between senses (allowing sounds to be tasted, smells to be heard), and experience hallucinations. Fatal overdose is possible.

Drawbacks. Suspicion exists that ibogaine harms brain function in humans. Rat experiments show that high doses of ibogaine can injure some types of brain cells but that lower doses do not cause such damage. High dosage has caused body tremors and heartbeat trouble in rats. Rat experiments also show that the drug can impair emotions, reaction times, and ability to move.

Abuse factors. Some persons trying to break drug addiction claim that ibogaine drastically reduces craving for **heroin**, **cocaine**, and other opioids and stimulants. Switching an abuser from one drug to another one is routine in substance abuse treatment, but supposedly just one ingestion of ibogaine is enough to stop another drug's withdrawal symptoms and to diminish craving for it, with no need to keep taking ibogaine. Scientific efforts to verify such claims were under way while this book was being written. Verification would make ibogaine unique in the history of substance abuse treatment and would also challenge much of what is known about why people abuse drugs.

Ibogaine was given to 33 heroin addicts who did not reside in a treatment center; 25 of them exhibited no effort to obtain heroin during the four days of subsequent observation. These 33 experiences were not, however, part of an experimental study but instead were individual instances noted from time to time over a 31-year period, an overall average of about one instance per year. A group of researchers reported that ibogaine not only suppressed desire for heroin and cocaine among residents being weaned off those drugs in a treatment facility but that ibogaine made the people less depressed as well— an improvement in mood that was still present 30 days after release from treatment. In another study 7 opiate addicts received a single dose of ibogaine. Although 1 addict shortly resumed opiate use, 3 avoided further opiate use for several weeks, and 3 avoided further drug abuse for at least 14 weeks. None of the 7 experienced an opiate withdrawal syndrome. Ibogaine reduces intake of **alcohol**, cocaine, heroin, **morphine**, **nicotine**, food, and water by rats. Lowered consumption of food and water raises question about whether ibogaine is affecting drug consumption per se or is exerting some broader action. An ibogaine derivative, however, reduces rats' drug intake without reducing water intake.

Results are inconsistent on whether the drug improves or impedes learning in rats, an effect related to memory. One theory holds ibogaine allows humans to remember why they started using drugs, thereby helping abusers to stop. The instant results claimed for ibogaine, however, are inconsistent with the time necessary for memories to liberate persons from other psychiatric afflictions. And the memory theory also assumes that the reason an abuser started using drugs was either invalid in the past or is no longer valid in the present, an assumption inconsistent with much that is known about drug abuse. Nor does the memory theory explain why ibogaine reduces drug consumption in rats. The memory aspect is commonly mentioned by users, however, and some claim to achieve major positive realignment of their lives through ibogaine-induced insights into past experiences and allegorical interpretations of hallucinations. Nonetheless, some heroin addicts who initially announced themselves cured by ibogaine did not find the change permanent and resumed heroin use. One report says the ibogaine cure lasted less than a month for about 25% of heroin addicts who received it, longer for others who received supplemental therapy and who were dedicated to changing their lives.

A curiosity about the use of ibogaine in addiction treatment is that reported doses range from 500 mg to 1,800 mg. One authority says 1,000 mg is typical. An amount of 200 mg is considered sufficient to cause hallucinations. Additional effects of 200 mg are described as nervousness (perhaps bordering on fear), unpleasant feelings in arms and legs, difficulty in muscular coordination, tremors with rapid and repeated contraction and relaxation of muscles, and inability to sleep. Nausea and vomiting are sometimes reported, along with so much uncomfortable sensitivity to light that people cover their eyes. Such unwanted actions might be publicized as substantial drawbacks in a street drug but receive little, if any, mention in reports where ibogaine is adminis-tered as an addiction treatment. Individual personality and the circumstance in which a drug is taken can, of course, make a big difference in effects. So perhaps massive doses of ibogaine do not affect addicts in the same way that people are affected outside a therapeutic context.

Drug interactions. In rat experiments alcohol raised ibogaine's effects.

Cancer. Not enough scientific information to report.

Pregnancy. Not enough scientific information to report.

Additional information. "Iboga" is a nickname for **MDMA**, but they are not the same substance.

Additional scientific information may be found in:

Alper, K.R., D. Beal, and C.D. Kaplan. "A Contemporary History of Ibogaine in the United States and Europe." *The Alkaloids. Chemistry and Biology* 56 (2001): 249–81.

Mash, D.C., et al. "Ibogaine: Complex Pharmacokinetics, Concerns for Safety, and Pre-liminary Efficacy Measures." *Annals of the New York Academy of Sciences* 914 (2000): 394–401.

Mash, D.C., et al. "Medication Development of Ibogaine as a Pharmacotherapy for Drug Dependence." *Annals of the New York Academy of Sciences* 844 (1998): 274–92.

Popik, P., and S.D. Glick. "Ibogaine." *Drugs of the Future* 21 (1996): 1109–15.

Popik, P., R.T. Layer, and P. Skolnick. "100 Years of Ibogaine: Neurochemical and Pharmacological Actions of a Putative Anti-Addictive Drug." *Pharmacological Reviews* 47 (1995): 235–53.

Jimson Weed

Pronunciation: JIM-sn weed

Chemical Abstracts Service Registry Number: 8063-18-1

Formal Names: Datura, *Datura stramonium*

Informal Names: Angel Tulip, Devil's Apple, Devil's Trumpet, Green Dragon, Jamestown Weed, Locoweed, Mad Apple, Malpitte, Nightshade, Peru Apple, Sacred Datura, Stinkweed, Stinkwort, Thorn Apple

Type: Hallucinogen. *See* page 25

Federal Schedule Listing: Unlisted

USA Availability: Uncontrolled natural product

Pregnancy Category: None

Uses. This bad-smelling plant grows around the world in temperate and subtropical climates and thrives without cultivation. Jimson weed can cause hallucinations and has been a component of witches' potions and shaman experiences. Archaeological evidence exists for prehistoric spiritual use in North America, and accounts exist of such usage by native peoples into the twentieth century. Jimson weed is biologically related to several food plants including potato, pepper, eggplant, and tomato. Someone was able to graft a tomato plant onto jimson weed, with the resulting fruit so potent that consumers were hospitalized; one account described the incident as apparently "the first known instance of hallucinogenic tomatoes."

Effects are similar to those of **belladonna**. Drugs found in jimson weed leaves, flowers, and seeds include atropine, hyoscyamine, and scopolamine, which are often called "belladonna alkaloids." Folk medicine preparations from jimson weed flowers are put on bruises, wounds, or insect bites to diminish discomfort; leaves and roots are used in a similar way and also to treat boils. A drink from the plant is given to help people endure the pain of setting broken bones. Inhaling jimson weed smoke is a traditional remedy for asthma, sore breathing, or coughing. Vapor from boiling the substance is used for the same purposes. Scientific measurement has confirmed that jimson weed smoke improves airway function of asthmatics. The natural product is also a treatment against cramps, eye inflammation, and feverish infection. The plant has been used as an aphrodisiac.

Drawbacks. Jimson weed has anticholinergic actions, meaning it can change heartbeat, affect eyesight (including extreme and prolonged dilation of pupils), and halt progress of material through the intestines. Jimson weed should be avoided by persons with heart trouble, glaucoma, or slow bowels. Other body signs indicating that Jimson weed should be avoided include enlarged prostate, urination difficulty, fluid buildup in lung tissue, and obstruction that impedes movement of food from the stomach. The substance can raise blood pressure and body temperature while drying mucous membranes. Persons hospitalized following jimson weed ingestion have shown a flushed face, exaggerated reflexes, other reflexes consistent with a poison acting upon the brain, and changes involving prothrombin (a factor in blood clotting). Paranoia may be present. More than one report about jimson weed describes users with a saying such as this: "Blind as a bat, hot as a hare, dry as a bone, red as a beet, mad as a hatter, the bowel and bladder lose their tone, and the heart runs alone."

Fever and breathing difficulty may occur after using jimson weed. People can become fidgety and even manic, talk continuously, go into delirium (which may be combative), and fall into an exhausted sleep. Reportedly such responses to the plant inspired medical use in past times against epilepsy and psychotic behavior. The atropine component of jimson weed is powerful enough to agitate an elephant.

Intoxicated persons can be unaware of what they are doing and unaware of what is going on around them, additional hazards on top of the drug's sometimes dangerous physical effects. As with other substances accidental dosage can occur. Cases are documented of agricultural workers and gardeners being affected by apparently rubbing their eyes after contact with jimson weed or other datura plants; a case report also exists of absorption through the skin. Contamination of food is known, and unsuspecting persons have used wine and honey made from the plants. Rats on a 90-day diet including jimson weed seed experienced lower cholesterol levels, less weight gain, and increased weight of livers. Investigators running the experiment described the consequences of chronic jimson weed seed diet as undesirable, but of course humans do not eat the seeds as a regular food. In this experiment female rats were more affected by jimson weed than males. Jimson seed meal has also been found to harm development of chickens. Horses, cattle, and pigs react badly to jimson weed, but rabbits and sheep are relatively unaffected.

Abuse factors. Europeans were using *Datura* plants such as jimson weed in the 1500s; one account from that era mentions long-lasting intoxication with emotions ranging from euphoria to weeping, with people having amnesia about what they did while under the influence. The same account mentions prostitutes using *Datura* to make clients more pliable, and old reports speak of sexual frenzy induced by the substance. During the 1600s soldiers sent to suppress Bacon's Rebellion in colonial Virginia partook of jimson weed, and according to an account dating from 1722, some were incapacitated for days: "One would blow up a Feather in the Air; another would dart Straws at it with much Fury; and another stark naked was sitting up in a Corner, like a Monkey, grinning and making Mows [grimaces] at them; and a Fourth would fondly kiss, and paw his Companions, and snear [*sic*] in their Faces."[1] Such incidents still occurred in the twentieth century. In a three-week period during 1980 almost two dozen U.S. Marines at Camp Pendleton were treated for hallucinations from recreational jimson weed usage. A few years earlier a survey of drug users in the South African military found about 3% to be using jimson weed. U.S. military personnel have been known to "accidentally" inject themselves with the jimson weed component atropine, on hand as a nerve gas antidote but also able to create hallucinations.

Some jimson weed users describe sensations of flying, instant travel between one city and another, and communication with plants and inanimate objects. Although insects are a commonly reported visual hallucination from jimson weed, one uncommon sensation is a feeling of crawling insects, reminiscent of the "coke bugs" hallucination associated with **cocaine**. Jimson weed experiences have sometimes been likened to those from **LSD**, but reasons for that comparison are unapparent from accounts given by users of those substances. Both may be hallucinogens, but users relate very different observations. Descriptions of jimson weed experiences often have an ominous tone and lack LSD qualities such as striking down barriers between senses (hearing colors, seeing sounds). In keeping with an old but largely abandoned tradition of medicine, an articulate medical journal author engaged in *Datura* self-experimentation and produced a graphic account of interactions with charms of nineteenth-century Paris and with horrors of twentieth-century monsters. A witness later "told me that I fought the restraining devices so violently that he thought every blood vessel in my face and neck would explode."[2] The researcher did not repeat the experiment.

Drug interactions. Not enough scientific information to report.

Cancer. The Ames test, a standard laboratory procedure that screens substances for carcinogenicity, indicates jimson weed seeds have potential for causing cancer.

Pregnancy. Datura plants are suspected of causing birth defects in farm animals. Birth defects did not become more common in children of 450 pregnant women who received the atropine component of jimson weed. The same lack of effect on congenital abnormalities was observed in a similar number of pregnancies after the women used the scopolamine component of jimson weed, a finding consistent with a rodent study.

Additional information. Jimson weed is botanically classified as the *stramonium* species of the *Datura* genus. Other *Datura* genus plants around the world are used for similar effects, but they are not jimson weed.

Additional scientific information may be found in:

DiGiacomo, J.N. "Toxic Effect of *Stramonium* Simulating LSD Trip." *Journal of the American Medical Association* 204 (1968): 265–66.

Gowdy, J.M. "*Stramonium* Intoxication: Review of Symptomatology in 212 Cases." *Journal of the American Medical Association* 221 (1972): 585–87.

Jacobs, K.W. "Asthmador: Legal Hallucinogen." *International Journal of the Addictions* 9 (1974): 503–12.

Johnson, C.E. "Mystical Force of the Nightshade." *International Journal of Neuropsychiatry* 3 (1967): 268–75.

Keeler, M.H., and Kane, F.J., Jr. "The Use of Hyoscyamine as a Hallucinogen and Intoxicant." *American Journal of Psychiatry* 124 (1967): 852–54.

Thabet, H., et al. *"Datura Stramonium* Poisonings in Humans." *Veterinary and Human Toxicology* 41 (1999): 320–21.

Tiongson, J. "Mass Ingestion of Jimson Weed by Eleven Teenagers." *Delaware Medical Journal* 70 (1998): 471–76.

Notes

1. [R. Beverley], *The History of Virginia, in Four Parts*, 2nd ed. (London: F. Fayram and J. Clarke and T. Bickerton, 1772), 121.

2. C.E. Johnson, "Mystical Force of the Nightshade," *International Journal of Neuropsychiatry* 3 (1967): 272.

Ketamine

Pronunciation: KEET-a-meen

Chemical Abstracts Service Registry Number: 6740-88-1. (Hydrochloride form 1867-66-9)

Formal Names: Ketaject, Ketalar, Ketanest, Ketavet

Informal Names: Bump, Cat Valium, Green, Honey Oil, Jet, K, Kay, Kay-Blast, Kay Jay, Keets, Keller, Kellys Day, Ket, Kit Kat, Mauve, Purple, Rockmesc, Special K, Special LA Coke, Super Acid, Super C, Super K, Vitamin K

Type: Depressant. *See* page 19

Federal Schedule Listing: Schedule III (DEA no. 7285)

USA Availability: Prescription

Pregnancy Category: C

Uses. Ketamine is related to **PCP** and can produce a false-positive urine test for that substance. In contrast to the violent reputation of PCP, however, ketamine users are described as peaceful. Ketamine is likened to PCP, **alcohol**, and **LSD**—rather vague comparisons given the differences among those drugs. The substance was invented in the 1960s and was used as an anesthetic for Vietnam War combat casualties; it has been routinely used for war injuries ever since. Third World physicians report the drug is safe for surgical use outside high-tech environments. It is given as a pain reliever and, less commonly, to reduce convulsions. Ketamine is also a veterinary anesthesia drug used with wild animals ranging from giraffes and gazelles to polar bears and arctic foxes.

Success has been reported with using ketamine to supplement alcoholism therapy. Two researchers reported that ketamine therapy with 42 alcoholics produced a two-year abstinence from drinking in 15 of them, an outstanding result. Other researchers report one-year abstinence in almost 66% of 111 alcoholics who received ketamine therapy (perhaps a single dose), as opposed to 24% in 100 who did not receive ketamine. Among the 111 in the original group, 81 were tracked for two years, and 40% of the 81 remained abstinent. Of 42 who were tracked for three years, 33% remained abstinent.[1] Such results have prompted researchers to speculate that ketamine may also be useful in treating addiction to drugs other than alcohol. These reported beneficial effects of ketamine are surprising. Admittedly they are related to self-insights prompted by the substance and guided by psychotherapists, but in principle a single dose of a drug is unlikely to stop addiction to some other drug.

Experiments indicate ketamine may have potential for treating migraine headache and depression, and researchers have seen evidence that ketamine may improve asthma and shrink breast cancer cells. Ketamine can reduce phantom limb pain, a strange affliction in which a person senses that an amputated limb is still present and hurting. The drug has been used in psychotherapy to help persons face and deal with unpleasant memories, a process accompanied by what researchers described as "mind expanding effects." Ketamine has also been investigated as a potential defense against the chemical warfare agents soman and diisopropylphosphorofluoridate.

Healthy volunteers receiving ketamine in an experiment have experienced sensations reminiscent of LSD. Researchers have described such effects as "profound" among alcoholics, and illicit ketamine users have said such effects are "intense." The substance can prompt people to feel like they are becoming transparent, blending into nearby individuals, or becoming an animal or object. Users may feel like their bodies are transforming into harder or softer substances. Persons may think they remember experiences from a past life. Some users take the drug to enter the "K-hole," a semiparalytic state described as similar to near-death experiences in which people perceive their consciousness as floating above their bodies, sometimes accompanied by meaningful hallucinations and by insights about the user's life and its proper place in the cosmos.

Examination of deaths among recreational ketamine users in New York City in a two-year period during the 1990s found none in which ketamine was the only substance in the person's body. Children have accidentally been given 5 to 100 times the normal size dose and have survived with no apparent injury.

Drawbacks. A case report tells of recreational users experiencing temporary paralysis. Nausea and vomiting have been reported, and scientific literature contains several mentions of temporary breathing interruption caused by the drug. Increased pressure within the eye (a potential problem for glaucoma sufferers) has been measured following a ketamine dose, but not all researchers looking for that effect have found it. The drug can interfere with a male's physical ability to engage in sexual activity. Experiments show that ketamine can cause brain damage in rats and that simultaneous use of **nitrous oxide** worsens the damaging action. Ketamine can cause nervous agitation, extra salivation, blood pressure elevation, abnormal heartbeat, and muscle injury. Persons suffering from the body chemistry disorder porphyria should exercise caution about ketamine use.

The drug can change perceptions of one's surroundings. Tests indicate ketamine can alter visual perception for at least 24 hours, causing people to misjudge size and speed of objects (implying that driving skills may be impaired). Long-term use may cause persistent difficulties with attention, memory, and learning ability. The substance can create amnesia about what happens while a person is under the drug's influence.

Ketamine's psychological actions have been characterized as similar to temporary schizophrenia. A study examining persons who received the drug during surgery found that upon awakening some felt they were floating; some were euphoric; some screamed in apparent terror. A study found such effects to be twice as common in female patients as in males. Such effects are stronger among alcohol abusers. The floating sensation may occur as people regain consciousness before they regain sense of touch, a sequence that would temporarily eliminate awareness of gravity. One surgery patient experienced LSD-like effects that continued even after release from the hospital. Reports exist of patients experiencing psychological effects for a year after a dose. A reviewer who examined many years of scientific reports about ketamine, however, found a consensus that long-term psychological consequences from ketamine occur no more frequently than with other anesthetics—a conclusion about incidental effects from anesthetic use, not about deliberate effects induced as part of psychotherapy or illicit use.

One authority claims that the greatest physical hazard has a psychological base, as users sometimes become indifferent about death and take risks they would otherwise avoid. Persons intoxicated with ketamine may be woozy and have lower perception of pain, conditions that can cause or worsen accidents.

Female lemmings are more susceptible to the drug than males. While the male-female difference does not necessarily carry over to humans, use of ketamine's anesthetic properties by sexual predators seeking to weaken victims was publicized in the 1990s. Researchers using the drug to treat alcoholism have found that ketamine makes a person more susceptible to suggestions, perhaps making a person more vulnerable to manipulation.

Abuse factors. Tolerance and dependence can develop when rats and mice receive ketamine. Those traditional signs of addictive potential seem unconfirmed in human use, but people have been known to take the drug daily for no medical purpose and to feel they have a problem with that usage.

Drug interactions. In surgery patients administering **diazepam** simultaneously with ketamine has diminished unwanted psychological effects such as delirium and nightmares. **Midazolam** may also help.

In experimentation with rats and mice the actions of ketamine and alcohol have similarities, and the two have cross-tolerance (meaning one can substitute for the other in various ways). Human alcoholics report that ketamine produces sensations like those of alcohol. A small study found that ketamine has stronger effects on perceptions and thinking skills in alcoholics than in other persons.

In rats **morphine** can boost some pain relief from ketamine, and ketamine can reduce pain relief from morphine. In contrast, a human experiment found that patients needed less morphine for pain relief if they also received ketamine. In humans ketamine can boost opiate and barbiturate actions so much as to be fatal. **Lorazepam** can boost the sedative and amnesia qualities of ketamine in humans.

Cancer. Not enough scientific information to report.

Pregnancy. Experimentation on mice shows that birth defects can occur when ketamine and **cocaine** are used together, but the impact of just ketamine seems uncertain. Experiments on pregnant rats, rabbits, and dogs have produced no harm. Ketamine has harmed hamster genes when they are experimented upon outside the body. Research published as the twenty-first century began indicated that the drug may harm fetal brain development in humans.

Citing possible danger to fetus survival, one authority recommends caution about using ketamine as an anesthetic in childbirth. While the drug may pass into breast milk, nursing is considered safe for infants.

Additional scientific information may be found in:

Corrigan, I.J. "Ketamine—A New Anesthetic." *Canadian Nurse* 68 (April 1972): 43–44.

Curran, H.V., and C. Morgan. "Cognitive, Dissociative and Psychotogenic Effects of Ketamine in Recreational Users on the Night of Drug Use and 3 Days Later."*Addiction* 95 (2000): 575–90.

Hetem, L.A., et al. "Effect of a Subanesthetic Dose of Ketamine on Memory and Conscious Awareness in Healthy Volunteers." *Psychopharmacology* 152 (2000): 283–38.

Jansen, K.L. "A Review of the Nonmedical Use of Ketamine: Use, Users and Consequences." *Journal of Psychoactive Drugs* 32 (2000): 419–33.

Krupitsky, E.M., and A.Y. Grinenko. "Ketamine Psychedelic Therapy (KPT): A Review of the Results of Ten Years of Research." *Journal of Psychoactive Drugs* 29 (1997): 165–83.

Weiner, A.L., et al. "Ketamine Abusers Presenting to the Emergency Department: A Case Series." *Journal of Emergency Medicine* 18 (2000): 447–51.

Note

1. E.M. Krupitsky and A.Y. Grinenko. "Ketamine Psychedelic Therapy (KPT): A Review of the Results of Ten Years of Research." *Journal of Psychoactive Drugs* 29 (1997): 165–83; I.P. Sivolap and V.A. Savchenkov. "Opyt Primeneniia Preparatov Ketamina v Psikhoterapii Alkogolizma [Experience in Using Ketamine Preparations in the Psychotherapy of Alcoholism]." *Zhurnal Nevropatologii i Psikhiatrii Imeni S.S. Korsakova* 94 (1994): 76–79. (Abstract in English.)

Ketobemidone

Pronunciation: KEET-ah-behm-ih-dohn

Chemical Abstracts Service Registry Number: 469-79-4

Formal Names: Cetobemidone, Ketogan

Type: Depressant (opioid class). *See* page 24

Federal Schedule Listing: Schedule I (DEA no. 9628)

USA Availability: Illegal to possess

Pregnancy Category: None

Uses. This substance has no authorized medical use in the United States. Elsewhere, since the 1950s it has been used as a pain reliever for surgery, cancer, and other conditions. Figures for total legal usage of opioids/opiates in Denmark from 1981 to 1993 showed only **morphine** and **methadone** were used more than ketobemidone.

In an experiment ketobemidone caused less breathing difficulty than did **buprenorphine** (another opioid used for pain relief). Patients who receive morphine chronically may develop muscle twitches and experience more pain rather than less. After studying that problem one group of researchers recommended that such patients be switched to ketobemidone, methadone, sufentanil, or **fentanyl**. A case report indicates ketobemidone works in such a switch. Despite the drug's usefulness for pain relief, test results conflict on whether it is better than a placebo for easing anxiety before surgery.

Drawbacks. Unwanted effects include shivering, coughing, nausea, and vomiting. Pain may cause vomiting, so paradoxically ketobemidone can also prevent vomiting through pain relief. A study noted that ketobemidone lowers blood pressure, but not as much as morphine does.

Abuse factors. Although illicit use of this drug has received little attention in the United States, ketobemidone has been a prominent substance in the abuse scenes of Scandinavian countries. The drug is available in a pharmaceutical intravenous format, but some illicit users crush oral tablets containing ketobemidone and inject the powder. That practice is suspected of harming eyesight. The same practice can cause skin to harden around injection sites and also break open into sores. In one report of several such cases medical personnel expressed puzzlement that the ketobemidone users acted like they felt no discomfort and were unconcerned about skin conditions that would prompt most persons to seek immediate medical aid. Such indifference about physical well-being is typical among individuals engaged in self-destruction. A study of ketobemidone overdose deaths in Denmark was revealing in that respect as well; victims often had blood **alcohol** levels that would be fatal in themselves.

Drug interactions. A study comparing commercial intravenous pharmaceutical formats found morphine to be only half as strong as a combination product containing one part ketobemidone and five parts of a drug called A29. The latter drug is used to fight spasms. Experiments with rats and mice indicate that A29 boosts ketobemidone's pain-relieving effect, so the human research comparing the combination to morphine does not mean that ketobemidone alone is stronger than morphine. The same study did find, however, that when doses were adjusted for equivalent strength, the ketobemidone-A29 combination was still more effective at pain relief than morphine.

Cancer. Not enough scientific information to report.

Pregnancy. The drug passes into human milk. Based on a small number of cases involving 5,000 micrograms of ketobemidone given during childbirth, one study estimated that breast-fed infants would receive under 2 micrograms of ketobemidone from their first day's milk.

Additional scientific information may be found in:

Kjaer, M., et al. "Bioavailability and Analgesic Effect of Sustained Release Cetobemidone Capsules in Cancer Patients with Chronic Pain of Malignant Origin." *Acta Oncologica* (Stockholm, Sweden) 31 (1992): 577–83.

Ohqvist, G., et al. "A Comparison between Morphine, Meperidine and Ketobemidone in Continuous Intravenous Infusion for Postoperative Relief." *Acta Anaesthesiologica Scandinavica* 35 (1991): 44–48.

Steentoft, A., and K. Worm. "Cases of Fatal Intoxication with Ketogan." *Journal—Forensic Science Society* 34 (July–September 1994): 181–85.

Wolff, T., et al. "Analgesic Treatment in Acute Myocardial Infarction. A Double-Blind Comparison of Ketobemidone + the Spasmolytic A29 (Ketogan) and Morphine." *Acta Medica Scandinavica* 223 (1988): 423–30.

Khat

Pronunciation: kaht

Chemical Abstracts Service Registry Number: 71031-15-7 (cathinone component); 492-39-7 (cathine component)

Formal Names: *Catha edulis*

Informal Names: Abyssinian Tea, Arabian Tea, Goob, Jaad, Miraa, Qaad, Qat, Shat, Somali Tea

Type: Stimulant (amphetamine class). *See* page 12

Federal Schedule Listing: Schedule I (cathinone DEA no. 1235); Schedule IV (cathine DEA no. 1230)

USA Availability: Illegal to possess

Pregnancy Category: None

Uses. Although amphetamine is a laboratory creation and not a natural product, the khat plant is likened to a "natural amphetamine" due to the actions of the two scheduled substances found in it, cathinone and cathine. Because one of them is listed in Schedule I the plant is illegal to possess even though all other chemicals in it are legal. Cross-tolerance exists among amphetamine, cathinone, and cathine. One thorough chemical analysis of khat found that the natural product also contains **ephedrine**.

Khat has the same psychological effects as those associated with amphetamine, both positive and negative. An additional effect can be vivid hallucinations as people hover between wakefulness and sleep. In contrast to job performance benefits observed with true amphetamines, airplane crew members who use khat are found to have poorer visual memory and decision-reaction times when compared with nonusers. The substance is nonetheless used as a stimulant assisting physical labor, much as **coca** leaves are traditionally used in South America.

The shrub is mainly found in countries along the Red Sea and Indian Ocean region of eastern and northeastern Africa. Leaves are traditionally harvested in the morning and wrapped to slow their drying. Potency declines as they dry out. The main active component cathinone transforms into the less-active component cathine over time, reducing the strength of a particular batch of khat. That factor formerly limited the product's availability, but modern transportation and freezer technology allows khat to be exported around the world. The product has been a major cash crop in Ethiopia. Sometimes khat is used as a tea or in a paste format, but just like coca, users generally chew the leaves while (in the delicate phrase of one scientist) "rejecting the residues." Some people simultaneously drink sweet beverages to mask khat's bitter flavor. The natural product's potency is mild enough that dangerous overdose is unlikely. During the aftermath of the Persian Gulf War in the 1990s, concern was expressed that American military personnel in that region might use khat instead of beverage **alcohol**.

Although khat has no approved medical use in the United States, elsewhere it is used against depression, stomach problems, headaches, coughs, as a mild stimulant, appetite suppressant, bronchodilator, aphrodisiac, and as a gonorrhea remedy. An antiinflammatory compound has been found in the natural product. Khat raises body temperature, breathing rate, blood pressure, heart action, and muscle tension.

Drawbacks. Khat promotes constipation and may damage kidneys and liver. When fed to rabbits, khat lowers their vitamin C levels. The substance can raise diabetics' blood sugar.

Despite theoretical possibilities for afflictions, investigation of khat use in North Yemen discovered little or no evidence of physical harm. Some researchers find better dental health among persons who regularly chew khat, but other researchers find the opposite (such results suggest that khat may be an "invalid variable" actually having no impact). Investigators in London attributed very few illnesses to khat in a group of 162 users. Tuberculosis may be the main physical peril from khat, not from the substance itself but from disregard of Western hygiene in social use of the drug (spitting around, sharing a water pipe). Khat psychosis is rare, probably because of the natural product's relatively low strength. In two Israeli villages the mental illness rate for users was no worse than for nonusers; the same was found in Liverpool, England.

Abuse factors. Known as the "flower of paradise," khat has wide recreational use in countries of its traditional origin: A survey of over 10,000 Ethiopian villagers found that half were currently using the substance; a survey of Ethiopian high school students found a still higher percentage of users. In cultures where khat usage originated, it is a social drug used to lubricate conversation. Users feel more alert and confident and even a little contentious, making for lively gatherings. Persons who have a troubled relationship with khat are generally persons who disregard social customs about it. For example, users will feel a letdown as the drug wears off. People who use khat in its traditional social context are likely to experience that letdown as simply part of a genial gathering breaking up as members go about their individual business and are unlikely to have interest in taking more khat right then. Someone alone in an apartment who feels let down may see more khat as the answer instead of more friends. Also, using a drug in a social context differing from its traditional one can cause trouble. People who use khat at all-night high-energy rave dance parties are unlikely to experience the same sensations as are found in an intimate circle of mutually trusting acquaintances who interact with each other in daily life.

Despite khat's well-documented stimulant properties, the substance is considered a threat to economic productivity in countries where it has long tradition of use. The "threat" probably has less to do with chemistry and more to do with khat's traditional societal role—helping people pass time genially while they sit around and visit.

Around a century ago famed novelist Theodore Dreiser wrote a short story "Khat" about using the substance. The story is an atmospheric portrayal of the drug's cultural context, how khat aided the functioning of a society that had become archaic by the year 2000. The story is told from the perspective of a beggar, and ironically, the society that despised the beggar is now itself despised by Western modernists who condemn khat. A drug viewed as benevolent by a disappearing world is viewed as a threat in a new world possessing different values. Yet nothing about khat's chemistry has changed.

Tolerance appears to develop to some khat effects, such as elevations in pulse rate, blood pressure, body temperature, and respiration rate.

Drug interactions. The substance can interfere with amoxycillin and ampicillin antibiotics.

Cancer. A study searching for a link between khat chewing and precancerous conditions in the mouth found none, but some researchers feel the habit promotes oral cancer, and others suspect that khat causes cancer of the esophagus and stomach.

Pregnancy. Researchers have concluded that khat harms human sperm. Experiments on mice indicate that khat lowers male fertility and promotes fetal death from matings by those males. Rat experiments on females demonstrate that khat can cause fetal death and birth defects. Women who chew khat leaves tend to deliver lower-weight babies, but no birth defects were observed in infants from a sample of over 500 pregnant khat users. Nursing mothers can pass a psychoactive khat chemical into their milk, and the chemical can be measured in an infant's urine.

Additional information. Khat's main effects are attributed to the presence of the illegal drug cathinone (also called norephedrone), which is similar to **dextroamphetamine** and can be manufactured in a laboratory. Volunteers taking cathinone show higher blood pressure and pulse rate, feel pepped up, and have a brightened mood. Scientists believe the substance has pain-relieving properties when given to rats. Animal experiments indicate the drug has 50% or more of amphetamine's strength and that **caffeine** has a multiplier effect, boosting the impact of a cathinone dose. Animal experiments find no aphrodisiac qualities in cathinone but do find that it lowers **testosterone** levels and harms sperm and testes. Compared to the natural product khat, the pure laboratory drug has much more potential for harm. People can chew wads of khat for hours and get no more than mild effects, but a person using the pharmaceutical product can experience a much more powerful dose in an instant.

Khat also contains cathine. Cathine's effects are similar to cathinone but so much weaker that khat users disdain old leaves that have lost cathinone but still retain cathine. Laboratories can make cathine. The compound has been known to produce cranial tics (uncontrollable jerking of the head) among persons using it for weight loss. The drug has been found in **ma huang** food supplements. A professional athlete was disqualified from competition after consuming such a supplement without knowing it was cathine laced.

"Khat" is a nickname for **MDMA**, but they are not the same substance. Additional scientific information may be found in:

Brenneisen, R., et al. "Amphetamine-Like Effects in Humans of the Khat Alkaloid Cathinone." *British Journal of Clinical Pharmacology* 30 (1990): 825–28.

Kalix, P. "Cathinone, a Natural Amphetamine." *Pharmacology and Toxicology* 70 (1992): 77–86.

Kalix, P. "Khat, an Amphetamine-Like Stimulant." *Journal of Psychoactive Drugs* 26 (1994): 69–74.

Khattab, N.Y., and G. Amer. "Undetected Neuropsychophysiological Sequelae of Khat Chewing in Standard Aviation Medical Examination." *Aviation, Space, and Environmental Medicine* 66 (1995): 739–44.

Krikorian, A.D. "Kat and Its Use: An Historical Perspective." *Journal of Ethnopharmacology* 12 (November 1984): 115–78.

Nencini, P., and A.M. Ahmed. "Khat Consumption: A Pharmacological Review." *Drug and Alcohol Dependence* 23 (1989): 19–29.

Nencini, P., A.M. Ahmed, and A.S. Elmi. "Subjective Effects of Khat Chewing in Humans." *Drug and Alcohol Dependence* 18 (1986): 97–105.

LAAM

Pronunciation: ehl-ā-ā-ehm
Chemical Abstracts Service Registry Number: 1477-40-3. (Hydrochloride form 43033-72-3)
Formal Names: Levo-Alpha-Acetylmethadol, Levo-alphacetylmethadol, Levome-thadyl acetate, Orlaam
Type: Depressant (opioid class). *See* page 24
Federal Schedule Listing: Schedule II (DEA no. 9648)
USA Availability: Prescription
Pregnancy Category: C

Uses. LAAM has pain-relieving qualities, but its main medical use is for treatment of opiate/opioid addiction, typically switching addicts from illegal **heroin** to the legal substance LAAM.

Drawbacks. LAAM can produce heartbeat irregularity, and although this unwanted action has not been known to harm users, it is a factor in deciding between LAAM or **methadone** for drug addiction treatment. When used for addiction therapy LAAM is generally considered to produce no significant reduction in alertness, but persons new to the drug or who take high doses are told to be careful about engaging in dangerous activity such as driving a car. One study involving over 600 users found weariness to be a frequent undesired LAAM effect, also constipation, abdominal discomfort, anxiety, perspiration, and decreased male sexual ability. In one study scientists found that **testosterone** measurements in males declined to levels below normal when those persons used LAAM, but another study showed no change. In one study euphoria was an unusual effect, but another study typically found LAAM users to be "slightly euphoric" in comparison to methadone users. Researchers have noted aggressiveness in monkeys taking LAAM, but that effect is unconfirmed in humans. Rodent experiments measuring food intake have produced conflicting results showing increased, unchanged, and decreased appetite. One human study reported no appetite change in LAAM users.

Because oral LAAM's long-lasting effects are slow to start, some illicit users have taken more and more of the drug in order to feel expected effects and then died from a cumulative fatal overdose when LAAM's full actions finally kicked in.

Abuse factors. In drug abuse treatment programs, some addicts prefer

LAAM, and some prefer methadone. LAAM is related to methadone and is generally considered weaker, but some research has found LAAM stronger in certain ways. A dose of LAAM can last three times as long as one from methadone, making LAAM more convenient for addicts in a treatment program, as they can come less often to the clinic to receive LAAM than if they were receiving methadone. Convenience can influence an addict's decision on whether to continue with a program. Another LAAM advantage is that the long-lasting nature of a dose means that effects may be steadier over a given amount of time than those from methadone, allowing more consistent job performance by addicted employees. A case report mentions addicts who preferred LAAM over methadone because LAAM's steadiness reduced mood swings that occurred with methadone. One experiment, however, discovered that LAAM users are far more physically active on days when they receive the drug than on days when they don't—a finding that questions whether LAAM effects are as steady as commonly believed. Scientists know less about actions of LAAM than about those of methadone, so sometimes addicts with complicated medical conditions are given methadone instead of LAAM because methadone's influence on those conditions is better understood.

Experimentation with rhesus monkeys revealed that LAAM does not necessarily have uniform cross-tolerance with other opioids. Thus switching someone to LAAM from another opioid can be tricky; LAAM may closely match the other drug in some ways but not in others. For example, the same level of pain relief may be achieved by particular doses of LAAM or some other opioid, but those same doses will not necessarily affect breathing to the same extent.

LAAM is supposed to provide no drug high to persons on maintenance doses, but by definition a "maintenance" dose is only enough to hold off withdrawal symptoms and not enough to produce effects desired by drug misusers. So the lack of a high may be related to size of dose rather than to chemistry of the drug.

Dependence can develop.

Drug interactions. Because of oral LAAM's slow onset of effects, judging safe amounts to take with other depressants can be perilous. **Alcohol** is considered especially risky to use with LAAM. **Phenobarbital** is suspected of altering the effectiveness of an LAAM dose, and the same suspicion holds for the epilepsy drugs carbamazepine and phenytoin, the tuberculosis medicine rifampin, and the antacid-ulcer drug cimetidine.

Cancer. LAAM's potential for causing cancer is unknown. Data from laboratory tests are inconclusive. One two-year test of the drug on rats and mice produced no evidence of cancer, but another two-year test yielded some evidence of liver cancer in rats. A human LAAM study looking for chromosome mutations, which can lead to cancer, found none. Another human study found no evidence of tumor development.

Pregnancy. LAAM's impact on fetal development is unknown, but concern is high enough that women of childbearing age are supposed to have monthly pregnancy tests while on LAAM and to switch to methadone if pregnancy occurs. Upon examining results from chicken and rat experiments, however, some researchers suspect that more fetal damage may occur by stopping exposure to LAAM than by continuing it, and there has been speculation about whether the same applies to humans. Abnormal breathing is seen in puppies that had lengthy fetal exposure to LAAM. Rat experiments have attributed no physical birth defects to LAAM, but some researchers suspect that fetal exposure to the drug affects offspring behavior. Animal experiments also indicate that even if LAAM causes no birth defects, risk of miscarriage may increase. If pregnant rats routinely receive LAAM, their offspring quickly show withdrawal symptoms upon birth (an event that stops exposure to the drug) even though the drug is long-lasting in adults and would not produce withdrawal symptoms in adults for quite some time after the last dose.

Additional information. Scientific literature often refers to LAAM as methadyl acetate, short for levo-alpha-acetylmethadol. "Methadyl acetate," however, is also the name of a Schedule I substance occasionally called acetylmethadol, and some scientific literature uses acetylmethadol as a synonym for LAAM. Even the CAS Registry Numbers of these substances get mixed up, with articles sometimes assigning CAS RN 509-74-0 to LAAM. Adding even more confusion, LAAM and the Schedule I substances acetylmethadol, alphacetylmethadol, and betacetylmethadol all have the same molecular formula (and Orlaam is similar but with the addition of hydrochloride). Persons using this book as a starting point for more research about LAAM should look carefully at other information sources to be sure which drug is being discussed.

Additional scientific information may be found in:

Finn, P., and K. Wilcock. "Levo-Alpha Acetyl Methadol (LAAM). Its Advantages and Drawbacks." *Journal of Substance Abuse Treatment* 14 (1997): 559–64.
Prendergast, M.L., et al. "Levo-Alpha-Acetylmethadol (LAAM): Clinical, Research, and Policy Issues of a New Pharmacotherapy for Opioid Addiction." *Journal of Psychoactive Drugs* 27 (1995): 239–47.
Rawson, R.A., et al. "A 3-Year Progress Report on the Implementation of LAAM in the United States." *Addiction* 93 (1998): 533–40.
Sorensen, J.L., W.A. Hargreaves, and J.A. Weinberg. "Heroin Addict Responses to Six Weeks of Detoxification with LAAM." *Drug and Alcohol Dependence* 9 (1982): 79–87.
Tennant, F.S., Jr., et al. "Clinical Experiences with 959 Opioid-Dependent Patients Treated with Levo-Alpha-Acetylmethadol (LAAM)." *Journal of Substance Abuse Treatment* 3 (1986): 195–202.

Levorphanol

Pronunciation: lee-VOR-fa-nohl

Chemical Abstracts Service Registry Number: 77-07-6. (Tartrate anhydrous form 125-72-4; tartrate dihydrate form 5985-38-6)

Formal Names: Levo-Dromoran

Type: Depressant (opioid class). *See* page 24

Federal Schedule Listing: Schedule II (DEA no. 9220)

USA Availability: Prescription

Pregnancy Category: C

Uses. Unlike many pain relievers, levorphanol's oral formulation has an effectiveness almost as good as the intravenous version. An animal experiment demonstrated the drug can work when simply rubbed on an area of the skin that is hurting; that capability is an asset because it avoids the necessity of having the substance circulate through the entire body when only a particular spot needs treatment. Even severe pain can be successfully treated with the drug, which is used for conditions ranging from surgery to cancer. Studies have likened it to **fentanyl**, **meperidine**, and **morphine**. Levorphanol is considered 4 to 15 times stronger than morphine. Pain control doses of levorphanol take effect at about the same speed as morphine but last longer. Prolonged administration of morphine can reverse pain relief action and instead increase discomfort, while at the same time causing muscle spasms; morphine patients can be switched to levorphanol to avoid those outcomes.

Drawbacks. Levorphanol can cause dangerous and even fatal breathing difficulty. For that reason medical personnel are supposed to carefully adjust dosage to a patient's individual needs rather than depend upon customary amounts of the drug being safe. It is supposed to be used with special caution in patients with asthma, low thyroid function, urinary difficulty, or an enlarged prostate. Wariness is also prudent when using the substance to reduce heart pain, because the drug's influence on cardiac function has not been confirmed. The substance can lower blood pressure and may produce nausea, vomiting, and constipation. Levorphanol can make users woozy and harm skills needed for operating a car or other dangerous machinery. Although levorphanol is a depressant in humans, it increases leg activity in ponies—an effect that may not have escaped notice by persons seeking ways to improve the animals' performance in races.

Abuse factors. Tolerance and dependence can develop. When dependent rats were given a choice between water and a sweetened solution of levorphanol, they preferred the drug solution, but when the choice was between the same drug solution and sweetened water they preferred the sweet water. When experimenters offered another set of dependent rats straight water and unsweetened levorphanol solution, those animals preferred straight water. Such results imply that the drug has a low addiction potential, but an implication is not a fact. Also, animals do not always react to a substance in the same way humans do.

In humans the drug can improve spirits and even produce euphoria, and some users say they became addicted. A rat experiment demonstrated partial cross-tolerance with **alcohol**, suggesting that the two drugs appeal to the same kinds of people.

Some employer drug testing cannot distinguish between levorphanol and **dextrorphan**.

Drug interactions. Simultaneous use of levorphanol with alcohol or other depressants increases the possibility of cumulative overdose. In mice the anesthetic lidocaine boosts levorphanol's pain relief actions. Antihistamines and monoamine oxidase inhibitors (MAOIs, found in some antidepressants and other medicine) should be avoided when taking levorphanol. Levorphanol can also be dangerous when taken with **alprazolam, diazepam, flurazepam, lorazepam, phenobarbital,** or **temazepam**.

Cancer. Levorphanol's potential for causing cancer is unknown.

Pregnancy. Mice experiments with the drug have caused pregnancy failures and birth defects. Offspring from male mice exposed to the drug weighed less than normal, were slower to mature, and had abnormal motions in water. The potential for similar outcomes with humans is unknown. Rabbit experiments show the drug passing into the fetus of a pregnant animal, reducing fetal respiration. Milk from a nursing mother who uses levorphanol is assumed to contain enough of the drug to cause unwanted effects in a nursing infant, but that possibility may be minimized by waiting long enough after a dose before nursing (the delay can allow much of the drug to wash out of the woman's body).

Additional scientific information may be found in:

Chernin, T. "Use of Opioids for Chronic Nonmalignant Pain." *Pharmacy Times* 65 (1999): 18–20, 23–25.

Coniam, S.W. "Withdrawal of Levorphanol." *Anaesthesia* 46 (1991): 518.

Friedler, G. "Effects of Limited Paternal Exposure to Xenobiotic Agents on the Development of Progeny." *Neurobehavioral Toxicology and Teratology* 7 (1985): 739–43.

Fuchs, V., and H. Coper. "Development of Dependence on Levorphanol in Rats by Oral Intake of the Drug—The Influence of Taste on Drinking Behaviour in Rats Physically Dependent on Levorphanol." *Drug and Alcohol Dependence* 6 (1980): 373–81.

Knych, E.T. "Cross-Tolerance between Ethanol and Levorphanol with Respect to Stimulation of Plasma Corticosterone." *Life Sciences* 31 (1982): 527–32.

Lorazepam

Pronunciation: lor-A-ze-pam
Chemical Abstracts Service Registry Number: 846-49-1
Formal Names: Ativan, Temesta
Type: Depressant (benzodiazepine class). *See* page 21
Federal Schedule Listing: Schedule IV (DEA no. 2885)
USA Availability: Prescription
Pregnancy Category: D

Uses. This antianxiety drug is also known for its sedative properties and is used to promote sleep and to fight convulsions. The substance is given to treat status epilepticus, a dangerous condition in which people have one epileptic seizure after another, back-to-back. It can reduce and sometimes even eliminate vomiting from cancer chemotherapy. Lorazepam has been used to treat **LSD** and **methamphetamine** overdose and has been a standard medicine to help alcoholics through the **alcohol** withdrawal syndrome. Recreational sedative users report euphoria from lorazepam. When given experimentally in combination with other drugs, it has helped reduce depression. In contrast, experimentation using motion picture excerpts to evoke particular emotions found that lorazepam may reduce happy feelings and increase unhappy ones. One study found that lorazepam worked as well as **alprazolam** for treating panic attacks, and a case report tells of success in treating mania. Lorazepam has been used to cure both catatonia (in which people are frozen in place) and akathisia (compulsive moving around). Patients being prepared for surgery receive the drug to calm them and to cloud their memory of the event.

Lorazepam is 5 times stronger than **diazepam** and 15 times stronger than **oxazepam**, and one experiment showed that lorazepam is 370 to 783 times stronger than **meprobamate** in producing some effects, ranging from degraded performance in tests to amount of liking for one drug or the other.

Relatively little research seems to be done on whether members of different races respond differently to the same drug. This type of uncommon study has been done with lorazepam. The work found that although doses lasted about as long in young Americans as in young Japanese, a dose lasted about 20% longer in elderly Japanese than in elderly Americans—and a dose lasted about 20% longer in elderly Americans than in young Americans, so the difference became quite noticeable in Japanese subjects. ("American" and "Japanese" are nationalities, not races, but the research description stated that the issue of racial effect was being investigated; so those nationality labels were intended to have racial connotations.)

Drawbacks. Partial amnesia is a typical effect of the substance, and after using it for several days, people may have trouble gaining new memories. Investigators have also found that the drug interferes with detecting whether information is correct, while simultaneously reducing a person's awareness of memory trouble. Occasionally lorazepam temporarily stops respiration, and people suffering from serious breathing trouble should avoid the substance. The same goes for persons with acute narrow-angle glaucoma. The drug can reduce body temperature and, depending on circumstances in experiments, either raise or lower heart rate and blood pressure.

Researchers find that the substance interferes with recognizing common items shown in distorted pictures; such trouble is considered evidence of the brain suffering from weakened ability to understand what the eyes see. A case report notes that lorazepam may impede movements of the mouth and face. The drug somewhat garbles speech. Because of adverse impact on mental clarity and physical performance, people are advised to avoid operating dangerous machinery (such as cars) for at least 48 hours after using lorazepam. Driving tests have shown the drug to reduce vehicle control skill while increasing risk-taking. Other tests demonstrate worsened attention, slower reaction time, and delay in reasoning out the solution to a problem. An experiment demonstrated that users may be unaware of how much the drug is interfering with their abilities. Dizziness and weakness may occur. Typically a dose has greater impact on the elderly, and all persons risk falling down until the drug wears off. A case report notes that lorazepam can eliminate a person's interest in sexual activity. An unusual case report tells of someone who was hearing noises in an ear, and the noises became musical hallucinations of popular songs when the person began taking lorazepam. More typically, however, the drug is able to stop auditory hallucinations. Other case reports tell of visual hallucinations after taking the compound, and that response was also observed in 3 children among 112 who were given the drug. Although lorazepam is used to reduce anxiety, case reports and formal experimentation show that the substance can increase aggressiveness (perhaps because people are less afraid to do things). A schizophrenic who received the drug lost enough inhibitions to start acting out violent impulses, and similar reports exist. In formal experimentation volunteers receiving lorazepam became more aggressive but did not realize they were angrier than other persons in the experiment.

Abuse factors. Various psychological tests measure how much a drug appeals to someone. Among persons who already have a history of drug abuse (a population prone to like drugs much more than nonusers do), some results indicate lorazepam has about the same addictive potential as diazepam or meprobamate; some results simply show lorazepam to have an unspecified amount of appeal; and in one experiment abusers found the drug about as attractive as a placebo (indicating low addictive potential). Rats begin exhibiting tolerance to lorazepam after several days of dosing. If a person takes lorazepam enough to develop dependence on it, suddenly quitting the drug can produce a withdrawal syndrome. If drug use has been heavy the withdrawal can include confusion, depression, perspiration, cramps, tremors, vomiting, mania, and convulsions. Lighter use can produce lighter withdrawal such as insomnia and generally feeling out of sorts. Symptoms can be avoided altogether if a person gradually takes smaller and smaller doses rather than stopping abruptly.

Drug interactions. Lorazepam generally makes people more susceptible to effects of alcohol. If a person taking lorazepam simultaneously ingests other depressants (alcohol, barbiturates, opiates) the total depressant effects deepen. Although we might expect stimulants to counteract lorazepam's actions, research has found that **cocaine** can boost some of them, with sleepiness becoming particularly greater. Thus cocaine users receiving lorazepam for medical treatment may require lower doses than normal.

Cancer. Mice and rat studies have not yielded evidence that lorazepam causes cancer.

Pregnancy. In mice lorazepam increases incidence of eyelid malformation and cleft palate. Mice having fetal exposure to lorazepam exhibit lasting neurochemistry abnormalities, and rats with fetal exposure demonstrate brain difficulty. Extrapolating from rat test results, two researchers concluded that fetal exposure to the drug may result in male offspring having more anxiety than normal and females having less than normal. Pregnant rabbits receiving lorazepam in an experiment produced more birth defects than usual. Persuasive evidence indicates that the drug passes from a pregnant woman into the fetus. The drug is not recommended for pregnant women unless the need is dire. Analysts examining thousands of medical records concluded that lorazepam does not necessarily cause birth defects but found that the drug may be involved with a deformity blocking an infant's anal opening. Fetal exposure to lorazepam is suspected of slowing development of infants' abilities to move and think. Case reports say that infants can have withdrawal symptoms if the mother used the drug during pregnancy, symptoms accompanied by abnormal muscle tone and trouble with eating. Nursing mothers are told to avoid lorazepam, as infants might be drugged from the amount of lorazepam that passes into milk.

Additional scientific information may be found in:

Bond, A., and M. Lader. "Differential Effects of Oxazepam and Lorazepam on Aggressive Responding." *Psychopharmacology* 95 (1988): 369–73.

Funderburk, F.R., et al. "Relative Abuse Liability of Lorazepam and Diazepam: An Evaluation in 'Recreational' Drug Users." *Drug and Alcohol Dependence* 22 (1988): 215–22.

"Lorazepam." In *Therapeutic Drugs*, C. Dollery. 2d ed. New York: Churchill Livingstone, 1999. L98–L100.

O'Hanlon, J.F., et al. "Anxiolytics' Effects on the Actual Driving Performance of Patients and Healthy Volunteers in a Standardized Test. An Integration of Three Studies." *Neuropsychobiology* 31 (1995): 81–88.

Schweizer, E., et al. "Lorazepam vs. Alprazolam in the Treatment of Panic Disorder." *Pharmacopsychiatry* 23 (1990): 90–93.

Shader, R.I., et al. "Sedative Effects and Impaired Learning and Recall after Single Oral Doses of Lorazepam." *Clinical Pharmacology and Therapeutics* 39 (1986): 526–29.

LSD

Pronunciation: ehl-ess-dee

Chemical Abstracts Service Registry Number: 50-37-3

Formal Names: Lysergic Acid Diethylamide

Informal Names: A, Acid, Acido, Angel Tears, Animal, Backbreaker (combined with strychnine), Barrel, Battery Acid, Beast, Beavis & Butthead, Big D, Birdhead, Black Acid, Black Star, Black Sunshine, Black Tab, Blotter, Blotter Acid, Blotter Cube, Blue Acid, Blue Barrel, Blue Chair, Blue Cheer, Blue Heaven, Blue Microdot, Blue Mist, Blue Moon, Blue Vial, Boomer, Brown Bombers, Brown Dots, California Sunshine, Cap, Chief, Chocolate Chips, Cid, Coffee, Conductor, Contact Lens, Crackers, Crystal Tea, Cubes, Cupcakes, D, Deeda, Delysid, Domes, Doses, Dots, Double Dome, Electric Kool Aid, Ellis Day, Elvis, Felix the Cat, Fields, Flash, Flat Blues, Ghost, God's Flesh, Golden Dragon, Goofy, Grape Parfait, Green Double Domes, Green Single Dome, Green Wedge, Grey Shields, Hats, Hawaiian Sunshine, Hawk, Haze, Head Light, Heavenly Blue, Instant Zen, L, Lason Sa Daga, LBJ, Leary's, Lens, Lime Acid, Little Smoke, Live Spit and Die, Logor, Loony Toons, Lucy in the Sky with Diamonds, Mellow Yellow, Mickey, Microdot, Mighty Quinn, Mind Detergent, One Way, Optical Illusion, Orange Barrel, Orange Cube, Orange Haze, Orange Micro, Orange Wedge, Owsley, Owsley's Acid, Pane, Paper Acid, Peace, Peace Tablet, Pearly Gates, Pellet, Pink Blotter, Pink Panther, Pink Robot, Pink Wedge, Pink Witch, Potato, Pure Love, Purple Barrel, Purple Flat, Purple Haze, Purple Heart, Purple Ozoline, Rainbow, Recycle, Red Lips, Royal Blue, Russian Sickle, Sacrament, Sandoz, Smear, Snowman, Squirrel, Strawberry, Strawberry Fields, Sugar, Sugar Cubes, Sugar Lumps, Sunshine, Superman, Tab, Tail Light, Ticket, Trip, 25, Valley Dolls, Vodka Acid, Wedding Bells, Wedge, White Dust, White Lightning, White Owsley, Window Glass, Window Pane, Yellow, Yellow Dimples, Yellow Sunshine, Ying Yang, Zen, Zig Zag Man

Type: Hallucinogen. *See* page 25

Federal Schedule Listing: Schedule I (DEA no. 7315)

USA Availability: Illegal to possess

Pregnancy Category: None

Uses. When LSD was invented in Switzerland during 1938 no one realized that this chemical was a hallucinogen even though it was known to be related to **ergot**. Its inventor Albert Hofmann wanted to make a stimulant to help people push past weariness. Five years passed before he accidentally discovered the drug's ability to alter physical and mental perceptions. One element of his discovery was the drug's potency. A later estimate calculated that one ounce is enough for 300,000 doses. Authorities list the substance as 3,000 to 4,000 times stronger than **mescaline**. One authority lists LSD as 30 times stronger than **DOM**.

LSD strikes down barriers. Barriers between physical senses can disappear, allowing colors to be smelled and sounds to be seen. Psychological barriers can disappear, allowing insights that help people to cope with long-standing problems. Barriers between shared realities and personal fantasies can disappear, with people perceiving sights and sounds that no one around them is experiencing. Those perceptions can be so compelling that some people believe the drug strikes down barriers separating us from realities that are otherwise inaccessible. Some users report a mystical experience; some simply gain pleasure. Other possibilities include terrifying hallucinations and psychoses impelling persons to do things that may harm themselves or other individuals (a 1968 report from a government official about LSD users staring at the sun until they were blinded turned out to be a hoax, but similar reports have appeared since then). An LSD user's personality, expectations, and surroundings all influence outcome of a dose. The drug's effects are not invariable. Investigators have found that LSD is more rewarding for people who are spontaneous and inspired by impulses from within themselves than for people who are conforming and controlling.

Some results perceived by users turn out to be illusory. Artists who took the drug felt more creative for months afterward, but scientists who gave tests to detect elements of creativity found no change from predrug performance. On a test of sketching the human form the artists did worse than before, indicating that technical proficiency declined. An experiment involving word and image tests found LSD did not enhance creativity of normal persons.

Despite LSD's power, volunteers have typically been able to push through their intoxication and produce almost normal results in psychological tests given during the drug experience. One investigator noted that the experimental setting of such tests seemed to weaken the drug's effects. Ability to perform "almost" normally in a laboratory does not necessarily transfer to tasks of everyday life, however. For example, a person intoxicated by LSD should not attempt to engage in dangerous activity such as driving a car. During 1943 in one of the first recorded LSD experiences the drug's inventor was barely able to ride a bicycle, let alone drive a car, while under the influence. He had the illusion of being almost motionless, although he was actually traveling at normal speed, an indication that so many events were happening to him at once that his perception of time contracted—and an indication that he was in no condition to judge the speed of vehicles on the road. His feeling of time contraction in turn expanded his perception of space, a linkage that drug researchers can demonstrate, which probably made him feel he had a vaster distance to travel and was making little progress.

Before American government authorities certified LSD as having no medical value in 1970, the substance was used for a variety of therapeutic purposes. LSD has stimulant effects allowing it to be used as an antidote for barbiturate poisoning. With varying degrees of success LSD has been used to treat neuroses, sexual disorders, **heroin** addiction, alcoholism, and psychopathology. The drug has also been given to reduce cancer pain, to supplement drugs used for pain relief in surgery, and to treat phantom limb pain (a sensation that an amputated limb is still present and hurting). After legal LSD research was phased out in the 1970s, relatively little new information has emerged about the drug. In subsequent years even reports in scientific literature occasionally had a casualness not often associated with science. For example, in 1997 a medical journal published a report about "presumed LSD intoxications," but medical personnel did not confirm that their patients had taken the drug.

Drawbacks. Although LSD fatalities have been reported in animal experimentation, by the 1990s no human overdose deaths had been documented despite LSD's tremendous potency. An overdose nonetheless can produce a physical collapse requiring hospitalization. In a population of psychiatric patients who took the drug, only 2 in 1,000 had a resultant psychosis lasting more than 48 hours; such a result was even less frequent for psychologically normal persons. In the 1990s, however, one review of LSD research noted that lengthy psychoses can be instituted by the substance. Research found that the suicide rate for psychiatric patients who used the drug under medical supervision was the same as for other psychiatric patients, indicating LSD might present no peril in that regard—although this aspect might be different in uncontrolled circumstances.

The drug's physical effects can include headache, nausea, vomiting, hot or cold feelings, sweating, elevated body temperature, trembling, dizziness, blood pressure changes (up or down), increased heart rate, numb hands, sensitive hearing, and extra urine production. In dog experiments the substance reduced appetite.

Rat experimentation shows that administering LSD for a month can alter brain structure and chemistry. LSD has been reported to impair abstract thinking, but one commentary on those reports noted that alcohol abuse among the studied persons might also explain their thinking problems. Brief visual afterimages (such as happens when someone looks at a bright object and then sees an image of it in opposite colors for a few seconds after looking away) are normal for everyone, but a formal experiment and a few case reports note lengthy visual afterimages in proper colors among LSD users. These are not flashbacks, incidentally.

Flashbacks are one of the most publicized effects of LSD. Flashback is a reappearance of LSD actions without taking a dose. This phenomenon is normal in other contexts; something may remind a person of an event that had high emotional content, and the memory may flood one's consciousness and temporarily sweep aside awareness of one's surroundings. People are usually able to push out of an LSD flashback if they wish and are not taken over by it; a survey of 247 persons who experienced LSD flashbacks found only 1 who claimed to be unable to stop the experience at will. A case report indicates behavior therapy can stop LSD flashbacks, implying that their cause may have more to do with psychology than chemistry. Another case report notes additional evidence that personality affects likelihood of flashback. Still another case report says that some types of antidepressants appear to promote flashbacks among LSD users, and a research study concluded that phenothiazine tranquilizers worsen flashbacks after they start. Investigations have revealed that many persons who claim to have LSD flashbacks do not really have them, that people often use the term casually and incorrectly to describe other types of experiences. Psychiatrists call the LSD type of flashback "hallucinogen persisting perception disorder." Some persons, however, regard LSD flashbacks not as a disorder but as a sign they have learned to achieve altered states of consciousness without using a drug anymore.

Abuse factors. Tolerance has developed in rats and humans. Humans have shown LSD cross-tolerance with mescaline and **psilocybin** and slight cross-tolerance with **DMT**—meaning that the drugs can be substituted for one another, for some purposes at least.

Drug interactions. Two case reports indicate that LSD alone or in combination with **alcohol** may cause muscles to stiffen, accompanied by fever and insensibility. Some antidepressants can increase LSD's psychedelic effects; some others reduce them. Rat experiments show that various opioids in various doses can either increase or decrease LSD actions and that the schizophrenia medicine clozapine can reduce LSD effects. Case reports say that chlorpromazine (Thorazine) can cause an LSD psychosis among persons who have used LSD in the past. Ambroxol, a substance used to help people clear congested respiratory tracts, can give a false-positive urine test for LSD.

Cancer. LSD stopped breast cancer growth in a rat experiment. Researchers believe this result came not because of hallucinogenic activity but probably because LSD reduced amounts of a hormone called prolactin. Animal and plant experiments show that LSD can be a mutagen, meaning it might have a potential for causing cancer. A mutagen effect has not been observed in humans who took LSD under controlled conditions.

Pregnancy. Researchers have demonstrated that LSD passes from a pregnant mouse into the fetus. In other experiments pregnant mice that received LSD produced offspring with eye defects. The same happened with rats, but in that experiment investigators noted no significant statistical difference between LSD and non-LSD rats in malformations of any type, so the LSD may not have been responsible for the eye problems. Researchers who gave LSD to dozens of rats, mice, and hamsters found no proof that the drug caused malformations in their fetuses (which numbered in the hundreds). In the 1970s claims arose that LSD causes human chromosome damage and birth defects even if the drug use stops before pregnancy begins, but subsequent research failed to verify those claims. Some of the original laboratory tests involved conditions that do not occur in the human body, and early investigators typically did not know what drug a woman had actually taken, nor what the dose was, nor did they consider whether a woman's health problems promoted congenital malformations. The birth defect rate among children of LSD users is no higher than the general population's. A case report notes a woman who took an LSD dose during early pregnancy with no apparent ill effect on her infant. A study of pregnant women who attempted to commit suicide with drugs found no infant malformation attributable to LSD, but the investigators said data were too scanty to allow a conclusion about LSD's potential for causing developmental abnormalities. The rate of birth defects was not elevated in 121 pregnancies of women who took LSD under medical supervision. Another study of 27 pregnancies reached no conclusion on whether LSD causes miscarriage.

Additional scientific information may be found in:

Abraham, H.D., and A.M. Aldridge. "Adverse Consequences of Lysergic Acid Diethylamide." *Addiction* 88 (1993): 1327–34.

Cohen, S. "LSD: The Varieties of Psychotic Experience." *Journal of Psychoactive Drugs* 17 (1985): 291–96.

Hofmann, A. *LSD, My Problem Child*. Trans. J. Ott. New York: McGraw-Hill, 1980.

Li, J-H., and L-F. Lin. "Genetic Toxicology of Abused Drugs: A Brief Review." *Mutagenesis* 13 (1998): 557–65.

Mangini, M. "Treatment of Alcoholism Using Psychedelic Drugs: A Review of the Program of Research." *Journal of Psychoactive Drugs* 30 (1998): 381–418.

Masters, R.E.L., and J. Houston. *The Varieties of Psychedelic Experience*. A Delta Book. New York: Dell, 1966.

McGlothlin, W.H., and D.O. Arnold. "LSD Revisited." *Archives of General Psychiatry* 24 (1971): 35–49.

Novak, S.J. "LSD before Leary. Sidney Cohen's Critique of 1950s Psychedelic Drug Research." *Isis* 88 (March 1997): 87–110.

Ma Huang

See also **Ephedrine**

Pronunciation: mah-hwahng
Chemical Abstracts Service Registry Number: None
Formal Names: *Ephedra sinica*
Informal Names: Chinese Ephedra, Chinese Jointfir, Desert Tea, Herbal Ecstasy, Mexican Tea, Miner's Tea, Mormon Tea, Popotillo, Sea Grape, Squaw Tea, Teamster's Tea, Whorehouse Tea, Yellow Horse
Type: Stimulant (amphetamine class). *See* page 12
Federal Schedule Listing: Unlisted
USA Availability: Nonprescription natural product
Pregnancy Category: None

Uses. *Ephedra sinica* is one of several *Ephedra* species classified as the Chinese medical herb ma huang (loosely translated as "yellow drug that constricts the tongue"). Each species is a plentiful source of **ephedrine** and pseudoephedrine. A study found that the proportion of ephedrine to other mahuang components increased if the herb was boiled for two hours. A test comparing the natural herb to synthetic ephedrine (such as commonly found in medicines) revealed little difference in how the human body used ephedrine from those two different sources; investigators concluded that effects depend more on size of dose than source of drug.

The herb has been used in China for 5,000 years, principally to treat respiratory ailments. Ancient Greek utilization of *Ephedra* varieties is also noted. More recently ma huang has been used against narcolepsy. Though thought of as a Chinese herb, varieties of *Ephedra* plants also grow in Mexico and the American Southwest where they were once used to treat venereal disease. Mormon pioneers used the plants as alternatives to tea and coffee. Almost nothing is said of using the plants for food, although reports exist about bread made from the plants and about eating the berries, which are supposed to be a good source of vitamin C.

In Eastern medicine ma huang is administered as a tea to fight fever, asthma, and the common cold but has become popular in the Western world as a stimulant and for promotion of weight loss. One study found that people using a ma huang and cola nut combination lost over four times more weight than persons using a placebo. Ma huang is marketed as a muscle builder, as a means of improving sexual performance, and also as a legal substitute for **MDMA**. How well the product lives up to such advertising is debatable.

In the 1990s retail gross sales of ma huang products was estimated at over a half billion dollars a year. In the year 2000 surveys from 755 persons undergoing outpatient surgery were reported, saying that 18% were using ma huang.

Drawbacks. Purity of ma huang products is uncertain. Examination of 20 ma huang dietary supplements found them to vary widely in content of ephedrine and pseudoephedrine, and 4 even had inconsistency among various batches of the same product. One examined product lacked any ephedrine or pseudoephedrine at all. Many contained cathine, a Schedule IV prescription drug found in **khat**. Perhaps the most alarming finding was that actual contents of half the products did not match the label description. Another study of 9 ma huang products had similar results. In a separate instance, undeclared contents of a ma huang product was a factor causing an athlete to flunk when tested for drugs banned from competitive sports.

The herb is known to cause paranoia, delusions, combativeness, mania, and hallucinations similar to what amphetamine abuse can do. Someone with such behavior was diagnosed and medicated for mental illness because no one suspected ma huang use. Case studies offer vivid accounts of overdose causing users to direct violence against themselves and others. Psychiatric problems can persist for quite some time after drug use stops.

A study found that ephedrine did not account for all of ma huang's adverse effects and that unwanted actions increased if the herb was ground up. Herbalists commonly prescribe 5 or 6 grams of ma huang for steeping as one dose of tea, yielding (depending on potency) perhaps 38 to 75 mg of ephedrine. The U.S. Food and Drug Administration (FDA) has found many examples of hazard in an ephedrine dose exceeding 10 mg. Two studies found the substance to be safe in that amount, although one of those studies and a third one noted heartbeat irregularity, reduced salivation, and difficulty with sleep. Headache, dizziness, nausea, vomiting, skin rash, urinary retention, kidney stones, and heart inflammation have been associated with using ma huang. Persons with glaucoma should avoid the substance. Ma huang is suspected of causing liver disease, but investigators are uncertain. Stroke, heart attack, and death have been attributed to the substance, but those claims are disputed. An experiment measuring heart rate and blood pressure yielded unclear results about ma huang's influence. The herb may cause adverse reaction with monoamine oxidase inhibitors (MAOIs, commonly found in antidepressants). Persons with diabetes or thyroid disease should consult with a physician before using ma huang. Aircraft pilots have been advised to avoid the natural product.

Abuse factors. Stopping the usage of ma huang can cause a person to be tired, sleep a lot, be sad, and have trouble concentrating. Those are opposite of typical effects that the substance has, suggesting that a user's body has developed a dependence on ma huang (because withdrawal from dependence often produces effects opposite to what a drug does). Dependence is a traditional sign that a substance is addictive.

Drug interactions. The FDA considers combining ma huang with cola nut to be dangerous. The two prime drug components of those natural products are ephedrine and **caffeine**, and caffeine boosts ephedrine effects. Scientific study finds that ma huang with caffeine, but not ma huang alone, can improve functioning in physical exercise. The combination of ma huang with another medicinal herb called guarana may be particularly poisonous to dogs.

Cancer. Not enough scientific information to report.

Pregnancy. Ma huang is supposed to be avoided during pregnancy.

Additional scientific information may be found in:

Chen, K.K., and C.F. Schmidt. "Ephedrine and Related Substances." *Medicine* 9 (1930): 1–117.

Grauds, C. "Herbal Ephedra and the Pharmacist." *Pharmacy Times* 64 (March 1998): 60, 62.

Jacobs, K.M., and K.A. Hirsch. "Psychiatric Complications of Ma-Huang." *Psychosomatics* 41 (2000): 58–62.

Mack, R.B. " 'All But Death, Can Be Adjusted.' Ma Huang (Ephedrine) Adversities." *North Carolina Medical Journal* 58 (1997): 68–70.

Powell, T., et al. "Ma-Huang Strikes Again: Ephedrine Nephrolithiasis." *American Journal of Kidney Diseases* 32 (1998): 153–59.

Sprague, J.E., A.D. Harrod, and A.L. Teconchuk. "Pharmacology and Abuse Potential of Ephedrine." *Pharmacy Times* 64 (May 1998): 72–80.

Mandrake

Pronunciation: MAN-draik

Chemical Abstracts Service Registry Number: None

Formal Names: *Mandragora officinarum*

Informal Names: Satan's Apple

Type: Depressant. *See* page 19

Federal Schedule Listing: Unlisted

USA Availability: Nonprescription natural product

Pregnancy Category: None

Uses. In some cultures European mandrake has traditional association with the devil, perhaps because a little imagination can envision the plant's root as a small humanoid figure. The plant's ominous connotation is illustrated in *Romeo and Juliet* as Juliet approaches death and shudders about hearing "shrieks like mandrakes' torn out of the earth," referring to a belief that the plant screams if harvested. Witches reputedly made preparations from the plant that enabled them to fly.

Medicinal usage of European mandrake may date back as far as ancient Egypt, but in twenty-first-century Western medicine, only practitioners of homeopathy use the substance for healing. (Homeopathy uses extremely weak preparations of medicines.) Folk practitioners have given European mandrake to fight depression, asthma, hay fever, whooping cough, colic, and stomach ulcers. The plant has also been administered as a folk treatment to promote fertility, perhaps inspired by the story in Genesis 30: 14–17. Such usage is referred to by the line "Get with child a mandrake root" from John Donne's sonnet "Song: Go and Catch a Falling Star." The plant is linked with romance (Song of Solomon 7:13) and is a traditional aphrodisiac, although such a characteristic has not received scientific confirmation. Sedative and pain relief actions made the plant one of the first surgical anesthetics, and an image of it appears on the coat of arms of the British Association of Anaesthetists. European mandrake contains the so-called **belladonna** alkaloids atropine, hyoscyamine, and scopolamine; therefore, European mandrake produces actions similar to those of belladonna.

Drawbacks. Unwanted effects can include rapid heartbeat, elevated body temperature, decrease in sweat and salivation, and difficulty with urination and bowel movements. The natural product initially acts as a sedative, but a strong enough dose converts mandrake into a stimulant that can cause manic behavior, delirium, and hallucinations. An amount sufficient to bring on those latter effects may be an amount sufficient for dangerous poisoning. Expert guidance is recommended for anyone using the plant.

Abuse factors. Not enough scientific information to report about tolerance, dependence, withdrawal, or addiction.

Drug interactions. Not enough scientific information to report.

Cancer. Not enough scientific information to report.

Pregnancy. Not enough scientific information to report.

Additional information. *Podophyllum peltatum* (CAS RN 9000-55-9 for resin) is the American mandrake, a different plant from the European one and one that persons sometimes use accidentally when they are seeking the European variety. The American version is also known as Devil's Apple, Duck's Foot, Ground Lemon, Hog Apple, Indian Apple, May Apple, Peca, Raccoon Berry, Umbrella Plant, Vegetable Calomel, Vegetable Mercury, Wild Jalap, Wild Lemon, Wild Mandrake, and Yellowberry. American mandrake is not a controlled substance.

Odor from the flowers may be unpleasant, yet the small fruit is not only edible but enjoyed by some persons. Leaves and stems are described as poisonous.

American mandrake is a traditional Native American medicine, and in former times it was considered a substitute for mercury's medical employment. Folk medicine uses the plant to treat fever, worms, constipation, warts, syphilis, jaundice, liver disease, and cancer. Etoposide, a substance derived from the plant, is scientifically known to work against cancer. American mandrake contains podophyllotoxin, a substance that acts against viruses causing measles and herpes simplex type I. A study found podophyllotoxin and podophyllin (another American mandrake substance) to be effective against a type of wart. Application of American mandrake natural product preparations to the skin must be skillful because the plant can injure the skin and even be fatal if too much drug content is absorbed.

Animal experiments with the natural product have produced salivation, vomiting, pain, and straining to defecate. Those unwanted effects also appear in humans, with enough force to cause hemorrhoids and displacement of the rectum. One authority warns that if someone eats too much of the fruit, its laxative effect can become overpowering. Ulcers of the small intestine have developed in animals that ingest American mandrake. A case is known of damage to nerves providing sensation to limbs after a person drank an American mandrake preparation. Persons working in an environment containing American mandrake dust have suffered irritated eyes and noses, along with coldness in their hands and feet.

The plant is suspected of causing birth defects, and usage is supposed to be avoided during pregnancy. A case report tells of fetal death after American mandrake was used to treat warts on a pregnant woman.

Additional scientific information may be found in:

Frasca, T., A.S. Brett, and S.D. Yoo. "Mandrake Toxicity: A Case of Mistaken Identity." *Archives of Internal Medicine* 157 (1997): 2007–9.

Lust, J.B. *The Herb Book*. New York: Benedict Lust Publications, 1974. 259–60.

Millspaugh, C.F. *American Medicinal Plants*. Philadelphia: John C. Yorston & Company, 1892. Reprint, New York: Dover Publications, Inc., 1974. 61–64.

Morton, J.F. *Major Medicinal Plants: Botany, Culture and Uses*. Springfield, IL: Charles C. Thomas, 1977. 87–89.

Vlachos, P., and L. Poulos. "Case of Mandrake Poisoning." *Journal of Toxicology: Clinical Toxicology* 19 (1982): 521–22.

Weiner, M.A. *Weiner's Herbal*. New York: Stein and Day, 1980. 124–25.

Marijuana

See also **Dronabinol**

Pronunciation: mair-i-WAHN-uh (also pronounced mah-ri-HWAH-nuh)

Chemical Abstracts Service Registry Number: 8063-14-7

Formal Names: Cannabis, *Cannabis sativa*, Hashish, Marihuana, Sinsemilla

Informal Names: A-Bomb (with **opium** or **heroin**), Acapulco Gold, Acapulco Red, Ace, Afgani Indica, African Black, African Bush, Airplane, Alamout Black Hash (with **belladonna**), Alice B. Toklas (baked in brownie), AMP (with **PCP**, formaldehyde, or other substance), Angola, Ashes, Assassin of Youth, Astro Turf, Atomic Bomb (with heroin), Atshitshi, Aunt Mary, Baby, Baby Bhang, Bad Seed, Bamba, Bambalacha, Bammy, Banano (mixed with **cocaine**), Bar, Bash, Bazooka (with **coca** paste), Belyando Spruce, B-40 (mixed with tobacco and **alcohol**), Bhang, Black, Black Bart, Black Ganga, Black Gold, Black Gunion, Black Mo, Black Moat, Black Mote (with honey), Blanket, Blast, Block, Blonde, Blue de Hue, Blue Sage, Blue Sky Blond, Blunt, Bo, Bo-Bo, Bobo Bush, Bohd, Bomb, Bomber, Bone, Boo, Boo Boo Bama, Boom, Broccoli, Bud, Buda, Buddha (with opium), Burnie, Bush, Butter, Butter Flower, Cambodian Red, Cam Red, Cam Trip, Can, Canade (with heroin), Canadian Black, Canappa, Cancelled Stick, Candy Blunt (with **codeine**), Carmabis, Catnip, Caviar (with cocaine), Cavite All Star, Cest, Chamba, Champagne (with cocaine), Charas, Charge, Cheeba, Cheeo, Chiba Chiba, Chicago Black, Chicago Green, Chips (with PCP), Chira, Chocolate, Christmas Tree, Chronic, Chunky, Churus, Citrol, Clicker (with formaldehyde), Clickums (with PCP), Climb, Cochornis, Coli, Coliflor Tostao, Colombian, Colorado Cocktail, Columbus Black, Cosa, Crack Back (with crack cocaine), Crazy Weed, Cripple, Crying Weed, Cryppie, Cryptonie, CS, Cube (tablet form), Culican, Dagga, Dawamesk, Dew, Diablito (with crack cocaine), Diambista, Dimba, Ding, Dinkie Dow, Dirt Grass, Dirty Joint (with crack), Ditch, Ditch Weed, Djamba, Domestic, Dona Juana, Dona Juanita, Don Jem, Don Juan, Donk (with PCP), Doob, Doobee, Doobie, Doradilla, Draf, Drag Weed, Dry High, Dubbe, Dube, Duby, Durong, Duros, Dust (combined with other substances), Earth, El Diablito (with cocaine, heroin, and PCP), El Diablo (with cocaine and heroin), Elephant, Endo, Esra, Fallbrook Redhair, Fatty, Feeling, Fine Stuff, Finger, Finger Lid, Fir, Flower, Flower Tops, Fraho, Frajo, Frios (with PCP), Fry (with PCP or other substances), Fry Daddy (with crack cocaine), Fry Sticks (with PCP), Fu, Fuel (with insect poison), Gage, Gange, Gangster, Ganja, Garbage, Gash, Gasper, Gauge, Geek (with crack cocaine), Ghana, Giggle Smoke, Giggle Weed, Gimmie (with crack cocaine), Goblet of Jam, Gold,

Golden, Golden Leaf, Gold Star, Gong, Gonj, Good Butt, Good Giggles, Goody-Goody, Goofy Butt, Grass, Grasshopper, Grata, Green, Green Buds, Green Goddess, Greeter, Gremmies (with cocaine), Greta, Griefo, Griefs, Grifa, Griff, Griffa, Griffo, Gunga, Gungeon, Gungun, Gunja, Gyve, Haircut, Hanhich, Happy Cigarette, Harsh, Has, Hash, Hawaiian, Hawaiian Black, Hawaiian Homegrown Hay, Hay, Hemp, Herb, Herba, Hit, Hocus, Homegrown, Hooch, Hooter, Hot Stick, Hydro, Illies (with PCP), Illing (with PCP), Indian Boy, Indian Hay, Indian Hemp, Indo, Indonesian Bud, Instaga, Instagu, J, Jamaican Gold, Jane, Jay, Jim Jones (with cocaine and PCP), Jive, Joint, Jolly Green, Joy Smoke, Joy Stick, Juanita, Juan Valdez, Juice Joint (with crack cocaine), Juja, Ju-Ju, Jumbo (with crack), Kalakit, Kali, Kansas Grass, Kate Bush, Kaya, Kee, Kentucky Blue, Key, KGB (Killer Green Bud), Ki, Kick Stick, Kief, Kiff, Killer Weed (with PCP), Kilter, Kind, King Bud, Kumba, Lace (with cocaine), Lakbay Diva, Laughing Grass, Laughing Weed, Leaf, Leak (with PCP), Leno, Lid (quantity), Light Stuff, Lima, Liprimo (with crack), Little Smoke, LL, Llesca, Loaf, Lobo, Loco, Locoweed, Log, Love Boat (with formaldehyde or heroin), Love Leaf (with PCP), Lovelies (with PCP), Love Weed, Lubage, M, Machinery, Macon, Maconha, Mafu, Magic Smoke, Manhattan Silver, Mari, Marimba, Mary, Mary and Johnny, Mary Ann, Mary Jane, Mary Jonas, Mary Warner, Mary Weaver, Matchbox (quantity), Maui Wauie, Maui-Wowie, Meg, Megg, Meggie, Messorole, Mexican Brown, Mexican Green, Mexican Locoweed, Mexican Red, Mighty Mezz, M.J., M.O., Mo, Modams, Mohasky, Mohasty, Monte, Mooca, Moocah, Mooster, Moota, Mooter, Mootie, Mootos, Mor A Grifa, Mota, Mother, Moto, M.U., Mu, Muggie, Muggle, Muta, Mutah, Mutha, Nail, Nigra, Number, O.J., Oolies (with crack), Ozone (marijuana alone or with PCP and crack), Pack, Pakalolo, Pakistani Black, Panama Cut, Panama Gold, Panama Red, Panatella, Parsley, Pasto, Pat, P-Dogs (with crack), Pin, Pocket Rocket, Pod, Poke, Pot, Potlikker, Potten Bush, Prescription, Pretendica, Pretendo, Primo (with crack), Queen Ann's Lace, Ragweed, Railroad Weed, Rainy Day Woman, Rangood, Rasta Weed, Red Bud, Red Cross, Red Dirt, Reefer, Righteous Bush, Rip, Roach, Roacha, Rockets, Rompums (with horse tranquilizer), Root, Rope, Rose Marie, Rough Stuff, Rubia, Salt & Pepper, Sandwich Bag (quantity), Santa Marta, Sasfras, Scissors, Seeds, Sen, Sess, Sezz, Shake, Siddi, Sinse, Skunk, Smoke, Smoke Canada, Snop, Speedboat (mixed with crack cocaine and PCP), Spliff, Splim, Square Mackerel, Squirrel (with crack and PCP), Stack, Stems, Stick, Stinkweed, Stoney Weed, Straw, Sugar Weed, Super Grass (marijuana alone or with PCP), Super Pot, Sweet Lucy, Swishers, T, Taima, Takkouri, Tea, Texas Pot, Texas Tea, Tex-Mex, Thai Sticks, 13, 38 (combination with crack cocaine), 3750 (with crack), Thumb, Toke, Torch, Torpedo (with crack), Tray (quantity), Turbo (with crack), Tustin, Twist, Twistum, Unotque, Vega, Viper's Weed, Wac (with PCP), Wacky Weed, Wake & Bake, Water (with other substances), Water-Water (with embalming fluid or PCP), Weed, Weed Tea, Wet (with PCP), Whack (with insect poison), Whackatabacky, Wheat, White-Haired Lady, Wicky Stick (with crack and PCP), Wollie (with crack), Woolah (with crack), Wooly (with crack or PCP), X, Yeh, Yellow Submarine, Yen Pop, Yeola (with crack), Yerba, Yerba Mala (with PCP), Yerhia, Yesca, Yesco, Zacatecas Purple, Zambi, Zay (with other substances), Zig Zag Man, Zol, Zoom (with PCP).

Type: Hallucinogen. *See* page 25
Federal Schedule Listing: Schedule I (DEA no. 7360)
USA Availability: Illegal to possess
Pregnancy Category: None

Uses. As the twenty-first century began, the recreational use of marijuana was mainly for relaxation. The drug is often used in a social setting of mellow geniality. The drug can produce euphoria; in that context recreational usage can leak over into self-medication easing depression. One authority has said that psychological effects are facilitated by the substance, not caused by it. In other words, marijuana may help people achieve states of consciousness that they can learn to achieve in other ways.

When the federal government's drug scheduling system was adopted in the 1970s, marijuana was classified as Schedule I, certifying it as having no medical value. Like many other substances, over the years marijuana had been used for medical purposes that became obsolete as better treatments were discovered. Then, by accident, a glaucoma sufferer discovered that his condition improved when he smoked marijuana, and subsequent scientific tests confirmed that the natural product had a hitherto unknown ability to relieve that devastating eye disease that can cause blindness. Marijuana's long-known antinausea and appetite enhancement qualities also became publicized as a help to patients undergoing the rigors of AIDS (acquired immunodeficiency syndrome) and cancer treatments. As researchers began discovering other potential therapeutic actions of marijuana (including treatment of pain, multiple sclerosis, muscle spasticity, ulcerative colitis, and hiccups), medical use became a controversial issue in the 1990s. Among the debated points was whether the natural product had advantages over pharmaceutical **dronabinol** (containing delta-9-tetrahydrocannabinol, also called THC, which is marijuana's main active ingredient). Instead of swallowing dronabinol capsules, some patients prefer to smoke marijuana because they can fine-tune the THC dosage more easily, puffing just enough instead of taking a capsule that might have more THC than they need. Marijuana smoke may also reduce some of the unwanted actions of THC. Although **belladonna** and **jimson weed** cigarettes were used for many years to treat asthma, given what is known about the hazards of both tobacco and polluted air, few medical caregivers today are likely to favor inhaling any kind of smoke. Ancient Greeks reportedly put marijuana seeds on hot stones to release vapor, and modern efforts are devising other ways to produce vapor without igniting the substance, providing aerosol delivery without smoke.

Scientific debate aside, controversy about medical marijuana also had political components. Many powerful individuals and institutions had a vested interest in maintaining marijuana's Schedule I status. Also, many persons saw legalization for medical purposes as the first step toward lifting the ban on recreational use. Passionate claims and counterclaims about marijuana's medical value swirled as this book was written, and doctors could not prescribe marijuana.

Drawbacks. Although calling marijuana a hallucinogen stretches the definition of that type of drug, this book follows the governmental custom of classifying marijuana in that category. Despite that official classification, reports of hallucinations from marijuana are uncommon.

Physical effects can include reddened eyes, accelerated heartbeat, higher body temperature, lower **testosterone** level, and arousal of senses. In the 1970s reports began appearing from laboratory and animal experiments indicating that marijuana's active ingredient THC harms immune system functions, meaning infections may become more likely. Those experiments frequently involved conditions that are not duplicated in the human body, however, and by the 1990s fears about damage to the human immune system had quieted.

Marijuana is sometimes described as making people less interested in accomplishing tasks in life. Someone jokingly suggested that the substance instead creates insatiable ambition to hold elective office. In reality, marijuana does not make people unambitious. Such persons may be attracted to heavy marijuana use, but probably they were unambitious before using the substance. One research study found that marijuana users who lack ambition tend to be depressed and concluded that depression (not marijuana) was the underlying cause for these persons' diminished motivation. Case studies indicate that marijuana can worsen psychoses, neuroses, and phobias.

In one study a battery of thinking tests given to groups of marijuana users and nonusers found no difference in performance; in another study daily users did worse than occasional users. Long-term memory (the ability to recall many long-known things, such as remembering the year Columbus sailed to America) has been unaffected in experiments. Short-term memory performance (brief ability to recall a few newly known things, such as a list of random words) can decline during intoxication but afterward returns to normal. Some researchers have found marijuana to have no influence on muscular coordination, sensory perception, mental ability, or learning; other researchers have found that marijuana impedes muscular coordination and mental abilities. Driving skill tests have shown similar variation; some studies find that marijuana harms such skill, and some do not. Some research shows marijuana having no effect on users' performance the next day; some research shows impairment 24 hours after use. Such differing results may relate to intoxication levels, to volunteers' experience with handling the substance, and to how long persons have been using it (some researchers believe that long-term use produces long-term effects extending beyond the time of acute intoxication).

The most obvious unwanted physical effects of marijuana are caused or promoted by inhaling smoke, afflictions caused by the manner of dosing rather than by the substance itself. In an animal experiment primates that inhaled marijuana smoke were compared to those in a smoke-free group; the marijuana group developed lung damage that could have led to bronchitis or emphysema, had the smoking continued long enough. Among humans frequent marijuana smoking is known to produce coughing, wheezing, and sputum. Marijuana smoking reduces lung function in ways suggesting that chronic obstructive pulmonary disease (COPD) might develop if a person smokes four or five marijuana cigarettes daily for 30 years (with a lesser amount needed if a person also smokes tobacco). Certain kinds of lung damage have been seen in marijuana smokers but not in tobacco smokers. Marijuana smokers typically use big puffs and deep inhalations, held for a long period of time. Such a technique deposits larger quantities of damaging materials in lungs than the ordinary tobacco-smoking technique. Efforts to document lesser-known health risks have been flawed or outright unsuccessful. Reports of physical disease in marijuana users often fail to account for other possible (and perhaps more likely) causes.

Despite conceivable health hazards from marijuana, it seems safe in moderation, no more dangerous than many foods (such as items high in sugar, salt, fat, and cholesterol). The natural product is extraordinarily safe from a dosage standpoint.[1] No human fatality has been confirmed, although cattle deaths have been reported after consuming bales of dried marijuana.

Abuse factors. Tolerance and dependence have been reported. A marijuana abstinence syndrome is described as including physical and mental tenseness, peevishness, less happiness, and diminished appetite. Such symptoms, however, sound much like the reasons many persons use marijuana. If a chronic headache sufferer reported discomfort when pain relievers were unavailable, that would not be considered evidence of dependence on and withdrawal from pain relievers. Self-administration of a drug by laboratory animals is a traditional sign of addictive potential, but researchers have mixed success in getting animals to self-administer THC.

Drug interactions. Not enough scientific information to report, although it is reasonable to assume interactions could be similar to those occurring with dronabinol.

Cancer. Laboratory tests indicate that marijuana smoke can cause cancer. Oral and lung cancer is reported among marijuana users, although we must remember that typical users also smoke tobacco. One study did find that marijuana, even when tobacco use is accounted for, increases chances of getting head and neck cancer. One of the more impressive studies of marijuana's cancer-causing potential involved medical records of 64,888 persons and discovered that people who used marijuana, whether frequently or infrequently, were in general no more likely to get cancer than anyone else. That study did find evidence, however, that marijuana promotes prostate and cervical cancer. Researchers have found that children are more likely to develop acute non-lymphocytic leukemia if their mothers used marijuana during pregnancy. This is a rare disease; in a population of 1 million children, about 5 will have the affliction. The disease is also associated with pesticide exposure, and investigators are uncertain whether pesticide contamination of marijuana is a more important factor than marijuana itself.

Chromosome damage can indicate a potential for development of cancer. Some laboratory and animal experiments indicate marijuana causes chromosome damage, but a study found human chromosome abnormalities to be about the same in moderate users of marijuana and nonusers. Researchers conducting one human study sent the same samples to two laboratories, but neither lab was able to find chromosome damage attributable to marijuana.

Pregnancy. Normally we think of marijuana as a recreational substance, but some women use it to ease discomforts of pregnancy and childbirth. Marijuana chemicals pass from a pregnant woman into the fetus. Almost all research finds no evidence that marijuana causes human birth defects. A study examining infants of adolescent mothers who used marijuana during pregnancy noted some "minor" birth defects, but even these researchers did not conclude that marijuana was necessarily the cause. Studies of newborns' birthweights have been inconclusive about an impact from prenatal marijuana exposure. No major effect on muscular coordination and balance turned up in an examination of preschool children having prenatal marijuana exposure, but investigators cautioned that the tests lacked measures of subtle skills. Behavior problems have been reported among children who had prenatal marijuana exposure, but we do not know whether those problems were caused by marijuana or by years of exposure to a particular type of parent. Investigators watching development of children up to age 5 found no difference attributable to maternal marijuana use during pregnancy; differences existed but were ascribed to home environment and schooling. Examination of reading and language abilities in children aged 9 to 12 years found no significant impact from prenatal marijuana exposure. Some researchers believe they have found problems caused by prenatal marijuana, but most research is consistent with marijuana being benign.

Marijuana's THC passes into human milk, and researchers report deficient development of muscle and limb coordination among infants nursed on such milk. One case report noted the THC level in milk was eight times higher than the mother's blood level.

Additional information. Marijuana and hemp come from different portions of the same plant, *Cannabis sativa.* Leaves, flowers, and resin are the illegal drug marijuana; the resin is also called hashish. Stalks and seed (if processed so it will not germinate) are the legal commercial product hemp. The terms *hemp* and *marijuana* are sometimes used interchangeably, but such use is incorrect. After marijuana was outlawed in the 1930s, hemp raising continued to thrive because law enforcement authorities of the era were familiar with the industry and understood that crops were not entering the illegal drug market even though the plants had leaves and flowers and resin. During World War II the federal government subsidized hemp farming to replace natural fiber supplies cut off by the war. In the 1950s subsidies finally stopped, and the American hemp industry also stopped because it could no longer make money at the unsubsidized world market price.

Some food products contain hemp components and can cause false positives for marijuana in urine drug screen tests. Hemp lotions and creams rubbed on the skin produce marijuana chemicals in urine, but not enough to cause false positives in a drug screen.

"Locoweed" and "stinkweed" are nicknames for both jimson weed and marijuana, but the substances are different.

Additional scientific information may be found in:

Carlson, B.R., and W.H. Edwards. "Human Values and Marijuana Use." *International Journal of the Addictions* 25 (1990): 1393–401.

Fried, P., et al. "Current and Former Marijuana Use: Preliminary Findings of a Longitudinal Study of Effects on IQ in Young Adults." *CMAJ: Canadian Medical Association Journal* 166 (2002): 887–91.

Gruber, A.J., H.G. Pope, and P. Oliva. "Very Long-Term Users of Marijuana in the United States: A Pilot Study." *Substance Use and Misuse* 32 (1997): 249–64.

Hendin, H., et al. "The Functions of Marijuana Abuse for Adolescents." *American Journal of Drug and Alcohol Abuse* 8, no. 4 (1981–1982): 441–56.

Iversen, L. "Marijuana: The Myths Are Hazardous to Your Health." *Cerebrum* 1, no. 2 (1999): 37–49.

Labouvie, E.W. "Alcohol and Marijuana Use in Relation to Adolescent Stress." *International Journal of the Addictions* 21 (1986): 333–45.

Reilly, D. "Long-Term Cannabis Use: Characteristics of Users in an Australian Rural Area." *Addiction* 93 (1998): 837–46.

Sidney, S., et al. "Marijuana Use and Mortality." *American Journal of Public Health* 87 (1997): 585–90.

Solomon, D., ed. *The Marihuana Papers*. Indianapolis, IN: Bobbs-Merrill, 1966.

Taylor, D.R., et al. "A Longitudinal Study of the Effects of Tobacco and Cannabis Exposure on Lung Function in Young Adults." *Addiction* 97 (2002): 1055–61.

Thompson, K.M. "Marijuana Use among Adolescents: Trends, Patterns, and Influences." *Minerva Pediatrica* 53 (2001): 313–23.

U.S. Commission on Marihuana and Drug Abuse. *Marihuana, a Signal of Misunderstanding*. Washington, DC: Government Printing Office, 1972.

Von Sydow, K., et al. "The Natural Course of Cannabis Use, Abuse and Dependence over Four Years: A Longitudinal Community Study of Adolescents and Young Adults." *Drug and Alcohol Dependence* 64 (2001): 347–61.

Note

1. Decades of studies indicating marijuana's relative safety when used in moderation include Advisory Committee on Drug Dependence, *Cannabis* (Wooten Report) (London: HMSO, 1968); J. Brandt and L.F. Doyle, "Concept Attainment, Tracking, and Shifting in Adolescent Polydrug Abusers," *Journal of Nervous and Mental Disease* 171 (1938): 559; E.M. Brecher and the Editors of Consumer Reports, *Licit and Illicit Drugs: The Consumers Union Report on Narcotics, Stimulants, Depressants, Inhalants, Hallucinogens, and Marijuana—Including Caffeine, Nicotine, and Alcohol* (Boston: Little, Brown and Company, 1972), 395; N.Q. Brill and R.L. Christie, "Marihuana Use and Psychosocial Adaptation: Follow-up Study of a Collegiate Population," *Archives of General Psychiatry* 31 (1974): 713; Commission of Inquiry into the Non-Medical Use of Drugs (Le Dain Commission), *Interim Report* (Toronto, Canada: Addiction Research Foundation of Ontario, 1970); C.M. Culver and F.W. King, "Neuropsychological Assessment of Undergraduate Marihuana and LSD Users," *Archives of General Psychiatry* 32 (1974): 707; E. Goode, *Drugs in American Society* (New York: Alfred A. Knopf, 1972), 56, 59 n. 1; Jaffe, "Drug Addiction and Abuse," in L.S. Goodman and A. Gilman, *The Pharmacological Basis of Therapeutics*, 7th ed. (New York: The Macmillan Company, 1955), 560; *The Indian Hemp Drugs Commission Report* (Silver Spring, MD: Jefferson Press, 1969) (reprint of summary volume); T.H. Mikuriya, "Historical Aspects of Cannabis Sativa in Western Medicine," *New Physician* 18 (1969): 905; J.B. Murray, "Marijuana's Effects on Human Cognitive Functions, Psychomotor Functions, and Personality," *Journal of General Psychology* 113 (1986): 29, 40–41; National Commission on Marihuana and Drug Abuse, *Marihuana: A Signal of Misunderstanding* (Washington, DC: GPO, 1972) (SuDocs Y3.M33/2:2MM33, plus appendix volumes); H.G. Pope, Jr., A.J. Gruber, and D. Yurgelun-Todd, "Residual Neuropsychologic Effects of Cannabis," *Current Psychiatry Reports* 3 (2001): 507–12; H.G. Pope, Jr., et al., "Neuropsychological Performance in Long-Term Cannabis Users," *Archives of General Psychiatry* 58 (2001): 909–15; J.F. Siler, et al., "Mariajuana Smoking in Panama," *Military Surgeon* 73 (1933): 269–80; C. Stark-Adamec, R.E. Adamec, and R.O. Phil, "Experimenter Effects in Marihuana Research: A Note of Caution," *Psycho-

logical Reports 51 (1982): 203; D. Solomon, ed., *The Marihuana Papers* (Indianapolis: Bobbs-Merrill, 1966) (including the classic LaGuardia Committee Report); Swiss Federal Commission for Drug Issues (EKDF), *Cannabis Report* (1999); G. Teichner, et al., "The Relationship of Neuropsychological Functioning to Measures of Substance Use in an Adolescent Drug Abusing Sample," *International Journal of Neuroscience* 104 (2000):113–24; A.S. Trebach, *The Great Drug War and Radical Proposals That Could Make America Safe Again* (New York: Macmillan Publishing Company, 1987), 81; J.T. Ungerleider and T. Andrysiak, "Bias and the Cannabis Researcher," *Journal of Clinical Pharmacology* 21 (1981): 153 S-85 S; United Kingdom House of Commons, *Cannabis,* Library Research Paper 00/74 (2000); A. Weil, *The Natural Mind: An Investigation of Drugs and the Higher Consciousness,* Rev. ed. (Boston: Houghton Mifflin Company, 1986), 47; A. Weil, N.E. Zinberg, and J.M. Nelsen, "Clinical and Psychological Effects of Marihuana in Man," *Science* 162 (1968): 1234–42; R.C. Wert and M.L. Raulin, "The Chronic Cerebral Effects of Cannabis Use. I. Methodological Issues and Neurological Findings," *International Journal of the Addictions* 21 (1986): 602–28; R.C. Wert and M.L. Raulin, "The Chronic Cerebral Effects of Cannabis Use. II. Psychological Findings and Conclusions," *International Journal of the Addictions* 21 (1986): 629–42.

Mazindol

Pronunciation: MA-zin-doll (also pronounced MAYZ-in-dohl)

Chemical Abstracts Service Registry Number: 22232-71-9

Formal Names: Mazanor, Sanorex, Teronac

Type: Stimulant (anorectic class). *See* page 15

Federal Schedule Listing: Schedule IV (DEA no. 1605)

USA Availability: Prescription

Pregnancy Category: C

Uses. Mazindol reduces appetite, and the drug's main medical usage is short-term promotion of weight loss. For that purpose one study showed mazindol having about 10% to 20% of **dextroamphetamine**'s strength; another study noted that regardless of relative strength per milligram, patients on mazindol shed about twice as many pounds as those on dextroamphetamine. In studies examining diet drugs, persons using mazindol lost as many or even more pounds compared to persons using **phenmetrazine**. One 12-week experiment found mazindol considerably more effective than **diethylpropion** for human weight loss, although a rat study found those two drugs' effectiveness comparable. Some human studies put mazindol as about equal to **fenfluramine** for weight loss. Still other studies call mazindol's performance the same as a placebo. Perhaps these various findings are less a commentary on mazindol than on the unclear effectiveness of diet drugs in general.

Although mazindol appears to produce depression among some users, in others the drug works as an antidepressant. This antidepressant characteristic is considered helpful in promoting weight loss, as some overweight persons use food to compensate for sadness. As one condition improves, generally the other one does also. Mazindol's dual action as an anorectic and antidepressant can make it especially appropriate for persons struggling to lose both melancholy and weight.

Some mazindol effects are like those of amphetamine, but the two substances are described as chemically unrelated. Mazindol seems to pep up rats. In rat experiments the drug increases tendency to move around, more in females than in males. In humans the compound is used to combat narcolepsy and the decline of muscle tone sometimes associated with that affliction. Mazindol acts as a pain reliever in mice. One study found the drug made humans more sensitive to pain, but other experimental usage reduced pain in terminal cancer patients. Researchers believe mazindol can aid sufferers from Parkinson's disease. A case is reported of the drug acting as an aphrodisiac in a human female. The compound can reduce cholesterol levels.

Drawbacks. Mazindol increases pulse rate, may cause hallucinations, and disrupts sleep. In one study users complained of headache, skin rash, dry mouth, perspiration, tremor in heart and other muscles, nausea, and difficult urination and bowel movements. Users also report being wired, edgy, and dizzy. In human males mazindol can make the testes painful, interfere with erection and ejaculation, and cause urine retention. The latter effect has been exploited to treat incontinence. Mazindol may interfere with production of human growth hormone, a consideration when juveniles take the drug. When tested as a treatment for schizophrenia the drug at best had no effect and even worsened some symptoms. A medical journal article published in 2000 linked mazindol to pulmonary hypertension, the first time such an association was reported. Earlier reports noted development of heart disorder after taking mazindol in combination with fenfluramine or dexfenfluramine, but such affliction has been attributed to those latter two drugs by themselves, so mazindol's role is uncertain.

Abuse factors. In rhesus monkey experiments the animals show a liking for mazindol, but a review of clinical studies found no instances of patients becoming addicted. Although reports exist of mazindol inducing euphoria, human users show no particular liking for the drug. Volunteers comparing several diet drugs found mazindol to have the least appeal by far. Scientists evaluating another experimental study of the drug described it as a "punisher" that persons wanted to avoid.

Drug interactions. Researchers say mazindol and **alcohol** have a multiplier effect when used together, boosting each other's potency and producing an extra buzz for recreational users. Mazindol interferes with some **cocaine** effects, but studies examining mazindol's potential for treating cocaine addiction find a placebo to be about as good. One study even found the two drugs to have a hazardous multiplier effect raising blood pressure and pulse rate, and rat experiments find that mazindol reduces the size of a cocaine dose needed to cause death. Mazindol can react adversely with antimania drug lithium and can counteract drugs intended to lower blood pressure.

Cancer. Laboratory experiments show mazindol promoting cell mutations and chromosome breaks (traditional signs of cancer-causing potential), but that finding's real-life meaning is unclear.

Pregnancy. The drug's influence on fetal development is unestablished. Whether the drug passes into milk of nursing mothers is unknown. Doses that kill female rats while pregnant or after giving birth can leave males and nonpregnant females unscathed. Whether such findings mean that pregnancy increases human sensitivity to the drug is unknown.

Additional scientific information may be found in:

Alvarez, B., et al. "Mazindol in Long-Term Treatment of Narcolepsy." *Lancet* 337 (1991): 1293–94.
Bierger, P., F. Gawin, and T.R. Kosten. "Treatment of Cocaine Abuse with Mazindol." *Lancet* 1 (1989): 283.

Chait, L.D., E.H. Uhlenhuth, and C.E. Johanson. "Reinforcing and Subjective Effects of Several Anorectics in Normal Human Volunteers." *Journal of Pharmacology and Experimental Therapeutics* 242 (1987): 777–83.

Hagiwara, M., et al. "Delayed Onset of Pulmonary Hypertension Associated with an Appetite Suppressant, Mazindol: A Case Report." *Japanese Circulation Journal* 64 (2000): 218–21.

Preston, K.L., et al. "Effects of Cocaine Alone and in Combination with Mazindol in Human Cocaine Abusers." *Journal of Pharmacology and Experimental Therapeutics* 267 (1993): 296–307.

MDA

Pronunciation: em-dee-ā

Chemical Abstracts Service Registry Number: 4764-17-4

Formal Names: Amphedoxamine, 3,4-Methylenedioxyamphetamine

Informal Names: Chocolate Mescaline, Hug Drug, Love, Love Pill, Mellow Drug of America

Type: Hallucinogen. *See* page 25

Federal Schedule Listing: Schedule I (DEA no. 7402)

USA Availability: Illegal to possess

Pregnancy Category: None

Uses. This drug is a derivative of amphetamine and an analog to **MDMA**, with effects similar to the latter and to **MDEA**. MDA is stronger than those two hallucinogens. Researchers also report it to be three to five times stronger than **mescaline**, to which it is chemically related. MDA is legally defined as a hallucinogen, but its stimulant qualities put it in the entactogen pharmacological class—a type of drug with both stimulant and hallucinogenic qualities. MDA is an illicit drug designer's delight; by the 1970s thousands of offshoots had been made.

First produced in a laboratory in 1910, MDA was intended to help people lose weight. One authority believes the drug has potential for stopping allergic reactions to a variety of allergens. As the 1960s arrived the drug had been patented as a cough suppressant and as a tranquilizer, but MDA never went into legal commercial manufacture.

Reports of MDA's psychological effects date back to the 1930s, but not until three decades later did the substance become a recreational drug. It has the capability to change how a person views time and space. While under the influence a user's hearing and sense of touch can become more sensitive, and a person's sense of identity can alter. Emotions and caring about other persons can intensify, as can ability to communicate feelings. Such aspects allowed MDA to find a niche in psychotherapy as well as on the street. Strong doses can bring on hallucinations, with experiences so similar to **LSD** and mescaline that users cannot tell whether they were dosed with the latter drugs or with MDA.

Drawbacks. MDA raises heart rate, blood pressure, body temperature, and salivation. The substance can cause nausea, along with high acid levels in blood. Although one authority notes that the drug can relax muscles, nonetheless tremors and seizures are also possible; MDA is known to worsen Parkinson's disease. MDA can tense up jaw muscles and cause grinding of teeth. As drug effects go away, users may experience weariness and muscle aches accompanied by depression. Users coming off the drug may also be short-tempered, suspicious of others, and nervous. Typically the effects desired by a user decline with repeated use of the drug, while undesired postintoxication effects increase. MDA can cause organic brain damage in rats, in some aspects worse than what MDMA does.

Overdose symptoms resemble those of amphetamine and MDMA, including massive perspiration and strange conduct prone to combativeness. The percentage of fatalities among abusers is small, but the size difference between a recreational dose and a serious overdose can vary tremendously between individuals. What one person can tolerate without apparent ill effect can send another person to a hospital. Blood and urine tests in one fatal overdose case showed only MDA, demonstrating that this drug can be lethal even when it is not part of a polydrug abuse mix.

Men may suffer fewer ill effects from MDA than women do. In one animal study documenting a gender difference in effects, male rats showed a higher body temperature increase than female rats did, but blood levels of MDA stayed higher in the female.

Abuse factors. Not enough scientific information to report about tolerance, dependence, or withdrawal. In animal experiments self-administration is a traditional sign of addictive potential; rats show mild interest in self-administration of MDA.

Drug interactions. Animal experiments suggest that taking certain drugs along with MDA can reduce its toxicity.

Cancer. MDA causes cancer in mice and rats, with males being more susceptible than females.

Pregnancy. Not enough scientific information to report.

Additional information. At one time MDA was nicknamed Ecstasy, but that street name was later transferred to MDMA. An industrial chemical called MDA (methylene dianiline) is not the drug of abuse.

Additional scientific information may be found in:

Climko, R.P., et al. "Ecstacy: A Review of MDMA and MDA." *International Journal of Psychiatry in Medicine* 16 (1986–1987): 359–72.

Hegadoren, K.M., G.B. Baker, and M. Bourin. "3,4-Methylenedioxy Analogues of Amphetamine: Defining the Risks to Humans." *Neuroscience and Biobehavioral Reviews* 23 (1999): 539–53.

Poklis, A., M.A. Mackell, and W.K. Drake. "Fatal Intoxication from 3,4-Methylenedioxyamphetamine." *Journal of Forensic Sciences* 24 (1979): 70–75.

Richards, R.N. "Experience with MDA." *Canadian Medical Association Journal* 106 (1972): 256–59.

Richards, K.C., and H.H. Borgstedt. "Near Fatal Reaction to Ingestion of the Hallucinogenic Drug MDA." *Journal of the American Medical Association* 218 (1971): 1826–27.

MDEA

Pronunciation: em-dee-ee-ā

Chemical Abstracts Service Registry Number: 82801-81-8

Formal Names: 3,4-Methylenedioxyethylamphetamine, MDE

Informal Names: Eve, Intellect

Type: Hallucinogen. *See* page 25

Federal Schedule Listing: Schedule I (DEA no. 7404)

USA Availability: Illegal to possess

Pregnancy Category: None

Uses. This substance is related to **MDA**, **MDMA**, amphetamine, and **methamphetamine**. Drug laws call MDEA a hallucinogen, but it has stimulant effects also. Those dual properties put it in the entactogen pharmacological group, a type of drug with both stimulant and hallucinogenic qualities. Effects are similar to those from MDA and MDMA.

MDEA can create contentedness and feelings of intimacy with other persons. It may promote self-insight, gesturing, and articulate talking. Hallucinations can occur, described as less intense than those brought on by **psilocybin**. Volunteers had normal results in tests of numerical ability while using MDEA, indicating that people can force themselves to overcome at least some of the drug's effects if necessary. Even though users feel more relaxed after taking the substance, it has general stimulant effects—raising the pulse rate, blood pressure, and body temperature. It also elevates the level of cortisol, a hormone that increases blood sugar.

Drawbacks. Apparently MDEA inhibits secretion of human growth hormone. The drug disrupts sleep and dreaming. Psychosis is possible. In experiments with normal volunteers a minority had mental aftereffects including nervousness and discontent.

Some researchers describe MDEA as less toxic than MDMA, but damage is still possible to kidneys, liver, brain, and heart. Persons with heart disease may be in particular danger from MDEA. Overdose symptoms include hallucinations, excessive body temperature, massive perspiration, violent conduct, muscle spasms, difficulty moving arms and legs, convulsions, distress in breathing, and passing out. Fatalities have shown blood clots throughout the body and damage to skeletal muscle. Although deaths from "normal" doses are unlikely among healthy users, the same dose can have stronger effects on some users than on others.

In rat experiments comparing the strength of MDMA to MDEA, about twice as much MDEA is needed to induce excessive body temperature and about four times as much to cause one kind of organic brain damage. The experimenters note, however, that these findings do not extrapolate well to humans because people might take greater doses of MDEA than MDMA to get the desired psychological effects, so any net difference in harm to abusers may be nil despite difference in drug potency.

Abuse factors. Not enough scientific information to report about tolerance, dependence, withdrawal, or addiction.

Drug interactions. Medical investigators suspect that **heroin** and MDEA counteract each other's effects in humans.

Cancer. Not enough scientific information to report.

Pregnancy. Not enough scientific information to report.

Additional scientific information may be found in:

Gouzoulis, E., et al. "Neuroendocrine and Cardiovascular Effects of MDE in Healthy Volunteers." *Neuropsychopharmacology* 8 (1993): 187–93.

Gouzoulis-Mayfrank, E., et al. "Psychopathological, Neuroendocrine and Autonomic Effects of 3,4-Methylenedioxyethylamphetamine (MDE), Psilocybin and D-Methamphetamine in Healthy Volunteers. Results of an Experimental Double-Blind Placebo-Controlled Study." *Psychopharmacology* 142 (1999): 41–50.

Hegadoren, K.M., G.B. Baker, and M. Bourin. "3,4-Methylenedioxy Analogues of Amphetamine: Defining the Risks to Humans." *Neuroscience and Biobehavioral Reviews* 23 (1999): 539–53.

Hermle, L., et al. "Psychological Effects of MDE in Normal Subjects. Are Entactogens a New Class of Psychoactive Agents?" *Neuropsychopharmacology* 8 (1993): 171–76.

MDMA

Pronunciation: em-dee-em-ā

Chemical Abstracts Service Registry Number: 42542-10-9

Formal Names: Methylenedioxymethamphetamine, 3,4-Methylenedioxymethamphetamine

Informal Names: A, Adam, Baby Slits, B-Bomb, Bens, Benzedrine, Biphetamine, Blue Kisses, Blue Lips, California Sunrise, Chrystal Methadrine, Clarity, Cristal, Debs, Decadence, Dex, Dexedrine, Diamonds, Disco Biscuit, Doctor, Dolls, Domex, Draf, Drivers, E, E-Ball, E-Bomb, Ecstasy, Ekies, Elaine, Essence, Euphoria (combined with **mescaline** and **methamphetamine**), Everclear, Fastin, Gaggler, Go, Greenies, Hamburger, H-Bomb (with **heroin**), Honey Flip (with **2C-B**), Hug Drug, Hydro, Iboga, Ice, Khat, Kleenex, Love Doctor, Love Drug, Love Potion Number 9, Lovers' Speed, Love Doves, Love Trip (with mescaline), Lucky Charmz, M&M, MAO, MDM, Methedrine, Mini Beans, Mitsubishi, Molly, Monoamine Oxidase, Morning Shot, M25, New Yorkers, 19, Number 9, Orbit, Pikachu (mixed with **PCP**), Pink Studs, Pollutants, Rave, Road Runner, Rolling, Running, Scooby Snacks, Shabu, Slamming, Spivias, Strawberry Shortcake, Sweeties, 10, USP, Venus, Vitamin E, West Coast Turnarounds, Wheels, Whiffledust, White Dove, Whiz Bombs, Wigits, X, XTC, Yuppie Drug, Zen

Type: Hallucinogen. *See* page 25

Federal Schedule Listing: Schedule I (DEA no. 7405)

USA Availability: Illegal to possess

Pregnancy Category: None

Uses. MDMA was discovered and patented in Europe as World War I began, intended to make soldiers feel less hungry. In civilian usage the drug was supposed to help people lose weight, but other effects portended the product's commercial failure, and it never went on the market. Those other effects attracted attention in the 1960s and 1970s among therapists and recreational drug users alike.

MDMA intensifies sensory sensations (taste, touch, etc.), alters old understandings of what people observe, and allows people to feel distant from themselves. Some users experience self-insights and closer emotional attachment to other persons. Generally the drug does not appear to act as an aphrodisiac, but users report enhanced sexual experiences while under the influence. In therapeutic doses, which may be lighter than those taken by recreational abusers, effects occur without hallucinations and without causing apparent mental cloudiness while intoxicated. Before being banned by the U.S. Drug Enforcement Administration (DEA), doses were given to encourage patients to participate more freely in psychotherapy discussions—a usefulness that still found advocates in the 1990s—and to facilitate understandings among patients, understandings that helped reduce their problems. Underground knowledge of psychiatric usage persists despite an absolute legal prohibition against using the compound: Medical literature reports someone illegally taking the drug for self-medication of posttraumatic stress disorder.

In the history of abused drugs, psychological benefits claimed by proponents have often been deflated by scientific investigation. MDMA is no exception. Psychological tests have compared polydrug users who have or have not taken MDMA and also persons who have abstained from any illicit drug. These tests find no difference among these groups in anger, anxiety, or mood. Whatever feelings of peacefulness that recreational MDMA users experience while intoxicated, those results do not seem to persist afterward. Indeed, experimenters who gave these tests found the MDMA group to have more psychological trouble than the nondrug group. In such findings a key question is whether the drug caused psychic problems or whether problems caused the drug use. Staff members at a Spanish hospital's psychiatric service reviewed a substantial amount of medical literature about MDMA users and observed that the case reports did not sustain a conclusion that MDMA was the primary cause of users' psychiatric problems.

One significant exception exists in findings about MDMA's limited value in promoting personal insight and healthy integration with the world. That exception comes with persons using the drug for spiritual purposes rather than recreationally. Here the all-important influence of set and setting are demonstrated. Spiritual users tune in to certain kinds of psychic effect promoted by the drug and apparently are able to focus their attention so intensely that they can disregard and be unaffected by psychological effects that trouble recreational abusers. This situation appears to demonstrate a principle familiar to historians of drug use, who find that a substance can be beneficial in a particular cultural context and yet have catastrophic consequences when used by someone who disregards that context. Any spiritual purpose for which MDMA may be used will, of course, have no impact on the drug's physical actions, although persons who seldom use it may be spared various hazards documented by scientists.

MDMA is legally classified as a hallucinogen, but it is pharmacologically classified as an entactogen—a type of drug with both stimulant and hallucinogenic qualities. MDMA is recreationally used more for its hallucinogenic actions than for stimulant actions. It is an analog to **MDA** and related to **MDEA**, amphetamine, **methamphetamine**, and **mescaline**. MDMA is described as mellower than MDA, and some users experience MDMA as less potent than mescaline. MDMA can alter perceptions of time and space and induce feelings of peacefulness. Users typically understand that MDMA hallucinations (such as floating in midair or seeing geometrical designs) are unreal; users normally do not undergo a temporary psychosis in which the sensations are misperceived as objective reality.

After recreational use became publicized, MDMA was made a Schedule I controlled substance. Despite that ban, during the 1990s MDMA was popular at high-energy all-night rave dance parties, not only for psychic actions but for enabling people to go without sleep, food, and drink while physically exerting themselves. A person using MDMA in that way will likely feel complete exhaustion when the drug experience ends. The compound reduces pain and promotes talkativeness, factors that might be appealing at raves.

The Drug Abuse Warning Network (DAWN) tracks "mentions" of illicit drugs in hospital emergency room cases. A "mention" means that examination of a patient showed traces of a drug, not that the drug caused injury. DAWN thereby helps track a drug's popularity. In 1993 MDMA had 196 DAWN mentions; in 1998 the total was 143,600. As the twenty-first century began, the DEA reported 750,000 doses being consumed each week in just the New Jersey and New York City areas.

Drawbacks. Scientific literature portrays MDMA as a drug of extremes, producing pleasures and afflictions that either enrapture or kill users. Compared to many other drugs, much more is known about MDMA's hazards simply because so many persons have used it and received medical aid when things went badly. The volume of medical emergencies, however, is more than just a statistical phenomenon caused by sheer numbers of users. Some drugs used even more widely do not generate nearly as many medical complaints. MDMA really is more dangerous than many other substances.

One problem in evaluating MDMA dangers, a problem openly acknowledged by some scientists, is the challenge of confirming that a sick person indeed ingested MDMA a month ago rather than a fake substitute. All sorts of substances can produce effects similar to those of MDMA, which is why illicit dealers can so easily sell fake merchandise. Nonetheless, researchers investigating drug actions can often enough verify that MDMA is the actual substance. The following information reflects the scientific consensus about MDMA.

It has the physical and mental actions typical of amphetamine. A group of persons who at one time or another used amphetamine, **LSD**, and MDMA said they felt most pepped-up with amphetamine, least so with LSD, but had the greatest euphoria and contentedness with MDMA. Another group comparing amphetamine and MDMA reported MDMA to have fewer drawbacks. The DEA considers the drug less addictive than **cocaine** or **heroin**.

The substance degrades thinking processes. In tests of alertness, memory, learning, and intelligence a group of marijuana users performed as well as nonusers of marijuana, while a group that had used both marijuana and MDMA did worse. MDMA causes persistent and even permanent organic changes in the brain. Grand mal brain seizures have been attributed to the substance. Brain damage observed in MDMA users is consistent and is related to how much drug has been used (size of dose and frequency with which the drug is taken). Psychological tests verify that persons with such damage have trouble remembering things that are seen and heard, although the brain damage has not been proven to cause the memory difficulty. Whatever the precise cause, in memory tests polydrug users who have taken MDMA do worse than those who have never taken the compound. Evidence exists that MDMA reduces attention span and interferes with reasoning. The drug produces brain injury suspected of increasing someone's impulsiveness. In tests comparing polydrug users who have used MDMA with those who have not, MDMA users show increased impulsiveness correlating with how much they have used the drug. Interviews comparing polydrug users find the MDMA group more prone to paranoia, to physical complaints lacking any apparent bodily cause, to nervousness and unfriendliness, to phobias, and to obsessing on various things. Panic disorder with agoraphobia (fear of open spaces) can occur.

MDMA has various influences on blood. The drug is suspected of causing anemia. Under the influence of MDMA, blood components may block vessels, having the effect of tiny clots that can cause internal bleeding, evidenced by purple spots on the skin. Blood clots in the brain and death of cerebral tissue have been credited to MDMA. Autopsies have shown massive blood clotting throughout organs, accompanied by skeletal muscle deterioration.

Many other hazards exist. MDMA increases body temperature, sometimes enough to mimic heat stroke, and animal experiments indicate that temperatures in surroundings or inside the body can affect the amount of brain damage caused by MDMA. The drug boosts pulse rate. Initially a dose increases blood pressure (sometimes enough to burst vessels in the brain), but later, as the effects of a dose proceed, blood pressure falls below the user's original reading (a decline that can promote fainting). MDMA can create heart malfunction, kidney failure, and liver disease. Liver cirrhosis and failure can result—sometimes treatable, sometimes fatal. Cramps and muscle tics have been observed, even including one case where Parkinson's disease developed. Cases are reported of MDMA causing pneumomediastinum, an ailment involving severe breathing difficulty. The drug promotes nausea. Hazy eyesight and a case of temporary double vision caused by MDMA have been reported. Jaw clenching and grinding after taking the drug result in excessive tooth wear; one study of teeth in MDMA users found enamel completely worn away from some areas, an affliction seen far less often in people who did not use the drug. MDMA can cause skin rash and pimples.

Gender difference in drug effect is possible. One survey of case reports noted that men tended to use more MDMA than women did, and an experiment found that at any given dose the drug seemed to harm verbal memory more in men than in women. Another experiment showed male users having more change in two measures of brain chemistry function than females did. An experiment with rats showed males maintaining higher blood levels of the drug than females did, while females experienced more increase in body temperature than male rats did.

Abuse factors. In a survey of 100 American university students, two thirds said that desirable actions declined and undesirable ones increased as MDMA use continued; similar results came from a survey of 100 users in Australia, and scientists studying the drug concur with those survey findings. As with other potent stimulants, abusers are known to use MDMA in binges, taking one dose after another before the previous ones wear off. Heavy MDMA users have scored low in measures of harm avoidance, and MDMA use correlates with unprotected male homosexual conduct. Such findings raise the question of cause and effect: Does MDMA promote reckless behavior, or are self-destructive users simply indifferent about all sorts of life hazards, of which MDMA is only one?

Flashbacks are reported, with case reports mentioning time lengths ranging from less than one minute to two hours.

Drug interactions. Taking MDMA together with the drug saquinavir (used against human immunodeficiency virus [HIV] in AIDS [acquired immunodeficiency syndrome]) may be dangerous; usage with the HIV/AIDS drug ritonavir can be fatal. Untoward reaction with the antidepressant fluoxetine (Prozac) is suspected, and reaction with the antidepressant phenelzine sulfate (a monoamine oxidase inhibitor—MAOI) can produce excessive blood pressure, heavy sweating, muscle tics, and rigidity. Such perils are quite possible with any other MAOI. Keeping in mind the need to be cautious about extrapolating animal experiments to humans, we can note that taking MDMA with LSD (candyflipping) produces a multiplier effect intensifying MDMA actions in rats. **Chloral hydrate** permits some MDMA action in rats while reducing subsequent organic brain change. Also in rats MDMA boosts pain relief provided by **morphine**. In male rats the malaria and heart drug quinidine can increase MDMA's tendency to raise body temperature. **Alcohol** allegedly reduces some effects sought by MDMA users, but that belief has not received general scientific sanction. Scientists have confirmed that alcohol increases MDMA's reduction of immune system function, which may increase risk of infections. Physicians treating MDMA overdose find that water can worsen dangerous effects, and these doctors have concluded that people should not drink much liquid of any sort while using the drug (hard advice for sweaty and overheated dancers).

Cancer. Not enough scientific information to report.

Pregnancy. Scientists who studied what happened with 49 women who used MDMA while pregnant were unable to reach any conclusions about influence on fetal development. The researchers did conclude that the women's lifestyles routinely included assorted factors perilous to achieving healthy offspring—tobacco smoking, consuming alcohol to excess, unwanted pregnancy. A study of 136 women who used MDMA while pregnant noted an incidence of birth defects much higher than normal (15.4% versus normal 2% or 3%), but the usual confounding factors, such as polydrug abuse and unwanted pregnancy, hindered conclusions about effect on fetal development. Rat experiments confirm maternal brain damage but have not found brain damage in offspring even though their behavior differs in some respects from rats whose mothers receive no MDMA during pregnancy. An experiment with chickens found no MDMA effect on measured aspects of embryo development.

Additional information. "Benzedrine," "biphetamine," "dexedrine," "iboga" (**ibogaine**), and "**khat**" are nicknames for MDMA, but none of those substances is MDMA.

Additional scientific information may be found in:

Downing, Joseph. "The Psychological and Physiological Effects of MDMA on Normal Volunteers." *Journal of Psychoactive Drugs* 18 (1986): 335–39.

Gouzoulis-Mayfrank, E., et al. "Impaired Cognitive Performance in Drug Free Users of Recreational Ecstasy (MDMA)." *Journal of Neurology, Neurosurgery, and Psychiatry* 68 (2000): 719–25.

Greer, G., and R. Tolbert. "Subjective Reports of the Effects of MDMA in a Clinical Setting." *Journal of Psychoactive Drugs* 18 (1986): 319–27.

McGuire, P. "Long Term Psychiatric and Cognitive Effects of MDMA Use." *Toxicology Letters* 112–13 (2000): 153–56.

Rochester, J.A., and J.T. Kirchner. "Ecstasy (3,4-Methylenedioxymethamphetamine): History, Neurochemistry, and Toxicology." *Journal of the American Board of Family Practice* 12 (1999): 137–42.

Shulgin, A.T. "The Background and Chemistry of MDMA." *Journal of Psychoactive Drugs* 18 (1986): 291–304.

Vollenweider, F.X., et al. "Psychological and Cardiovascular Effects and Short-term Sequelae of MDMA ("Ecstasy") in MDMA-Naive Healthy Volunteers." *Neuropsychopharmacology* 19 (1998): 241–51.

Meperidine

Pronunciation: me-PER-i-deen

Chemical Abstracts Service Registry Number: 57-42-1. (Hydrochloride form 50-13-5)

Formal Names: Centralgin, Demer-Idine, Demerol, Dolantin, Dolosal, Mepergan, Pethidine, Pethoid

Informal Names: Demmies

Type: Depressant (opioid class). *See* page 24

Federal Schedule Listing: Schedule II (DEA no. 9230)

USA Availability: Prescription

Pregnancy Category: B

Uses. This drug has been used since the 1930s for easing pain in many conditions, including migraine headaches, surgery, gallbladder attack, sickle cell anemia crisis, childbirth, and emergency treatment of injury on mountaineering expeditions. The drug is also used to manage porphyria, a body chemistry disorder that can make a person extremely sensitive to light and that can include violent outbursts. The substance is used to bring persons out of a **PCP** psychosis. Experimental usage of meperidine and **dextroamphetamine** together has reduced symptoms of mental depression, but the test was too brief to measure how long benefits might continue. Oral meperidine dosage can partly numb a person's mucous membranes, and the drug is used as one element of general and local anesthesia. The substance has a calming action but is not considered to be a sleep inducer at medical dosage levels. Upon prolonged usage the calming action can be replaced by depression and uneasiness. Depending on specifics of use, **morphine** is 6 to 10 times stronger than meperidine.

Drawbacks. Meperidine can reduce blood pressure and can make a person feel faint upon suddenly standing up. Itching, perspiration, muscle tremors, nausea, and vomiting are other unwanted effects. Although constipation is a classic unwanted action of opiates/opioids, meperidine may produce less than morphine does. Meperidine can cause cardiac and breathing difficulty and has been known to cause seizures, delirium, and hallucinations. The drug may promote convulsions in persons who are already susceptible to such affliction. Some tests show the drug to have slight influence on eye-hand coordination and no effect on other voluntary physical movement. Tests oriented specifically toward driving skills, however, led researchers to conclude that people should not operate a motor vehicle for 24 hours after an intramuscular injection of meperidine. Anyone with enlarged prostate, urinary difficulty, Addison's disease, or underactive thyroid should be wary about using the drug. An unusual case report tells of a patient developing Parkinson's disease symptoms from meperidine; more commonly such reports arise from contaminated illicit substances related to meperidine. Another illicit peril occurs when persons grind up and inject oral meperidine tablets; the talc in those tablets can block tiny blood vessels throughout the body and also cause those vessels to bleed—serious business in the eyes or brain. Illicit intramuscular injection of the drug over a period of years can cause muscle damage. Injecting into an artery can lead to gangrene.

Abuse factors. Meperidine tolerance occurs. Dependence may develop faster than with morphine, but meperidine's withdrawal syndrome may be briefer; symptoms also tend to be more limited than with morphine, perhaps just muscle spasms and unrest. When medical personnel are withdrawing addicts from **heroin**, meperidine has enough cross-tolerance to control withdrawal symptoms.

Drug interactions. Meperidine should be avoided by persons taking monoamine oxidase inhibitors (MAOIs, found in some antidepressants). That combination can be dangerous or even fatal. **Alcohol** and other depressants should be used carefully with meperidine in order to avoid cumulative overdose. Amphetamines boost pain relief provided by meperidine. The HIV/AIDS (human immunodeficiency virus/acquired immunodeficiency syndrome) drug ritonavir is believed to lengthen a meperidine dose, meaning that too much of the opioid could build up in a person who is on a normal meperidine medication schedule. Experiments with the ritonavir-meperidine combination, however, have shown the risk to be less than expected. Air pressure affects a meperidine dose; the higher the altitude, the longer a dose lasts. **Phenobarbital**, the antipsychotic drug chlorpromazine (Thorazine), and the heartburn-ulcer medicine cimetidine interfere with meperidine. Brewer's yeast is said to produce a bad reaction with meperidine, such as raising blood pressure so high that a medical emergency occurs.

Cancer. One analysis of medical records in Great Britain found a statistical association between receiving meperidine at birth and subsequent development of childhood cancer. A statistical association, however, simply provides guidance for future research and does not demonstrate cause and effect. Analysis of a different and smaller set of records found no association.

Pregnancy. An experiment on pregnant mice produced no birth defects definitely attributable to the drug, but meperidine has caused congenital malformations in hamsters. Medical records from a few dozen women who used meperidine during pregnancy revealed no congenital malformations attributable to the substance. If a pregnant woman takes the drug, it will pass into the fetus, where the substance tends to build up. Difficulties have not been seen in infants from such women unless the drug has been administered during childbirth. In those latter cases a respiratory emergency can occur in infants who acquired the drug during birth, and less serious newborn behavioral abnormalities are common. Rhesus monkeys who received fetal exposure at time of birth were tested for perception and thinking ability. On one test they did worse than monkeys who had no meperidine exposure, and on another test they did better. In humans, meperidine enters the milk of nursing mothers, but the level is low enough to be considered safe for the infant.

Additional information. An injectable format of the drug called Mepergan is intended for deep intramuscular administration. Intravenous injection can diminish breathing and stop the heart. Subcutaneous administration can cause sores at the injection site and even kill patches of skin. The product ingredients include sodium metabisulfite, to which some persons have a dangerous allergy. Mepergan is to be used cautiously by asthmatics.

Additional scientific information may be found in:

Clark, R.F., E.M. Wei, and P.O. Anderson. "Meperidine: Therapeutic Use and Toxicity." *The Journal of Emergency Medicine* 13 (1995): 797–802.

Henderson, M.E. "Central Nervous System Effects of Meperidine." *Hospital Pharmacy* 20 (1985): 934.

Korttila, K., and M. Linnoila. "Psychomotor Skills Related to Driving after Intramuscular Administration of Diazepam and Meperidine." *Anesthesiology* 42 (1975): 685–91.

Miller, R.R., and H. Jick. "Clinical Effects of Meperidine in Hospitalized Medical Patients." *Journal of Clinical Pharmacology* 18 (1978): 180–89.

Zacny, J.P., et al. "Subjective, Behavioral and Physiological Responses to Intravenous Meperidine in Healthy Volunteers." *Psychopharmacology* 111 (1993): 306–14.

Mephobarbital

Pronunciation: mef-oh-BAR-bi-tal

Chemical Abstracts Service Registry Number: 115-38-8

Formal Names: Mebaral, Methylphenobarbital, Methylphenobarbitone

Type: Depressant (barbiturate class). *See* page 20

Federal Schedule Listing: Schedule IV (DEA no. 2250)

USA Availability: Prescription

Pregnancy Category: D

Uses. Mephobarbital has both sedative and anticonvulsant effects. Anticonvulsant properties make the drug a standard treatment for epilepsy. When used for that condition, stoppage of the drug must be handled carefully lest a person start having a streak of seizures one after another (a potentially fatal condition called status epilepticus). Sedative qualities make mephobarbital an effective tranquilizer, with users feeling lighthearted and mellow without getting very sleepy. Men metabolize the drug faster than women do, meaning a dose will last longer in women. After ingestion the drug metabolizes into **phenobarbital**, which seems to be a more potent sedative. Health care practitioners sometimes administer those two drugs together.

Drawbacks. In an experiment comparing mephobarbital to phenobarbital in epileptic children, parents reported fewer unwanted behavioral effects with mephobarbital, and some pediatricians agree with that observation. The most typical behavior problem in such children is hyperactivity. A formal test comparing the two drugs, however, found no difference in either unwanted conduct or therapeutic power.

Mephobarbital is to be avoided if a person has porphyria, a disease reflecting a body chemistry disorder and in which a person may be harmed by exposure to light. The drug should also be avoided if a person has a muscle-weakening disease called myasthenia gravis, or a thyroid deficiency causing an affliction called myxedema.

Persons using this drug may need extra vitamin D, due to possible deficiency that might be caused by faster metabolism of the vitamin.

Abuse factors. Not enough scientific information to report on tolerance, dependence, withdrawal, and addiction.

Drug interactions. Taking mephobarbital with acetaminophen (Tylenol and similar products) may promote liver injury. Mephobarbital can interfere with effectiveness of birth control pills and with actions of medicines used to control epilepsy and blood clotting. Drugs used to treat asthma, blood pressure, and heart ailment may not work as well if a person also takes mephobarbital.

Cancer. Not enough scientific information to report.

Pregnancy. Additional vitamin K is recommended for pregnant women using mephobarbital as childbirth approaches, in order to reduce bleeding in the women and offspring. Mephobarbital can help reduce fetal pulse rate irregularity but has been found to cause birth defects, with the risk malformations increasing if other antiepileptic drugs are also used. The drug is found in breast milk of nursing mothers who use the substance.

Additional scientific information may be found in:

De Haan, J., and L. Stolte. "Drugs and the Fetal Heart Rate." *British Medical Journal* 4 (October 16, 1971): 171.

Willis, J., et al. "Barbiturate Anticonvulsants: A Neuropsychological and Quantitative Electroencephalographic Study." *Journal of Child Neurology* 12 (1997): 169–71.

Young, R.S., et al. "A Randomized, Double-Blind, Crossover Study of Phenobarbital and Mephobarbital." *Journal of Child Neurology* 1 (1986): 361–63.

Meprobamate

Pronunciation: meh-proh-BA-mait

Chemical Abstracts Service Registry Number: 57-53-4

Formal Names: Deprol, Equagesic, Equanil, Micrainin, Miltown, Stopayne, Tenavoid

Informal Names: Mother's Little Helper

Type: Depressant. *See* page 19

Federal Schedule Listing: Schedule IV (DEA no. 2820)

USA Availability: Prescription

Pregnancy Category: D

Uses. This drug became available in the 1950s as an alternative to barbiturates. It works as a sleep aid and muscle relaxant, the latter property perhaps a result of the drug's antianxiety property rather than a direct effect. Meprobamate's muscle relaxant action improved breathing in experimental treatment of tetanus. A person's appetite may get better with the drug, but again as a result of anxiety reduction rather than direct appetite stimulation—an agricultural experiment using meprobamate to encourage weight gain in chickens was unsuccessful. The drug may lessen petit mal epilepsy seizures but worsen grand mal seizures. Meprobamate has also been used against neuroses and attention deficit hyperactivity disorder (ADHD), against a type of muscular discomfort called myofascial pain, and as part of therapy treating skin lesions brought on by worry. Meprobamate has helped improve stubborn cases of gastrointestinal afflictions, which may have a component of stress. An experiment showed that persons using the drug can fool a lie detector test.

Meprobamate became perhaps the most highly regarded tranquilizer in the United States. In some research during that era of meprobamate's popularity the question was no longer whether the drug worked but how much better it worked for some groups of people (married, widowed, overweight) than for others. Nonetheless, meprobamate's medical uses declined after benzodiazepine class depressants became available. In retrospect skepticism arose about whether meprobamate had ever been as beneficial as its reputation indicated. Some experts decided that its muscle relaxant and antianxiety actions were no stronger than those inherent to any sedative. One team of scientific investigators concluded that in some circumstances patients' therapeutic reactions to meprobamate were "no worse than to placebo"—faint praise indeed. Transformation of the medical establishment's attitude toward meprobamate is, however, a social history study beyond the scope of this book.

Drawbacks. Meprobamate can cause euphoria and, even though it is a depressant, can have stimulant actions in some circumstances—indeed, mania has been known to occur after a dose. Unwanted actions include headache, vision trouble, nausea, diarrhea, dizziness, slurred speech, burning or prickling sensations, rashes or other skin outbreaks, severely reduced body temperature, low blood pressure, accelerated heartbeat, fainting, and difficulty in moving around. Users should avoid operating dangerous devices such as automobiles. Tests have measured worsened learning ability, physical coordination, and reaction time while a person is under meprobamate's influence—although such problems are not found with all tests designed to detect them.

During meprobamate's medical popularity in the 1960s military tests explored the drug's influence on performance under stress. One test series simulated aircraft pilot situations involving simultaneous tracking of locations in two dimensions, monitoring changes in audio signals, and decoding messages—while exposed to reduced oxygen levels simulating altitudes up to 17,000 feet. In another test series civilian experimenters adapted techniques used by the Swedish air force in a task where persons had to push buttons, pull levers, and press pedals in response to lights and sounds. Investigators basically found that the drug acted as a distraction; people could perform adequately when low levels of skill were required, but as more and more tasks had to be accomplished at higher speeds, the drug interfered with performance. Such a result was hardly surprising, although details may have been relevant to military decision makers.

In mice the drug promotes amnesia. Experimenters gave the drug to rats for 12 weeks and found it reduced the amount of DNA in brain cells. Meprobamate may aggravate porphyria, a blood chemistry disorder that can make people violent and sensitive to light. Although some persons use the drug for years without untoward effect, case reports note uncommon instances where the drug may have caused serious and sometimes fatal blood diseases such as agranulocytosis and aplastic anemia.

One disquieting effect of meprobamate is its ability to produce flat brainwave readings, which could cause medical personnel to cease vital treatment in a mistaken belief that the patient has died.

Abuse factors. Meprobamate's abuse potential has been described as similar to benzodiazepine depressants. Dependence on meprobamate can develop if excessive amounts are routinely used. Abuse of this drug is considered a particular risk with addicts to **alcohol** or other drugs. Symptoms of withdrawal from meprobamate have been likened to delirium tremens of alcohol withdrawal and can include tremors and twitches, trouble in controlling movement, insomnia, headache, vomiting, anxiety, confusion, and hallucinations. Convulsions are possible but uncommon. On rare occasion death has been attributed to withdrawal, but not all authorities agree that meprobamate is the sole cause. For sure, however, dogs that are dependent on the substance can go into convulsions and die if their supply is suddenly cut off.

Drug interactions. In mice **nicotine** reduces the time they are physically uncoordinated after a meprobamate dose, just as we might expect when a stimulant (nicotine) is taken after a depressant. In contrast, injection of **marijuana**'s main active component THC increases the power of a meprobamate dose in animals. Meprobamate has been used in combination with **dextroamphetamine** for human weight loss, a combination that had uncertain effectiveness but that produced fewer unwanted actions than dextroamphetamine alone. Alcohol and meprobamate each have similar unwanted effects, and in that regard using both together can be the equivalent of taking extra doses of one or the other. Among steady drinkers, however, blood levels of meprobamate decline faster than in nondrinkers, meaning a meprobamate dose lasts a shorter time in the drinkers. A mice study indicated that poisonous effects of meprobamate worsen if either alcohol or **phenobarbital** is also used. Phenobarbital and other barbiturates have cross-tolerance with meprobamate, meaning that the barbiturates can substitute for meprobamate in at least some respects.

Cancer. Not enough scientific information to report.

Pregnancy. Meprobamate administered into chicken eggs results in embryo malformations, and skeletal deformity has been observed with fetal development in rats exposed to the compound. The drug passes into a human fetus. A study of over 50,000 pregnancies, including many women who used meprobamate, found no evidence of birth defects linked to the drug, findings duplicated by another analysis of outcomes in more than 6,000 pregnancies. Nonetheless, meprobamate is suspected of causing birth defects. Indeed, in a study of almost 20,000 pregnancies, birth defects were over twice as common among women using meprobamate during early pregnancy than among women who used other antianxiety drugs and more than four times as common compared to women who took no drug at all in early pregnancy. One study found that congenital heart lesions occurred more often if meprobamate was used during pregnancy. Rats with fetal exposure to meprobamate show learning difficulties, and tests of five-year-old children who had prenatal exposure to the substance reveal impaired reasoning ability. The meprobamate level in milk of nursing mothers has been measured as up to four times higher than the level in their blood.

Additional scientific information may be found in:

Carson, J. "Meprobamate Revisited." *New York State Journal of Pharmacy* 2 (1989): 45–46.

Gomolin, I. "Meprobamate." *Clinical Toxicology* 18 (1981): 757–60.

Greenblatt, D.J., and R.I. Shader. "Meprobamate: A Study of Irrational Drug Use." *American Journal of Psychiatry* 127 (1971): 1297–1303.

Logan, B.K., G.A. Case, and A.M. Gordon. "Carisoprodol, Meprobamate, and Driving Impairment." *Journal of Forensic Sciences* 45 (2000): 619–23.

McNair, D.M. "Antianxiety Drugs and Human Performance." *Archives of General Psychiatry* 29 (1973): 611–17.

"Meprobamate." *Medical Letter on Drugs and Therapeutics* 7 (1965): 36.

Mescaline

Pronunciation: MES-kuh-lin (also pronounced MES-kuh-leen)

Chemical Abstracts Service Registry Number: 54-04-6

Formal Names: 3, 4, 5-Trimethoxyphenethylamine

Informal Names: Beans, Big Chief, Blue Caps, Button, Cactus, Cactus Buttons, Cactus Head, Chief, Love Trip (combination with **MDMA**), Mesc, Mescal, Mescalito, Mescap, Mese, Mezc, Moon, Musk, Peyote, Topi

Type: Hallucinogen. *See* page 25

Federal Schedule Listing: Schedule I (DEA no. 7381)

USA Availability: Illegal to possess

Pregnancy Category: None

Uses. This is the main active drug in the **peyote** cactus. In addition to being found in that natural product, mescaline can also be manufactured in a laboratory. Researchers have noted that mescaline, **LSD**, and **psilocybin** have similar actions even though the substances have significant chemical dissimilarities. Effects are so alike that volunteers who took the drugs in experiments could not tell which of the three they received. Studies indicate cross-tolerance exists among the three. Mescaline is related to amphetamine.

Mescaline has been used to study mechanisms of schizophrenia, and at one time the substance was used in experimental psychotherapy. The drug encouraged self-examination in patients and helped them to see significance in ordinary things they had barely noticed before. Such effects have also been described by persons who took the drug simply to find out what it is like. When mescaline was used as an experimental drug in psychotherapy, therapists reported that the substance helped people recall repressed memories. Debate existed, however, about whether the apparent memories were real and whether the recollection experience turned out to have therapeutic benefit. One experiment found that mescaline could help persons achieve creative answers to work-related problems that had resisted resolution for months. Research designed to measure whether the drug promotes creativity has found that volunteers' feelings of increased creativity were supported in general and as a group by higher test scores on elements of creativity. "In general" and "as a group" may be important qualifiers about the results, however.

Users have reported expansion of color perception, but a test designed to detect such a phenomenon produced mixed results. A rabbit study found that mescaline could relieve pain. In a human experiment mescaline promoted growth hormone levels. In rats appetite may increase.

Drawbacks. Individuals with a personal or family history of serious mental illness may be particularly vulnerable to lengthy psychosis from mescaline, although a study of former and current users of mescaline, LSD, or psilocybin found that they scored normally on psychological tests—with the exception that persons who engaged in current hallucinogen use were more depressed and nervous and prone to risk-taking.

Visual hallucinations during a mescaline dose are common; auditory ones less so. Aside from visual hallucinations, users not only may have trouble recognizing faces but may see startling transformations of their own faces in a mirror, viewing the image as not only something apart from themselves but as something ominous. People may feel like their bodies are changing in shape and be unable to detect portions of their bodies. Perceptions of time and space may also change. The drug intoxication typically begins with euphoria, but in a laboratory setting, the euphoria often converts to nervousness and suspicion, possibly ending in depression. Subjects have been known to say and do things they did not want to but were unable to stop themselves. Persons under the drug's influence may be very open to suggestions, a state that could be exploited by unscrupulous persons.

Research shows that the drug can cause headache, perspiration, hot or cold sensations, feelings of prickling or burning, dizziness, cramps, nausea, and vomiting accompanied by small increases in pulse rate and blood pressure. In a sufficient dose mescaline can impair breathing, increase body temperature, and lower pulse rate and blood pressure. Hearing may become so sensitive that ordinary noises are painful. Other senses may have abnormal reactions also.

Tests of reasoning and mental focus produce low scores while people use the drug. Mescaline-related deaths are usually not caused by the chemical itself but by things people did while their judgment was impaired. After rats receive mescaline they appear to forget how to navigate a maze and also take longer to solve problems (figuring out how to get past obstacles). The drug promotes fighting among rats; one group of researchers described the aggression as "robust." Debate exists about whether the drug makes rats fiercer or simply reduces inhibitions in stressful situations. Aggression and wild behavior are not seen as consequences of the drug among human users, and in some circumstances mescaline makes rats lethargic.

Dogs assume odd body stances after receiving the drug and act so lethargic as to be almost insensible. Monkeys seem fascinated as they look at ordinary objects, a reaction that may indicate visual hallucinations. Monkeys first act excitable after dosage, then lethargic. Rats, dogs, and monkeys all exhibit repetitive convulsivelike movements at high doses. In monkeys a fatal dose may not kill them until three or four days have passed.

Abuse factors. A rat experiment found evidence of tolerance, but investigators surmised that the rats might simply have been learning how to compensate for drug effects on performance as the experiment continued. Rather than dosage effectiveness declining, the effects may have been unchanging as rats pushed through them by strength of will. Investigators running a rabbit experiment reported tolerance. Evidence exists for tolerance in animals and humans who receive the drug daily, but such tolerance dissipates quickly once the drug is stopped; two or three days later a dose can produce the same level of effects as before. Dependence does not seem to occur.

Drug interactions. Not enough scientific information to report.

Cancer. Not enough scientific information to report.

Pregnancy. The drug will pass into the fetus of a pregnant monkey. In hamsters mescaline has caused birth defects and delayed development of bone structures, along with reducing the number of offspring in litters. Human birth defects are suspected.

Additional information. "Mescal" is both a nickname for mescaline and the name of an alcoholic beverage; they are different substances.

Additional scientific information may be found in:

Adlaf, E.M., et al. "Nonmedical Drug Use among Adolescent Students: Highlights from the 1999 Ontario Student Drug Use Survey." *CMAJ: Canadian Medical Association Journal* 162 (2000): 1677–80.

Hermle, L., et al. "Mescaline-Induced Psychopathological, Neuropsychological, and Neurometabolic Effects in Normal Subjects: Experimental Psychosis as a Tool for Psychiatric Research." *Biological Psychiatry* 32 (1992): 976–91.

Hoch, P.H., J.P. Cattel, and H.H. Pennes. "Effects of Mescaline and Lysergic Acid (D-LSD-25)." *American Journal of Psychiatry* 108 (1952): 579–84.

Hollister, L.E., and A.M. Hartman. "Mescaline, Lysergic Acid Diethylamide and Psilocybin: Comparison of Clinical Syndromes, Effects on Color Perception and Biochemical Measures." *Comprehensive Psychiatry* 3 (1962): 235–42.

Huxley, A. *The Doors of Perception, and Heaven and Hell.* New York: Harper and Row, 1963.

Kapadia, G.J., and M.B.E. Fayez. "Peyote Constituents: Chemistry, Biogenesis, and Biological Effects." *Journal of Pharmaceutical Sciences* 59 (1970): 1699–1727.

Unger, S.M. "Mescaline, LSD, Psilocybin and Personality Change." *Psychiatry: Journal for the Study of Interpersonal Processes* 26 (May 1963): 111–25.

Methadone

Pronunciation: METH-a-dohn (also pronounced METH-a-don)

Chemical Abstracts Service Registry Number: 76-99-3. (Hydrochloride form 1095-90-5)

Formal Names: Amidone, Dolophine, Eptadone, Heptanal, Ketalgin, Mephanon, Methadose, Physeptone, Symoron, Tussol

Informal Names: Balloons, Breeze, Burdock, Buzz Bomb, Cartridges, Dollies, Dolls, Done, Fixer, Fizzies, Juice, Juicer, Jungle Juice, Medecina, Meth-A-Done, Mud, Phyamps, Pixie, Red Rock, Tootsie Roll, Wafers

Type: Depressant (opioid class). *See* page 24

Federal Schedule Listing: Schedule II (DEA no. 9250)

USA Availability: Prescription

Pregnancy Category: B

Uses. This drug was invented by Germany's Nazi regime in 1941 as a substitute for inadequate **morphine** supplies. Today methadone is best known as a legal substitute for **heroin**. In addition to that use in addiction treatment programs, methadone is given to adults and children as a pain reliever for surgery, cancer, burns, and other conditions. The substance is used as a cough suppressant and also has calming qualities. In racehorses the drug can promote running ability and is banned from the sport. A human dose can last for 24 hours, rather long for a drug of this type and class. For pain relief a dose of methadone may be roughly 2.5 to 14.3 times stronger than morphine, depending on how and why the drug is administered.

Drawbacks. Some persons experience euphoria from methadone. Unwanted effects can include vitamin deficiency, constipation, sleepiness, breathing difficulty, and low blood pressure. People may feel faint if they suddenly stand up from a sitting or prone position. Nausea, vomiting, constipation, urinary difficulty, sweating, lowered sex drive, and impaired sexual performance are other well-known problems. Liver disease may allow dangerous buildup of methadone levels from normal doses.

Abilities to operate dangerous machinery such as automobiles may be reduced. Tests of persons undergoing methadone maintenance therapy indicate they may be able to drive satisfactorily if they use no other drugs, but most methadone maintenance patients also use other drugs that worsen driving performance and exhibit assorted types of personality problems that leak over into driving habits.

In the 1970s methadone was suspected of causing memory trouble, but a group of researchers who investigated the question found no such difficulties. In 2000 a study reported significant memory problems in a group of methadone maintenance recipients, but the same group also had confounding conditions such as head injury and alcoholism that may have affected memory test performance. Another 2000 study comparing methadone users to nonusers concluded that life factors other than methadone were the best explanation for differences in scores on thinking tests.

Abuse factors. Although methadone is sometimes described as blocking heroin's effects, the two drugs simply have cross-tolerance, meaning one of them can substitute for the other in some ways. In addition, persons who find one of the drugs pleasant will probably find the other one just as appealing. For those reasons, heroin addicts can often be switched to methadone in order to maintain their drug habit legally, but the switch does not cure their drug addiction. Some heroin users even like methadone better; some methadone recipients continue using heroin on the side. On the basis of death statistics, some authorities feel methadone is more dangerous than heroin.

Addicts in methadone maintenance programs have chaotic lives. One study of program participants found 7% were likely to be pathological gamblers; another study of methadone program participants found 16% to be pathological gamblers and an additional 15% to have a gambling problem. Researchers have noted that violent traumas are more frequent among methadone program participants than among the average population. In one survey 34% of patients said they received treatment for mental disorder, 64% of the women said they used psychoactive drugs during pregnancy, 80% of parents said they were arrested while their children were growing up, and parents reported that 30% of their children were suspended from school and 41% failed at least one grade in school and had to take that year of education again. For methadone maintenance patients and their families, drug abuse is simply one element in multiproblem lifestyles.

A rhesus monkey experiment showed the animals having no preference between water and a methadone solution. Such lack of interest is consistent with human experience. Some persons find opiates or opioids attractive, but most do not. Personality and life circumstances have much to do with such choices.

Methadone's calming qualities dissipate if tolerance occurs, so some other antianxiety medicine must then be used. Methadone's abstinence syndrome is reminiscent of morphine's but is generally described as more gradual in development and disappearance, longer lasting but with symptoms of lesser severity. Some research, however, has found no difference in morphine and methadone withdrawal, and some addicts say withdrawal from methadone is more difficult than withdrawal from heroin. Evidence suggests that methadone withdrawal symptoms are harsher in nonblack infants than in blacks.

Drug interactions. Using other depressants (including **alcohol**) or tricyclic antidepressants with methadone can increase the risk of a cumulative overdose—each individual dose may be safe, but all together may be dangerous.

Methadone should be used cautiously if a person is also taking monoamine oxidase inhibitors (MAOIs, found in some antidepressants and other medicine). Blood levels of methadone can be drastically altered by **phenobarbital**, by the epilepsy medicines phenytoin and carbamazepine, and by the tuberculosis medication rifampin. A case report notes that the HIV/AIDS (human immunodeficiency virus/acquired immunodeficiency syndrome) drug ritonavir reduces methadone blood levels, and methadone interacts with other HIV/AIDS drugs as well. Taking doses of methadone along with the psychiatric medicine fluvoxamine (Luvox) can be fatal. Depending on how a person uses alcohol, that drug can raise or lower blood levels of methadone. Data from one study showed that methadone did not decrease likelihood for alcohol abuse and that persons already abusing alcohol drank even more while on methadone. Other drug combinations common among illicit users can be hazardous with methadone, and methadone alone can be dangerous if a person who once had tolerance resumes usage at the old high-dose level. Experiments have found that consumption and enjoyment of tobacco cigarettes increase after volunteers use methadone, and another experiment found that methadone consumption increases after volunteers use **nicotine** (in gum or cigarettes).

Cancer. Chromosome damage is one measure of a drug's potential for causing cancer. A study of persons receiving methadone for 40 weeks found no more chromosome damage than a nondrug population would have.

Pregnancy. Safety for use during pregnancy is unknown. Researchers who gave various opioids to pregnant hamsters described methadone as one of the most powerful inducers of birth defects. Mice research shows that offspring are smaller than normal but have ordinary brain development. Compared to morphine, much more of a maternal methadone dose reaches a fetus. One group of investigators developed findings implying that methadone may harm human fetal central nervous system development. Those discoveries are consistent with research demonstrating abnormal development of neurons in rats that had prenatal methadone exposure; researchers speculate that such abnormalities may explain various behaviors in human infants who had prenatal methadone exposure. Use of methadone for easing pain of childbirth is not recommended because newborns can suffer breathing difficulty after picking up the drug from the maternal blood supply. Infants from women who use methadone chronically can be born with dependence to the drug.

A study compared pregnant women on methadone maintenance to a pregnant group on morphine maintenance and discovered that the morphine group used fewer benzodiazepine class drugs and fewer opiates than the methadone program participants. Another study noted that pregnant addicts in a methadone program received better prenatal care than addicts who were not in such programs, but program participants typically continued illicit drug use, their infants weighed no more than infants from pregnant addicts not in a methadone program, and infants from both those drug groups (program and nonprogram) weighed less than those of women who were not drug abusers. Such results have led more than one group of researchers to ask whether methadone maintenance helps pregnancy outcomes, but those researchers do not offer an answer. Nonetheless, some authorities report that pregnancy outcomes are substantially better for addicts in methadone programs.

A group of clinical observations found that infants from mothers addicted to heroin had better sucking ability than infants from methadone addicts (including those in methadone maintenance programs). Research finds that breast-feeding by methadone-using mothers does no harm to infants, and one investigator concluded that methadone in the milk helps ease a dependent child's withdrawal symptoms. Investigators have found that infants with fetal exposure to methadone eat more than normal but do not gain more weight than normal, a finding that suggests defective ability to use nutrition from food. A study of two-year-old children found that fetal exposure to methadone had no influence on ability to focus attention. Examination of school-age children who had fetal exposure to methadone found them to have normal scores in thinking tests and somewhat lower IQs than normal and to be more nervous and aggressive than typical children. How much of this is related to the drug and how much is related to tumultuous family life is uncertain. Another follow-up study found that girls had normal gender behavior, but boys had more female characteristics in their conduct.

A study found pregnancy outcomes to be much the same among methadone and **cocaine** users.

Additional scientific information may be found in:

Darke, S., et al. "Cognitive Impairment among Methadone Maintenance Patients." *Addiction* 95 (2000): 687–95.

De Cubas, M.M., and T. Field. "Children of Methadone-Dependent Women: Developmental Outcomes." *American Journal of Orthopsychiatry* 63 (1993): 266–76.

Fainsinger, R., T. Schoeller, and E. Bruera. "Methadone in the Management of Cancer Pain: A Review." *Pain* 52 (1993): 137–47.

Jarvis, M.A., and S.H. Schnoll. "Methadone Treatment during Pregnancy." *Journal of Psychoactive Drugs* 26 (1994): 155–61.

Martin, W.R., et al. "Methadone—A Reevaluation." *Archives of General Psychiatry* 28 (1973): 286–95.

Rossler, H., et al. "Methadone-Substitution and Driving Ability." *Forensic Science International* 62 (1993): 63–66.

Schneider, J.W., and S.L. Hans. "Effects of Prenatal Exposure to Opioids on Focused Attention in Toddlers during Free Play." *Journal of Developmental and Behavioral Pediatrics* 17 (1996): 240–47.

Specka, M., et al. "Cognitive-Motor Performance of Methadone-Maintained Patients." *European Addiction Research* 6 (2000): 8–19.

Methamphetamine

Pronunciation: meth-am-FET-uh-meen

Chemical Abstracts Service Registry Number: 537-46-2

Formal Names: Anadrex, Desoxyn, Norodin, Pervertin, Stimulex

Informal Names: Bambita, Bathtub Crank, Batu, Blue Meth, Boo, Bump, Chalk, Chicken Feed, Crank, Crink, Cris, Cristina, Cristy, Croak, Crossles, Crypto, Crystal, Crystal Meth, Desocsins, Desogtion, Geep, Glass, Go-Fast, Granulated Orange, Hanyak, Hironpon, Hiropon, Hot Ice, Ice, Jet Fuel, Kaksonjae, L.A. Glass, L.A. Ice, Lemon Drop, Load of Laundry, Maui-Wowie, Meth, Methlies Quik, Mexican Crack, Motorcycle Crack, Nazi Vitamins, Peanut Butter, Quartz Smokable, Quill Cocaine, Red Devils, Redneck Cocaine, Schmiz, Scootie, Shabu Ice, Sketch, Smoke, Soap Dope, Sparkle, Speed, Spoosh, Stove Top, Super Ice, Tick Tick, Trash, Twisters, Water, Wet, White Cross, Working Man's Cocaine, Yellow Bam, Yellow Powder

Type: Stimulant (amphetamine class). *See* page 12

Federal Schedule Listing: Schedule II (DEA no. 1105)

USA Availability: Prescription

Pregnancy Category: C

Uses. Methamphetamine was first manufactured in 1919. This stimulant of the central and sympathetic nervous systems is comparable to **dextroamphetamine**. Psychic effects are the same as for any amphetamine class drug.

Methamphetamine is used to treat narcolepsy, attention deficit hyperactivity disorder (ADHD), and adult obesity. Typically the drug is not recommended for juvenile obesity. Although patients lose more weight than if they use a placebo, the difference is only a few ounces per week. Researchers do not know how the drug promotes weight loss. Scientists are even unsure if the drug is responsible or if diet, coaching, attitude, and other factors explain the difference. In general, the longer patients take the drug, the lower their rate of weight loss. Standard practice is to stop the drug when weight benefits decline, rather than increase dosage.

To achieve top performance during World War II, pilots of the German Luftwaffe and the British Royal Air Force used methamphetamine. In 1953 Hermann Buhl was the first person to climb the mountain Nanga Parbat in the Himalayas, and during that feat he used methamphetamine tablets. Some observers wonder if that pharmaceutical aid was crucial. A person who climbed Mt. Everest without using supplementary oxygen noted, "Because mountaineering is, thank God, not an organized Olympic sport, there are no regulations about the use of drugs, so the choice is up to the individual." When methamphetamine was tested on champion cyclist athletes, they could not achieve a higher level of performance than normal, but they could extend top performance far longer than normal, a feat made possible in part by the drug's apparent ability to mask the body's normal signals of exhaustion. Researchers speculate that the drug could cause athletes to overextend themselves, collapse, and die. Another experiment found that the drug could improve work performance, but performing a few tasks under controlled conditions cannot be extrapolated to the whole world of real-life work.

The human body metabolizes assorted medical drugs into dextroamphetamine and methamphetamine, so if a body fluid test is used to accuse someone of unauthorized use, a blameless person should check whether any over-the-counter or prescribed drugs might be the explanation.

Drawbacks. Measurements have found damage to brain neurons correlated with amount of methamphetamine abuse, damage that does not seem to recover upon cessation of drug dosage. Some of that damage may promote Parkinson's disease. Tests show normal scores for methamphetamine abusers on some psychological perception tests, below normal scores on others. Animal experiments confirm that methamphetamine can alter DNA molecules, and some researchers ask whether these changes may invalidate DNA identifications made by law enforcement authorities.

Methamphetamine raises blood pressure; the most catastrophic consequence can be rupture of the aorta. The compound raises body temperature. Euphoria and overdose symptoms are similar to those of **cocaine** but last longer. Methamphetamine overdose can cause convulsions, heart attack, kidney failure, and stroke. Stroke can occur days after overdosage. Temporary blindness has developed. The drug can severely and permanently impair vision, apparently by temporarily cutting blood flow to the optic nerve. Serious ulcers may develop in the cornea. Although methamphetamine can slightly stimulate breathing and help open lung airways, the substance can also produce temporary emphysema. Animal experiments and human experience indicate that conccaled heart damage caused by the drug can repair itself if methamphetamine administration ceases.

Methamphetamine's smokable format is considered twice as strong as dextroamphetamine, can produce pulmonary edema, and has been identified as causing skin affliction. Smoking methamphetamine can narrow blood vessels, which will increase blood pressure. Another suspected consequence of the narrowing is acidosis found among methamphetamine users, a condition in which levels of acid in blood rise high enough to make a person sick. Studies of patients suffering from harm to bones and to skeletal muscles have found possible association with methamphetamine. Ischemic colitis, a bowel problem normally associated with old age, has been seen among young methamphetamine users. The substance is also associated with duodenal ulcers and malignant giant gastric ulcers. Inhaling the drug (as opposed to smoking, injecting, or swallowing) promotes excessive wear on teeth.

Methamphetamine affects insulin needs of diabetics. Persons with the same physical afflictions that make dextroamphetamine inadvisable should also avoid methamphetamine.

Abuse factors. Experiments with intravenous injection of pure pharmaceutical methamphetamine found that recipients did not experience the almost instantaneous rush of effect that would normally be expected from such a path of administration. Recipients instead began experiencing significant effects hours later. A study of Japanese abusers receiving treatment for their drug habit compared injectors to smokers. Injectors had less schooling and more criminality and were more likely to have alcoholic parents. Such background is typical in persons having a bad relationship with drugs. Contented people rarely fall victim to drug abuse.

Methamphetamine flashbacks are possible. Someone who experienced a threatening situation while undergoing frightening psychosis brought on by methamphetamine can have a flashback when later confronted with a mildly stressful situation. In one study of abusers methamphetamine was blamed for long-term psychosis, in one case lasting 38 years after abuse stopped, but most of those patients also had other troubles (broken homes, criminality) promoting maladjustment.

Persons who abuse methamphetamine are typically disappointed with their lives. The drug is sometimes blamed for causing "amotivational syndrome" in which abusers lack much interest in life, but abusers typically have much to be discouraged about regardless of drug use. One study of Japanese alcoholics compared those who had also abused methamphetamine to those who had not. The abusers were more afflicted with **alcohol** hallucinations, were much less likely to live together with someone, and were twice as likely to collect welfare and three times as likely to live in slums. (And about one fourth of the abusers had tattoos versus none of the nonabusers—the researchers called the variation "significant," but that term was surely meant in its statistical sense.) Another study of Japanese abusers found that only 5% came from an upper income background, in contrast to 71% of marijuana users. Still another study of Japanese abusers found that they ended their schooling early, hung out with gangs or other groups, and experienced effects typical of amphetamine class drugs (restlessness, irritability, low appetite, suspicion of other persons). Some negative aspects seemed to depend on how much the drug users perceived themselves as victims of society. Pepped-up feelings and drug-induced happiness declined as methamphetamine abuse continued over the years. One authority has noted that persons who get drunk on alcohol every day are five times more prone to smoke methamphetamine than persons who consume alcohol either moderately or not at all. This does not mean that alcohol itself promotes methamphetamine use, but a person who is so miserable as to get drunk daily will also be likely to seek additional ways to obliterate perception of problems. One of those choices may be methamphetamine.

Compared to persons who don't abuse methamphetamine, abusers are known for more frequently engaging in risky sexual practices (no condoms, partners with sexually transmitted diseases, multiple casual partners). Less is known about whether such conduct is promoted by the drug or whether the drug is simply one component of a life filled with risk-taking.

Methamphetamine abusers tend to get injured more often in accidents than nonusers. That correlation, however, does not tell us whether the cause is the drug or a reckless lifestyle that happens to include drug abuse—one study of methamphetamine user deaths found that over 25% were murders. Types of accidents experienced by methamphetamine users are similar to those suffered by alcohol abusers, with road mishaps being most common. A study of violent emergency room patients requiring "chemical restraint" (that is, involuntary administration of a sedating drug) found that 72% were intoxicated with methamphetamine, and many were also drunk on alcohol. Violent patients requiring restraint are, of course, a small minority; those figures do not mean that 72% of all patients were using methamphetamine. The figures do, however, indicate that persons who lose control of themselves cannot handle methamphetamine well, or alcohol either.

As for the drug's popularity, a 1999 analysis found that deaths related to methamphetamine in San Francisco had not particularly risen over a 13-year period. In contrast, toxicology tests at a California hospital (not involving all patients) showed 3% positive for either dextroamphetamine or methamphetamine or both in 1978, 10% in 1986 and 1987. Another California hospital found that 7.4% of trauma patients had been using the drug in 1989, 13.4% in 1994. As the drug promotes medical problems, we can expect evidence of methamphetamine abuse to be higher in a hospital patient population (composed of people seeking medical help) than in the general population. When the twenty-first century began, about 2% of the general American population was estimated to have used methamphetamine one or more times in their lives, and the percentage of regular users would be lower than that. Patients in medical cases examined in California, Taiwan, and Japan tend to be male, perhaps indicating a gender preference in use of this drug. Evidence exists for a gender difference in psychic reaction to the drug, with males feeling pepped up and happy while under the influence and postmenopausal women feeling tired and sad. The substance causes more brain changes in male mice than in female.

Drug interactions. Methamphetamine can have serious interactions with anesthesia and opioid drugs given in dentistry. Animal research indicates that smoking tobacco cigarettes can create a multiplier effect in which the **nicotine** and methamphetamine interact, boosting each other's potency. Opiate addicts receiving oral **methadone** report that injecting themselves with methamphetamine produces a **heroin**-type high lasting a full 24 hours.

A hospital emergency room study found that persons admitted for the same cause of injury had lower alcohol level in their blood if they had also been taking methamphetamine. Combining the two drugs allows mice to tolerate a higher methamphetamine dose than normal, but research on humans finds just the opposite, that alcohol can transform a normal dose of methamphetamine into a fatal one. Laboratory research on humans shows that using the two drugs together adds strain on the heart, while reducing pleasure gained from the alcohol and maintaining mental satisfaction from the methamphetamine. An unusual report tells of that drug combination rupturing a bladder, the alcohol helping to fill it up as the methamphetamine narrowed the bladder neck while taking away the normal sensation of pain that would warn a person to seek medical help.

Cancer. Not enough scientific information to report.

Pregnancy. Pregnant methamphetamine abusers tend to produce full-term babies having characteristics of premature infants. While such a problem merits attention, a California study of 563,573 women who gave birth in 1992 helped put a perspective on the situation: Only 774 used methamphetamine during their pregnancies. Pooling results from seven California hospitals provided still another perspective. Among one group of mothers in 1996 and 1997, 0.5% had positive drug tests for methamphetamine during pregnancy, and those women typically used other drugs as well. And that percentage is not from the total population of pregnant women but only from those whose infants required assistance in breathing, a group where drug abuse was more prevalent.

Animal studies involving many times the normal human medical dose have produced birth defects. Confirming fetal harm from methamphetamine in humans is difficult because of other drugs the women use (particularly alcohol), nutrition, amount of prenatal care, and other factors that simultaneously affect fetal development. Methamphetamine accumulates in the fetus where blood level can be two and even six times higher than elsewhere in the woman's body. One study measuring pregnancy outcome where umbilical blood showed misuse only of methamphetamine found the infants to be normal.

Additional scientific information may be found in:

Anglin, M.D., et al. "History of the Methamphetamine Problem." *Journal of Psychoactive Drugs* 32 (2000): 137–41.

Beebe, D.K., and E. Walley. "Smokable Methamphetamine ('Ice'): An Old Drug in a Different Form." *American Family Physician* 51 (1995): 449–53.

Boe, N.M., et al. "Methamphetamine Use during Pregnancy Increases the Risk of Adverse Maternal and Neonatal Outcomes." *American Journal of Obstetrics and Gynecology* 180 (January 1999, pt. 2): S71.

Lan, K.C., et al. "Clinical Manifestations and Prognostic Features of Acute Methamphetamine Intoxication." *Journal of the Formosan Medical Association* 97 (1998): 528–33.

Logan, B.K. "Methamphetamine and Driving Impairment." *Journal of Forensic Sciences* 41 (1996): 457–64.

Mayfield, D.G. "Effects of Intravenous Methamphetamine." *International Journal of the Addictions* 8 (1973): 565–68.

Mendelson, J., et al. "Methamphetamine and Ethanol Interactions in Humans." *Clinical Pharmacology and Therapeutics* 57 (1995): 559–68.

Simon, S.L., et al. "Cognitive Impairment in Individuals Currently Using Methamphetamine." *American Journal on Addictions* 9 (2000): 222–31.

Methandriol

Pronunciation: meth-AN-dree-ol

Chemical Abstracts Service Registry Number: 521-10-8

Formal Names: Andris, Arbolic, Crestabolic, Drive, Durandrol, Filibol Forte, Geld-abol, Hybolin, Methylandrostendiol, Methylandrostenediol, Novandrol, Spec-triol

Type: Anabolic steroid. *See* page 24

Federal Schedule Listing: Schedule III (DEA no. 4000)

USA Availability: Prescription

Uses. Although the substance is banned from sports, some bodybuilders and other athletes use it. A rat study found augmented muscle protein among animals receiving the drug. Researchers have noted that chickens gain more weight when getting methandriol. Other researchers, however, found no weight alteration after giving the drug to mares daily for 18 months. The compound has been tested as a treatment for excessive menstrual bleeding, but results left investigators rather unimpressed.

Drawbacks. Methandriol can masculinize women's body signs and behavior, though to a lesser degree than many drugs of this type. Indeed, when tested on horses, no change was seen in mares' conduct. Nonetheless, women's voices can deepen, and facial hair can appear—effects that may be permanent. Among bodybuilders there is a claim that the drug feminizes men's body signs and behavior. Boys and girls receiving the drug may undergo premature sexual maturity and stop growing in height. Reduced fertility may occur in men. Unwanted effects can include acne, hair loss, and tissue swelling due to fluid retention. Researchers noted development of high blood pressure in rats that steadily dosed on methandriol for several weeks. The drug is not recommended for persons with high blood pressure, heart trouble, or prostate disorder. Methandriol is suspected of causing liver damage.

Abuse factors. Not enough scientific information to report on tolerance, dependence, withdrawal, or addiction.

Drug interactions. Not enough scientific information to report.

Cancer. Not enough scientific information to report.

Pregnancy. Pregnant women are supposed to avoid methandriol. Bisexual fetal development in rats has been attributed to the drug. Other research has noted that genetic females can have outward male appearance after fetal exposure. The drug may interfere with milk production.

Additional scientific information may be found in:

Rendina, G.M., and D. Patrono. "The Use of a Biological Preparation in the Treatment of Some Gynaecological Diseases." *Current Medical Research and Opinion* 4 (1976): 151–57.

Rogozkin, V. "Metabolic Effects of Anabolic Steroid on Skeletal Muscle." *Medicine and Science in Sports* 11 (1979): 160–63.

Turner, J.E., and C.H. Irvine. "Effect of Prolonged Administration of Anabolic and Androgenic Steroids on Reproductive Function in the Mare." *Journal of Reproduction and Fertility*, no. 1 (1982, Suppl.): 213–18.

Methandrostenolone

Pronunciation: meth-an-droh-STEN-oh-lohn

Chemical Abstracts Service Registry Number: 72-63-9

Formal Names: Anabolin, Dianabol, Methandienone, Nerobol

Type: Anabolic steroid. *See* page 24

Federal Schedule Listing: Schedule III (DEA no. 4000)

USA Availability: Prescription

Uses. Medical uses of methandrostenolone include promoting growth in small boys, although with the risk of accelerating increase in height for awhile and then stopping further increase permanently. The drug has also been used to bring on male puberty when that development is delayed. A research study found that the substance increases sexual desire in men while simultaneously reducing their fertility. The drug has been given to control hereditary angio-edema, a disease producing giant hives on the skin. A lung disease called silicosis has been treated with the drug, and so have burns, cancer, and a type of anemia. Using the substance against a brittle bone condition called osteoporosis has been tried, with mixed results. Protection against lead poisoning was noted in a rat experiment. Levels of triglycerides, which are associated with heart attack and stroke, declined in diabetic humans who received the drug.

The substance is forbidden in sports competitions, but some athletes continue to use it, either because they will not be tested for it or because they hope to evade tests. Experiments have compared athletes using methandrostenolone to others not receiving the drug (either two different groups of athletes were compared, or the same volunteers were tested under both drug and nondrug conditions). In one study the drug group showed higher increase in weight and strength. In another experiment the drug group gained more weight than the drug-free group, but the scientists noted that water retention could have been the reason. Blood pressure also increased in the drug group. In still another comparison experiment the methandrostenolone users gained more weight and achieved more muscle development, but despite additional muscle mass their strength and performance did not differ from the drug-free group—scientists running those tests were unsure that anabolic steroid actions explained physical development in the drug group; as with an experiment mentioned above, a plausible alternative explanation was that methandrostenolone simply caused fluid swelling in tissues. Yet one more experiment measured increase in muscle mass among athletes using the substance but detected no increase in strength.

Stock raisers administer methandrostenolone to promote sheep and cattle growth.

Drawbacks. A case report warns that using the substance on girls can produce male qualities in voice while reducing female sexual characteristics; these changes can be long-lasting and perhaps permanent. Although a skin cream containing **nandrolone** is used to combat eczema, the same use of a cream containing methandrostenolone has had serious consequences when applied to girls, causing some female physical characteristics to diminish while masculine ones appeared.

A case report attributed a 28-year-old bodybuilder's heart disease and hardening of the arteries to a dozen years of using methandrostenolone and other steroids. Another case report blamed methandrostenolone alone for blockage of blood vessels between heart and lungs in a 26-year-old bodybuilder. Attempts to treat the condition with the anti–blood clot drug warfarin became complicated when the steroid boosted that drug's actions.

When taking methandrostenolone daily, a person experienced delusions and paranoia. Excessive self-confidence created by the drug inspired one user to buy a $17,000 automobile on credit despite his inability to make payments. After going off methandrostenolone the person sold the car, but upon resuming the drug, he purchased a $20,000 vehicle. Medical literature also records that a 22-year-old athlete using methandrostenolone and **stanozolol** developed feelings of powerfulness and aggression, accompanied by impatience.

Methandrostenolone apparently causes acne and is suspected of worsening tics in Tourette's syndrome. Men may experience urinary difficulty and lowered testosterone levels. The substance can bring on an attack of porphyria in persons who suffer from that body chemistry disease, an affliction that sometimes involves violence and sensitivity to light.

Abuse factors. An opiatelike dependence was reported in a 23-year-old bodybuilder who had been on a steady regimen including methandrostenolone, **oxymetholone**, and **oxandrolone**. When given a drug that counteracts opiate actions he quickly exhibited nausea, chills, dizziness, and headache—classic flulike opiate withdrawal symptoms. When his supply of steroids ceased he craved them and felt weary and depressed. Another case report notes a bodybuilder who dosed extensively on methandrostenolone and other steroids and experienced severe depression when he stopped.

Drug interactions. Not enough scientific information to report.

Cancer. Researchers examining reported deaths from a type of liver cancer called hepatic angiosarcoma found a total of 168 throughout the United States from 1964 to 1974, of which the investigators associated 1 with methandrostenolone (this individual was also a former **alcohol** abuser, conduct that is notoriously hard on the liver). Methandrostenolone and other steroids are suspected of causing kidney cancer in a 38-year-old bodybuilder.

Pregnancy. Mice studies indicate that the drug can produce lethal mutations in sperm, causing pregnancy failure.

Additional scientific information may be found in:

Freed, D.L.J., et al. "Anabolic Steriods in Athletics: Crossover Double-Blind Trial on Weightlifters." *British Medical Journal* 2 (1975): 47–73.

Hervey, G.R., et al. "Anabolic Effects of Methandienone in Men Undergoing Athletic Training." *Lancet* 2 (1976): 699–702.

Holma, P.K. "Effects of an Anabolic Steroid (Metandienone) on Spermatogenesis." *Contraception* 15 (1977): 151–62.

Johnson, L.C., and J.P. O'Shea. "Anabolic Steroid: Effects on Strength Development." *Science* 164 (1969): 957–59.

Kilshaw, B.H., et al. "Effects of Large Doses of the Anabolic Steroid, Methandrostenolone, on an Athlete." *Clinical Endocrinology* 4 (1975): 537–41.

Madea, B., and W. Grellner. "Long Term Cardiovascular Effects of Anabolic Steroids." *Lancet* 352 (1998): 33.

Robinson, R.J., and S. White. "Misuse of Anabolic Drugs." *British Medical Journal* 306 (1993): 61.

Methaqualone

Pronunciation: meth-a-KWAY-lohn

Chemical Abstracts Service Registry Number: 72-44-6

Formal Names: Dormutil, Hyminal, Mandrax, Melsed, Melsedin, Mequelone, Mequin, Methadorm, Mozambin, Optimil, Parest, Quaalude, Revonal, Somnafac, Sopor, Toquilone Compositum, Triador, Tuazole

Informal Names: Bandits, Beiruts, Blou Bulle, Blue Bulls, Drunken Monkey, Ewings, Flamingos, Flowers, Four Strokes, Genuines, Germans, Golfsticks, Humbles, Knoppies, Lizards, Loss of Memory, Love Drug, Ludes, Luds, Lula, Magwheels, Mandies, Mind Benders (with **heroin**), Pressouts, Pupumala, Q, Randy Mandies, 714, Shiny Tops, Sopes, Sporos, Strawberries, Wagon Wheels, White Pipe (Mandrax and marijuana)

Type: Depressant. *See* page 19

Federal Schedule Listing: Schedule I (DEA no. 2565)

USA Availability: Illegal to possess

Pregnancy Category: None

Uses. Methaqualone was invented in India during the 1950s as part of a program seeking substances for treating malaria. Experiments suggest methaqualone has anticonvulsant properties. Although the substance does little to relieve pain, experimentation indicates it might boost pain relief provided by **codeine**. Methaqualone may have cough suppression qualities but has not received general medical usage for that purpose. When introduced into American medicine in the 1960s, the compound was used to calm people and help them sleep and was welcomed as an alternative to barbiturates. The drug's actions have been likened to those of **pentobarbital**.

A clinical experiment found that a bedtime dose of the drug did not affect users' ability to move around after awakening the next morning, which is not always the case with insomnia medicine. Those results were supported by another experiment where volunteers did so well on tests the next day and the following day that the researchers optimistically speculated that job performance might improve among people using the drug against insomnia. Britain's Royal Air Force even thought the drug had potential to help pilots get proper rest on long missions.

Drawbacks. Unwanted actions of methaqualone may include tingling sensations in hands and feet, weariness, sweating, rashes, dry mouth, nausea, vomiting, and diarrhea. Instances are known of methaqualone causing people to act as if injury has occurred to nerves affecting the arms and legs. Poisoning by methaqualone is associated with bleeding, and a case report revealed that an overdose can even cause bleeding inside the eye. Research with rats showed the drug impeded learning ability.

Although fatal overdose with methaqualone or any other drug is possible, a 1983 study found that methaqualone users in that era were primarily dying from accidents involving poor decisions while under the drug's influence rather than from the poisonous effects of the drug itself. Also, if someone is intoxicated with the compound, driving skills are known to be impaired, an effect that does not involve poisoning but can have serious consequences. A study of emergency room admissions found that methaqualone poisoning cases typically involved some other substance as well, a finding indicating a certain recklessness among abusers. The same polydrug habit was observed among methaqualone abusers in the U.S. Army during the 1970s. That finding is unsurprising; most drug abusers use more than one substance.

The drug is fast acting, and persons unprepared for the speed with which methaqualone takes effect have been injured while engaged in ordinary activity that becomes dangerous if a person passes out, such as taking a bath or being near a fire. Methaqualone has the disturbing capability of causing flat brainwave readings, a standard sign that medical caregivers rely upon to verify a person's death and that could therefore cause them to stop efforts that are keeping the methaqualone patient alive.

Abuse factors. In Europe methaqualone was initially a nonprescription item. In the United States the drug was first put in Schedule V, but as methaqualone became popular among illicit users seeking euphoria and relaxation, more restrictions were placed on its legal accessibility. The drug became a Schedule II substance in 1973. When President Jimmy Carter's drug policy adviser Dr. Peter Bourne wrote a methaqualone prescription that violated regulations, that incident started a series of events that hounded Bourne out of office. Eventually concern about the drug grew so high that it was reclassified in 1984 as a Schedule I substance having no recognized medical function.

One study found that patients using methaqualone against insomnia readily changed to some other drug on advice from a medical practitioner; apparently they did not find methaqualone particularly attractive. Tolerance and dependence can develop, although one study was able to confirm tolerance only among heavy abusers. Withdrawal symptoms are similar to those with barbiturates and can include weakness, nausea, vomiting, heartbeat abnormality, tremors, seizures, and delirium tremens.

In the 1970s researchers surveyed college students who were using methaqualone, a broader population group than persons who have so much trouble with the drug that they seek medical treatment. Survey answers showed drug use to be the main difference between students who used methaqualone and those who did not; as a whole the methaqualone users were ordinary people. Investigators found that a cross section of Midwestern users had positive attitudes about themselves.

An exception to such a self-portrait emerged when someone interviewed users who claimed to be using methaqualone as an aphrodisiac. They turned out to be loners with a cold family background: Fully 10% said their closest family relationship was with the dog; 30% said they weren't close to any family member at all. Almost all the persons using methaqualone as an "aphrodisiac" had previously been using other drugs for the same purpose. None of the persons seemed capable of intimacy while sober, and all used methaqualone and other substances simply to get intoxicated enough to permit some form of temporary superficial imitation of intimacy. Such drug use has an air of desperation and sadness inconsistent with the normal understanding of what an aphrodisiac does.

One study found that emergency psychiatric hospital patients who abused methaqualone (definitely not a population of ordinary individuals) tended to menace other persons.

Drug interactions. Animal research shows that injection of THC, the main active component of **marijuana**, reduces the amount of methaqualone that is normally needed to get the drug's effects, which can make an overdose more likely. Animal and human studies using **alcohol** have had the same effect on a methaqualone dose—such findings are supported by examination of hospital emergency room cases, where analysis showed that methaqualone emergencies typically involved simultaneous ingestion of alcohol. Using alcohol and methaqualone simultaneously is a practice called "luding out." Indulgers in that technique say it makes them feel relaxed, interferes with their ability to move, makes them more tolerant of pain, and produces tingling in their fingers, lips, and tongue.

Tests can detect methaqualone in the body days after a dose, and alcohol lengthens the time that a methaqualone dose lasts. That combination can influence performance on various behavior and performance tests even three days after methaqualone is taken.

A woman's menstrual cycle can affect her body's ability to metabolize methaqualone; a dose can last a much shorter time when she is ovulating, but oral contraceptives can eliminate that effect.

Cancer. Not enough scientific information to report.

Pregnancy. The drug has produced birth defects in rats, and offspring had a death rate four times higher than that of a matched group receiving no drug. Researchers doing that work cautioned that the results do not necessarily carry over to humans. In rabbit studies the rate of birth defects from pregnant females receiving methaqualone did not significantly differ from drug-free females, but there was a big difference in death rates of offspring. Rabbits with fetal exposure to methaqualone died three times as often as those without exposure, a 6% death rate for those with exposure and 2% for those without. Analysts of such experiments note that in order to harm a fetus the methaqualone dose has to be high enough to poison the pregnant female, so the practical meaning of such results may be that normal doses of the drug are safe during pregnancy. Effects on human fetal development are unclear. Human reports tend to involve combinations with other drugs, making it hard to determine methaqualone's role. Given the uncertainties, pregnant women are advised to avoid the drug.

Combination products. Mandrax and Toquilone Compositum contain both methaqualone and the antihistamine diphenhydramine. Some research indicates that diphenhydramine boosts the actions of methaqualone; some research indicates that the antihistamine lengthens the time that a methaqualone dose lasts. Adverse reactions have occurred when persons take the combination along with tricyclic antidepressants.

Additional information. Methaqualone and **diazepam** each have the nickname "Ludes," but the drugs are different substances.

Additional scientific information may be found in:

Bailey, D.N. "Methaqualone Ingestion: Evaluation of Present Status." *Journal of Analytical Toxicology* 5 (1981): 279–82.

Brown, S.S., and S. Goenechea. "Methaqualone: Metabolic Kinetic and Clinical Pharmacologic Observations." *Clinical Pharmacology and Therapeutics* 14 (1973): 314–24.

"Evaluation of a Sedative-Hypnotic Agent; Methaqualone (Quaalude)." *Journal of the American Medical Association* 199 (1967): 749.

Falco, M. "Methaqualone Misuse: Foreign Experience and United States Drug Control Policy." *International Journal of the Addictions* 11 (1976): 597–610.

Gerald, M.C., and P.M. Schwirian. "Nonmedical Use of Methaqualone." *Archives of General Psychiatry* 28 (1973): 627–31.

Ostrenga, J.A. "Methaqualone—A Dr. Jekyll and Mr. Hyde?" *Clinical Toxicology* 6 (1973): 607–9.

Perry, C.D., et al. "The South African Community Epidemiology Network on Drug Use (SACENDU): Description, Findings (1997–99) and Policy Implications." *Addiction* 97 (2002): 969–76.

Roden, S., P. Harvey, and M. Mitchard. "Influence of Alcohol on the Persistent Effects on Human Performance of the Hypnotics Mandrax and Nitrazepam." *International Journal of Clinical Pharmacology, Therapy and Toxicology* 15 (1977): 350–55.

Wetli, C.V. "Changing Patterns of Methaqualone Abuse. A Survey of 246 Fatalities." *Journal of the American Medical Association* 249 (1983): 621–26.

Methcathinone

Pronunciation: meth-KATH-i-nun

Chemical Abstracts Service Registry Number: 5650-44-2

Formal Names: Ephedrone, Methylcathinone

Informal Names: Bathtub Speed, C, Cadillac Express, Cat, Crank, Gager, Gagger, Go Fast, Goob, Jeff, Khat, Qat, Quicksilver, Slick Superspeed, Somali Tea, Star, Stat, Tweak, Tweek, Tweeker, Wild Cat (with **cocaine**), Wonder Star

Type: Stimulant (amphetamine class). *See* page 12

Federal Schedule Listing: Schedule I (DEA no. 1237)

USA Availability: Illegal to possess

Pregnancy Category: None

Uses. The substance is derived from cathinone (the most potent drug ingredient in **khat**) and is related to **methamphetamine**. A U.S. patent was granted for methcathinone in 1957, but because of adverse actions described below the drug never went into commercial medical production.

Despite methcathinone's many drawbacks noted below, some drug abusers have found appealing aspects in the compound. These users experience euphoria accompanied by strong and prolonged feelings of sexual pleasure, along with an ability to use more **alcohol** than normal. Such characteristics can transform an otherwise unappealing substance into a party drug. Apparently these characteristics were discovered in the Soviet Union; at least that is where the drug first surfaced as a popular item, accounting for perhaps one fifth of illicit drug use in that territory during the late 1980s and early 1990s. In the 1990s the drug took hold in Michigan and spread elsewhere in America.

Drawbacks. At high doses the drug exhibits classic amphetamine effects: appetite loss, insomnia, hallucinations, paranoia, restlessness, and impaired ability to focus attention and to get along with people. Users have said methcathinone is more prone to produce paranoia than methamphetamine. In animal experiments methcathinone interferes with breathing, promotes trembling and epilepticlike seizures, and impedes limb control. In humans a dose may increase body temperature, cause irregular heart rate, excessively reduce blood pressure, bring on nosebleeds, produce red and blue spots in extremities accompanied by cold sweating, promote tics and cramps along with nausea and headaches, generate evidence of liver and kidney damage, and cause infected facial cysts that can leave scars. Heart impairment has been discovered among current users. Examination of former users reveals brain damage that may lead to Parkinson's disease. Autopsies find widespread blood vessel damage throughout the body, from skin to vital organs.

Abuse factors. When effects from a dose ebb, the drug's initial elevation of mood converts into the opposite, and abusers lacking in self-confidence may rely more and more on additional doses of the drug to restore a positive mood instead of seeking to build and rely upon inner resources. As mental spirits level off or decline, abusers respond with binge behavior—rather than gradually increasing their dosage, they alternate between heavy use and no use. They may take the drug every hour or so for days even though users report that effects of a dose can last for almost a week.

A group of 19 users compared methcathinone with other drugs. Those persons described methcathinone's stimulation as more of a physical jolt and cocaine's as more of a mental jolt. None of cocaine's physical numbing was noticed with methcathinone. The latter drug was described as stronger, cheaper (at least in the 1990s), and having better duration than cocaine. The 19 persons all misused methcathinone in ways that added turmoil to their lives and said their need for the drug was psychological, not physical. The users mostly said the drug had ruined their lives. Those lives seemed troubled before methcathinone entered, however. Only 4 of the persons were employed when they started using the substance. Relationships with family and friends declined, but that decline was accelerated by explosive anger and by deliberately avoiding friends and relatives. The employed persons got into conflicts with coworkers or stayed away from the workplace. All lost their jobs. No doubt the drug made things worse, but abusers seemed to be struggling with sad lives before adding methcathinone to other drugs they abused.

Drug interactions. Users claim that eating sugar can worsen methcathinone's undesirable psychological effects.

Cancer. Not enough scientific information to report.

Pregnancy. Not enough scientific information to report.

Additional information. "Qat" and "Somali tea" are nicknames for both methcathinone and khat, but those are different substances.

Additional scientific information may be found in:

Calkins, R.F., G.B. Aktan, and K.L. Hussain. "Methcathinone: The Next Illicit Stimulant Epidemic?" *Journal of Psychoactive Drugs* 27 (1995): 277–85.

Emerson, T.S., and J.E. Cisek. "Methcathinone: A Russian Designer Amphetamine Infiltrates the Rural Midwest." *Annals of Emergency Medicine* 22 (1993): 1897–903.

Goldstone, M.S. " 'Cat': Methcathinone—A New Drug of Abuse." *Journal of the American Medical Association* 269 (1993): 2508.

Zhingel, K.Y., et al. "Ephedrone: 2-Methylamino-1-Phenylpropan-1-One (Jeff)." *Journal of Forensic Sciences* 36 (1991): 915–20.

Methylphenidate

Pronunciation: meth-ill-FEN-i-dait

Chemical Abstracts Service Registry Number: 113-45-1. (Hydrochloride form 298-59-9)

Formal Names: Concerta, Metadate CD, Metadate ER, Methylin, Ritalin

Informal Names: Pellets, Rities, West Coast. *Combination with **pentazocine***: Crackers, 1s & 1s, Poor Man's Heroin, Ritz & Ts, Sets, Ts & Rits, Ts & Rs. *Combination with **heroin***: Speedball

Type: Stimulant (amphetamine class). *See* page 12

Federal Schedule Listing: Schedule II (DEA no. 1724)

USA Availability: Prescription

Pregnancy Category: C

Uses. Methylphenidate became available in the 1940s. The drug is fast acting and long lasting. Although not a true amphetamine, methylphenidate has properties similar to **dextroamphetamine** (including appetite suppression and sleep disruption) but is less potent.

Methylphenidate's prime medical use is for managing attention deficit hyperactivity disorder (ADHD), a condition in which people are so excitable that they have severe problems with social interactions. The affliction is more common in children than adults, and methylphenidate seems more effective against ADHD in children, though one study finds the drug to have little influence on long-term outcome. Limited success is seen in experimental usage of the drug to help autistic children. A case report says a regimen of that drug and the antidepressant sertraline (Zoloft) cured a young kleptomaniac. Among adults methylphenidate is typically prescribed for narcolepsy and has also been used successfully against apathy and depression. Despite the drug's occasional tendency to increase blood pressure, studies find the substance promising for rehabilitation of persons recovering from stroke and other brain injuries, not only improving mood but also helping ability to move.

In volume of use, methylphenidate has been called the predominant medically prescribed psychoactive drug among American juveniles. A survey of approximately 200,000 prescription records of preschool children found about 1% of them to be receiving stimulants in the 1990s, and almost all those prescriptions were for methylphenidate. By the decade's end, two medical authorities put the school-age population's stimulant prescription figure as high as 6%. In the mid-1990s approximately 1.5 million American school-age children were taking stimulant medications just for ADHD, compared to 50 children receiving methylphenidate for any purpose in Great Britain in 1991. Another comparison: A 1999 report said 1.65% of students in one South African urban area were receiving methylphenidate, but none of these children were Afrikaans. Such dramatic differences in prescribing practices suggest strong cultural influence on what is considered acceptable medical treatment. During the mid-1980s great debate arose in the United States about the custom of routinely prescribing methylphenidate to juveniles. The debate was based on ethical values rather than strictly medical concerns, with some persons arguing that the drug was being used as an agent of social control instead of treating disease. After a flurry of lawsuits, the controversy eased.

A review of 23 studies evaluating ADHD drug effectiveness found little distinction among methylphenidate, dextroamphetamine, and **pemoline**.

Drawbacks. Children with ADHD may also experience muscle tics, which methylphenidate and other stimulants can worsen. Such a dual condition is challenging, but in short-term usage, methylphenidate has been found effective for lessening ADHD without increasing tics, even though one study found that almost 10% of ADHD children may develop temporary tics when taking methylphenidate. A case report notes that a child began stuttering when dosage started, with the stutter ceasing when dosage ceased.

Amphetamine class drugs can promote psychosis and other psychiatric disability, and such unwanted results have been observed with methylphenidate, including paranoia and hallucinations. In youngsters methylphenidate has been known to bring on obsessive-compulsive behavior.

Among juveniles the compound has caused skin rash, stomach distress, mild headaches, and sleep difficulties. In juveniles the compound can at least temporarily reduce appetite, although in elderly users the drug has been observed to increase appetite. Controversy exists about whether the drug affects growth. The substance is associated with stroke suffered by two boys.

Methylphenidate is not recommended for persons suffering from seizures. The drug has been reported to cause anemia and is suspected of worsening allergies. The substance has been known to impair vision and is not recommended for persons with glaucoma. Methylphenidate tends to increase immune system activity; in theory that might affect vaccinations and also harm HIV (human immunodeficiency virus)-positive persons. In some humans abnormal liver activity has been seen, but whether the drug *caused* or *revealed* the problem is uncertain. The drug appears to cause heart damage in rats and mice, and a human case has been reported.

Despite potential drawbacks, however, with proper precautions the drug is considered generally safe for medical utilization.

Abuse factors. In primates **cocaine** and methylphenidate seem to work in similar ways; indeed, some illicit substance users have been unable to tell whether they received a dose of cocaine or methylphenidate. Although methylphenidate is a Schedule II substance, abuse of the drug is uncommon. Demand is small enough that the U.S. Drug Enforcement Administration reports no illicit manufacturing. A large review of scientific literature covering the years 1966 to 1998 was unable to substantiate news media claims about wide abuse. A survey of 161 children receiving the medication found none who believed they were at risk of becoming abusers (a belief sustained by general experience nationwide), although about 25 had encountered situations where someone wanted access to their drug supply. The oral format has little ability to produce euphoria. The drug has been called a more potent hallucinogen than **LSD**, but support for that claim seems nonexistent in scientific journals.

Adults suffering from ADHD are routinely found to be cocaine abusers. An experiment showed methylphenidate effective for improving both problems, but the treatment was also accompanied by several weeks of individual counseling, which in itself might have been a major factor in any improvement. Some drug abuse treatments seek to switch abusers from one drug to another. Results of an experiment were unencouraging for shifting cocaine abusers to methylphenidate but had intriguing findings nonetheless. For example, cocaine addicts are generally considered particularly susceptible to addictive properties in other drugs, but methylphenidate had little appeal to subjects in this experiment. The experiment also found mental effects of methylphenidate to include irritability, worry, sadness, and a general mood of dissatisfaction. Physical effects included quivering and accelerated pulse rate. Still, even though these cocaine users found methylphenidate unappealing, methylphenidate is not recommended for any medical treatment in persons with a history of substance abuse.

Experimenters using methylphenidate to help smokers give up tobacco found the results encouraging.

Methylphenidate abusers sometimes grind up oral tablets and inject the material. A preparation designed to go through the digestive system can have untoward consequences in the circulatory system. The talc in oral methylphenidate can lodge in small blood vessels, cutting off blood flow to portions of the lungs, eyes, or brain. Respiratory difficulty, vision damage, and crippling paralysis can result. Studies of such injuries sometimes refer to autopsy results; such reference implies that this type of drug abuse is dangerous indeed.

Tolerance has been noted from illicit usage. Intense depression can emerge when an abuser stops using the drug.

Drug interactions. Apparently methylphenidate interacts with valproic acid, a substance used to treat epilepsy in ADHD children; the interaction can cause teeth grinding and interfere with body movement. Interaction with serotonin reuptake inhibitors found in some antidepressants is suspected of causing heartbeat irregularity in a teenager, and methylphenidate is not recommended for persons taking monoamine oxidase inhibitors (MAOIs, found in some antidepressants). High blood pressure can occur if tricyclic antidepressants are used with methylphenidate, and methylphenidate also seems to reduce time needed for tricyclic antidepressants to show results; lower doses of those drugs are advised when a person is taking methylphenidate. Interactions with **phenobarbital** have been observed. Methylphenidate has allowed terminal cancer patients to tolerate higher doses of opiates, thereby improving pain management.

Cancer. Scientists looking for evidence that methylphenidate causes cancer in rats and humans have instead found lower-than-normal incidence of the disease. In one experiment mice developed liver tumors after receiving many times the therapeutic dose, but the strain of mice used is prone to such tumors, so scientists are uncertain about what the experiment means.

Pregnancy. An experiment using mice found the drug to have no effect on reproduction. Studies of pregnant women abusing methylphenidate find no birth defects associated with the drug, but babies tend to be small and premature. A one-year follow-up found the infants to be in the normal range of development, although some were at the low end of normal. In one study all the pregnant women abusing methylphenidate were cigarette smokers; some were alcoholics; some had sexually transmitted disease; few received much prenatal care. In another study the methylphenidate-abusing mothers' situations were so grim that over half the infants were put into immediate foster care after delivery and did not go home with their mothers. Such confounding factors cloud any conclusions about the drug's effect on fetal development. Whether levels in breast milk are safe for infants is unconfirmed.

Additional scientific information may be found in:

Cox, D.J., et al. "Effect of Stimulant Medication on Driving Performance of Young Adults with Attention-Deficit Hyperactivity Disorder: A Preliminary Double-Blind Placebo Controlled Trial." *Journal of Nervous and Mental Disease* 188 (2000): 230–34.

Crutchley, A., and J.A. Temlett. "Methylphenidate (Ritalin) Use and Abuse." *South African Medical Journal* 89 (1999): 1076–79.

Debooy, V.D., et al. "Intravenous Pentazocine and Methylphenidate Abuse during Pregnancy. Maternal Lifestyle and Infant Outcome." *American Journal of Diseases of Children* 147 (1993): 1062–65.

Efron, D., F.C. Jarman, and M.J. Barker. "Child and Parent Perceptions of Stimulant Medication Treatment in Attention Deficit Hyperactivity Disorder." *Journal of Paediatrics and Child Health* 34 (1998): 288–92.

Jadad, A.R., et al. "Treatment of Attention-Deficit/Hyperactivity Disorder." *Evidence Report/Technology Assessment,* no. 11 (1999): 1–341. Issue no. 11 is available online at: http://hstat.nlm.nih.gov/ftrs/dbaccess/adhd

Llana, M.E., and M.L. Crismon. "Methylphenidate: Increased Abuse or Appropriate Use?" *Journal of the American Pharmaceutical Association* 39 (1999): 526–30.

Parran, T.V., Jr., and D.R. Jasinski. "Intravenous Methylphenidate Abuse. Prototype for Prescription Drug Abuse." *Archives of Internal Medicine* 151 (1991): 781–83.

Scarnati, R. "An Outline of Hazardous Side Effects of Ritalin (Methylphenidate)." *International Journal of the Addictions* 21 (1986): 837–41.

Methyltestosterone

Pronunciation: meth-ill-tess-TOSS-ter-ohn

Chemical Abstracts Service Registry Number: 58-18-4

Formal Names: Android, Estratest, Methitest, Testred, Virilon

Type: Anabolic steroid. *See* page 24

Federal Schedule Listing: Schedule III (DEA no. 4000)

USA Availability: Prescription

Pregnancy Category: X

Uses. Methyltestosterone is a synthetic drug manufactured from **testosterone**. Methyltestosterone's medical uses include supplementation of testosterone in males with low levels of that hormone and treatment of female breast cancer. Scientists report unsatisfactory results from a test of whether the compound might work as a male contraceptive and mixed results when the substance was used to treat male impotence. Impotence improvement was better when methyltestosterone was taken in combination with a **yohimbe** preparation. Methyltestosterone has provided pain relief and occasionally fertility enhancement to women suffering from a reproductive disorder called endometriosis externa. Therapeutic regimens to build up bone strength in older women may include methyltestosterone, as may therapies designed to compensate for hormonal changes caused by menopause. In research projects height increase occurred when the drug was administered to boys of short stature. Experimenters describe the drug as effective treatment for hereditary angioedema, an affliction involving tissue swelling. The drug also has agricultural uses such as illegally promoting pig and cattle growth.

Drawbacks. Volunteers who took methyltestosterone in an experiment showed slight changes in thinking ability, and 2 of the 20 subjects had maniclike episodes that might be attributable to the drug. A report noted that someone receiving the drug experienced visual and auditory hallucinations, and a case report indicated that methyltestosterone and **methandrostenolone** were likely causes of psychotic incidents experienced by two bodybuilders. A human experiment attempted to document the drug's psychological effects but was unable to correlate behavioral changes with volunteers' usage of the substance. The substance is suspected of causing liver damage, sometimes resulting in jaundice, lesions, tumors, or other conditions. The compound may cause fluid retention, which can be risky for persons with kidney, liver, or heart malfunction. Like many drugs of this type, methyltestosterone can cause females to develop masculine characteristics such as facial hair or coarser voice. Such effects can become permanent if dosage is not swiftly stopped upon first appearance of the changes. Other unwanted actions of the drug can include acne, headache, uneasiness, burning or prickling sensations, menstrual disturbances, nausea, and high blood levels of calcium and cholesterol. In rats high blood pressure has been traced to methyltestosterone.

Abuse factors. Methyltestosterone is banned from athletic competitions, but some athletes are tempted to use it, nonetheless. Claims that the compound produces gains in weight and muscle strength have been difficult to document in humans, partly because experimenters cannot subject humans to experimental conditions that are as brutal as can be used with laboratory animals. A robust experiment on rats demonstrated increased strength and stamina from methyltestosterone.

Drug interactions. A case report mentions that a person using the hormone along with the anticholesterol medicine clofibrate developed extremely low levels of high-density lipoprotein (the so-called good cholesterol), a development attributed to methyltestosterone. A similar result occurred in an experiment tracking women using this anabolic steroid along with female hormones called esterified estrogens. Methyltestosterone interferes with blood clotting, which can be a serious problem for persons taking anticlotting medicine. A case report indicates that the substance interacts badly with cyclosporine, an immunosuppressive agent used to fight rejection of organ transplants. A small experiment using methyltestosterone to increase benefits from the tricyclic antidepressant imipramine went awry when almost all patients became paranoid, a condition that rapidly disappeared when methyltestosterone dosage stopped.

Cancer. Researchers have noted liver cancer in mice that received methyltestosterone. Other case reports indicate strong suspicion that the drug causes human liver cancer. The substance has been associated with a person's development of prostate cancer, but "association" is not the same as cause.

Pregnancy. Women are advised to avoid the drug during pregnancy because the substance may masculinize a female fetus, a discovery made in the 1950s when methyltestosterone was a standard medication for reducing the likelihood of miscarriage. Nursing mothers are advised to avoid the drug because it might pass into milk and masculinize a female infant. These effects of the drug are powerful enough that methyltestosterone is used in tilapia farming to change females of this fish into males. The drug has also been used to change female flounder into male fish. Research on rats has demonstrated that masculinizing effects on females can persist into a subsequent generation that did not receive the drug. Human males who use the substance may produce more male offspring than usual.

Additional scientific information may be found in:

Black, J.A., and J.F. Bentley. "Effect on the Fetus of Androgens Given During Pregnancy." *Lancet* 1 (1959): 21–24.

Greene, R., and L.S. Carstairs. "Effect of Anabolic Hormones on the Growth of Undersized Boys." *British Journal of Clinical Practice* 27 (1973): 3–7.

Regestein, Q.R., et al. "Neuropsychological Effects of Methyltestosterone in Women Using Menopausal Hormone Replacement." *Journal of Women's Health & Gender-Based Medicine* 10 (2001): 671–76.

Richardson, J.H., and S. Smith. "A Comparison of the Effects of Dianabol and Methyltestosterone on Muscle Contraction and Fatigue." *Journal of Sports Medicine and Physical Fitness* 21 (1981): 279–81.

Simon, J.A. "Safety of Estrogen/Androgen Regimens." *Journal of Reproductive Medicine* 46 (2001 Supp. 3): 281–90.

Su, T.P., et al. "Neuropsychiatric Effects of Anabolic Steroids in Male Normal Volunteers." *Journal of the American Medical Association* 269 (1993): 2760–64.

Westaby, D., et al. "Liver Damage from Long Term Methyltestosterone." *Lancet* 2 (1977): 261–63.

Wilson, I.C., A.J. Prange, and P.P. Lara. "Methyltestosterone with Imipramine in Men: Conversion of Depression to Paranoid Reaction." *American Journal of Psychiatry* 131 (1974): 21–24.

Midazolam

Pronunciation: mid-AZ-ah-lam

Chemical Abstracts Service Registry Number: 59467-70-8. (Hydrochloride form 59467-96-8; maleate form 59467-94-6)

Formal Names: Dormicum, Hypnovel, Versed

Type: Depressant (benzodiazepine class). *See* page 21

Federal Schedule Listing: Schedule IV (DEA no. 2884)

USA Availability: Prescription

Pregnancy Category: D

Uses. This quick-acting drug's common medical uses are to reduce anxiety, calm people, and help them sleep. Naturalists use the substance to knock out wildlife ranging from foxes to aardvarks. Effects do not last a long time, typically making the substance a good choice for weakened persons or animals who would be strained by a longer-acting drug. For example, weary mountaineers climbing Mt. Everest have used the drug to improve quality of sleep.

One study found the drug could help workers who must alter their sleep schedules for reporting to different work shifts. Experiments show the drug having potential for treating muscle spasms. Midazolam has been used successfully to alleviate status epilepticus, in which people have continual seizures, and to control seizures caused by high fevers in children. The U.S. Army has tested midazolam experimentally, but with limited success, to counteract seizures and other poisonous effects from the chemical warfare substance soman. A case report about treating a cobra snake bite victim notes that midazolam worked when another drug faltered. Midazolam reduces blood pressure. The compound is routinely given to people before surgical, dental, or uncomfortable medical procedures and is used to relieve pain in afflictions and after surgery. Midazolam can produce amnesia about events that occurred while under the drug's influence and may be able to interfere with remembering things that occurred shortly before the drug was received. That amnesia action can be beneficial in reducing stress from medical treatments but might also be used by unscrupulous persons wanting to exploit someone.

Drawbacks. When injected intravenously the drug can be so hazardous that in some instances a resuscitation specialist must be on hand with the exclusive duty of monitoring the patient's condition at all times. Without that precaution people have suffered crippling brain damage or death from respiratory arrest caused by the drug while a medical procedure was being performed. Respiratory emergencies have also occurred from oral dosage. Midazolam is not recommended for persons suffering from breathing trouble. Nonetheless, despite the drug's potential hazards, examination of 5,439 records of patients receiving the drug at one hospital revealed only 3 instances of respiratory arrest. Examination of 9,842 medical records of persons who received midazolam in 14 hospitals did not reveal serious respiratory events caused by the drug; indeed, the study concluded that people were more likely to die from **diazepam**. That conclusion, of course, was based on administration of the drugs in a medical setting, not misuse on the street.

A rat study found the drug to have "minimal" ability to cause brain damage, and then only in older rats, even after four months of daily dosing. In a subsequent and related report investigators stated flatly that the drug does not cause brain damage, although once again slight differences were observed when older rats were compared to others.

Researchers have noted that midazolam harms white blood cells. Other unwanted effects include headache, coughing and hiccups, nausea, and vomiting. Less commonly, the drug can prompt euphoria, hallucinations, tremor, rapid heartbeat, discomposure, and aggression. Two researchers tracking violent deaths in Finland concluded that the drug was found in victims more often than would be expected through chance occurrence. Hallucinations by surgical patients have occurred often enough and can be realistic enough (such as patients perceiving imaginary sexual assault by medical personnel) that medical staff have been advised to have someone witness all contact with patients receiving the drug.

Midazolam lengthens reaction times, although two experiments found that users performed normally 4 hours after a dose such as a patient would receive for outpatient surgery. Those findings are supported by other studies as well, including one using test equipment to measure performance of commercial airline pilots. Nonetheless, persons are supposed to avoid activity requiring careful vigilance (such as driving) for at least 24 hours after taking midazolam.

A small study found that a dose of midazolam produces higher blood levels of the drug and lasts longer in ethnic Mexicans than in ethnic whites.

Abuse factors. Among monkeys dependence has been established with the drug after 5 to 10 weeks of steady dosage. Sudden cessation of dosage can provoke a withdrawal syndrome: perspiration, tremors and cramps, vomiting, convulsions, and hallucinations. The syndrome can be avoided by gradually reducing drug use instead of stopping all at once. Some researchers believe tolerance has been demonstrated. The substance is considered to have at least the same addiction potential as diazepam, which is three or four times weaker than midazolam.

Drug interactions. In some circumstances midazolam can lower blood pressure drastically and cause seizures; administering the drug with **fentanyl** or other opiates can increase the likelihood of such severe actions. Rat experiments unexpectedly found that the stimulant **caffeine** boosts difficulties in movement caused by midazolam, and **cocaine** also worsened that performance. Opiates or **alcohol** can deepen some midazolam effects in humans, and rat experiments find that midazolam makes alcohol more appealing. The HIV/AIDS (human immunodeficiency virus/acquired immunodeficiency syndrome) drug saquinavir and the antibiotic erythromycin increase midazolam levels in the body and make effects last longer. The antacid and ulcer medication cimetidine (such as Tagamet) can lengthen sedation from a midazolam dose. Some research indicates that drinking grapefruit juice increases midazolam's ability to act upon a person, but other research does not support that finding. The tuberculosis medicine rifampin and the epilepsy drugs phenytoin and carbamazepine diminish midazolam's effectiveness.

Cancer. Rat and mice experiments have produced no cancer even when midazolam was given daily for two years at 25 times the recommended human dose. The same usage of the drug at about 225 times the recommended human dose, however, produced liver and thyroid tumors. Relevance of the latter outcome to human medical use, involving normal dosage and typically using the drug for one day, is unclear. Gene mutations are considered an element in causing cancer, and midazolam did not produce mutations in assorted standard tests, nor were they observed in a study of patients receiving the drug.

Pregnancy. The drug has been given to mice, rats, and rabbits at 5 to 32 times the normal human dose without producing birth defects. Researchers conducting one experiment concluded, however, that the drug altered behavior of mice after fetal exposure (making males more uneasy and females less uneasy) while slowing their development. Tests indicate that the drug will pass from a pregnant woman into the fetus. The substance has been successfully used to treat eclampsia, a serious disease of late pregnancy involving convulsions, but midazolam is generally not desirable for pregnant women. The drug passes into the milk supply of nursing mothers, and caution is recommended about breast-feeding in such circumstances.

Additional scientific information may be found in:

Curran, H.V., and B. Birch. "Differentiating the Sedative, Psychomotor and Amnesic Effects of Benzodiazepines: A Study with Midazolam and the Benzodiazepine Antagonist, Flumazenil." *Psychopharmacology* 103 (1991): 519–23.

Dundee, J.W. "Fantasies during Sedation with Intravenous Midazolam or Diazepam." *Medico-Legal Journal* 58 (1990, pt. 1): 29–34.

Gupta, A., et al. "The Effects of Midazolam and Flumazenil on Psychomotor Function." *Journal of Clinical Anesthesia* 9 (1997): 21–25.

Kelly, D.J., et al. "The Effects of Midazolam on Pure Tone Audiometry, Speech Audiometry, and Audiological Reaction Times in Human Volunteers." *Anesthesia and Analgesia* 88 (1999):1064–68.

Langlois, S., et al. "Midazolam: Kinetics and Effects on Memory, Sensorium, and Hemodynamics." *British Journal of Clinical Pharmacology* 23 (1987): 273–78.

"Midazolam." *Medical Letter on Drugs and Therapeutics* 28 (1986): 73–74.

Nordt, S.P., and R.F. Clark. "Midazolam: A Review of Therapeutic Uses and Toxicity." *Journal of Emergency Medicine* 15 (1997): 357–65.

Modafinil

Pronunciation: moh-DA-fih-nill
Chemical Abstracts Service Registry Number: 68693-11-8
Formal Names: Alertec, Modiodal, Provigil
Type: Stimulant. *See* page 11
Federal Schedule Listing: Schedule IV (DEA no. 1680)
USA Availability: Prescription
Pregnancy Category: C

Uses. This drug is a medical treatment for narcolepsy and other conditions involving difficulty in staying awake. The substance also improves vigilance. In the 1990s U.S. Air Force researchers called for exploration of the drug's potential in assisting military missions. Investigators have found that the compound may assist aircraft pilots in maintaining a better performance level when deprived of sleep for extended periods. An experiment indicated that the drug can help military personnel engage in sustained operations for 64 hours without sleep, with fewer unwanted effects than amphetamine has. A French military experiment showed the drug could be used along with short naps to permit extended operations without normal sleep periods. Additional study has shown, however, that people using the compound are less aware of reduced quality of performance; in comparison, sleep-deprived individuals who use **dextroamphetamine** or a placebo have a more accurate assessment of their capabilities. Thus, from a practical standpoint, sleep-deprived persons using modafinil may be overconfident and try to do things that should not be attempted.

Modafinil is used against obstructive sleep apnea, in which people have temporary breathing stoppages while asleep and which can make them sleepy the next day. Experiments find that although modafinil helps people stay awake, it does not interfere with the quality of their sleep, as dextroamphetamine does. Modafinil has helped patients respond better to antidepressant therapy while also reducing their feelings of weariness. Favorable results have been seen in experiments using the drug against attention deficit hyperactivity disorder (ADHD) and against organic brain problems caused by alcoholism. An animal study indicates the substance may have potential for treating Parkinson's disease. Some authorities speculate that the compound may reduce brain problems caused by aging. Modafinil makes animals more active.

Drawbacks. Modafinil can produce euphoria in humans. Headache, dry mouth, sore throat, appetite loss, nausea, diarrhea, uneasiness, depression, insomnia, fever, infection, and weakness have been reported by modafinil users. Among cardiac patients, unwanted actions may include heart palpitations, chest pain, and breathing difficulty. High doses have caused tremors, faster pulse rate, high blood pressure, peevishness, confusion, and aggression. Although the compound is a stimulant, it has a risk of adversely affecting skills needed for operating dangerous machinery such as automobiles.

A modafinil dose lasts a shorter time in young females than in young males.

Abuse factors. Modafinil's chemical properties reduce or even eliminate its effects if injected or smoked, reducing its convenience for abuse. Studies indicate the drug has less abuse potential than many other stimulants, but monkeys will self-administer modafinil, a traditional sign of addictive potential in a substance. Scientists running one monkey experiment noted, however, that only massive doses would interest the animals; even an amount of modafinil 200 times the size of a dextroamphetamine dose was not enough to get them to self-administer the two drugs at the same rate. In a rat test the rodents acted like modafinil has some effects reminiscent of **cocaine**. In one scientific study persons with a history of drug abuse found modafinil's actions pleasurable and similar to those of **methylphenidate**. People using modafinil daily for 9 weeks showed no dependence; and a study of 140 patients who used the drug for varying amounts of time, ranging from 1 month to almost 10 years, revealed no dependence. Tests of humans taking modafinil daily for 40 weeks indicated no development of tolerance.

Drug interactions. Modafinil can make birth control pills and implants less effective. A laboratory test indicated that the drug may reduce blood levels of cyclosporine, an immunosuppressant used to help organ transplant patients. Modafinil may raise blood levels of **diazepam**, tricyclic antidepressants, the anti–blood clot medicine warfarin, and the epilepsy medicine phenytoin.

Cancer. Laboratory tests have not found indications that modafinil causes cancer.

Pregnancy. Fetal injury emerged in pregnant rats receiving 10 times the normal maximum human dose of modafinil, but pregnant rabbits receiving the same dosage did not show fetal damage attributable to the substance. At lower doses rat offspring appeared normal, and milk from nursing rats receiving the drug did not seem to harm the pups. Effects on human pregnancy and milk are uncertain.

Additional scientific information may be found in:

Akerstedt, T., and G. Ficca. "Alertness-Enhancing Drugs as a Countermeasure to Fatigue in Irregular Work Hours." *Chronobiology International* 14 (1997): 145–58.

Baranski, J.V., and R.A. Pigeau. "Self-Monitoring Cognitive Performance during Sleep Deprivation: Effects of Modafinil, D-Amphetamine and Placebo." *Journal of Sleep Research* 6 (1997): 84–91.

Lyons, T.J., and J. French. "Modafinil: The Unique Properties of a New Stimulant." *Aviation, Space, and Environmental Medicine* 62 (1991): 432–35.

"Modafinil for Narcolepsy." *Medical Letter on Drugs and Therapeutics* 41 (1999): 30–31.

Rugino, T.A., and T.C. Copley. "Effects of Modafinil in Children with Attention-Deficit/Hyperactivity Disorder: An Open-Label Study." *Journal of the American Academy of Child and Adolescent Psychiatry* 40 (2001): 230–35.

Morning Glory

Pronunciation: MOR-neen GLOH-ree

Chemical Abstracts Service Registry Number: None

Formal Names: *Ipomoea hederacea, Ipomoea purpurea, Ipomoea sidaefolia, Ipomoea tricolor, Ipomoea violacea*

Informal Names: Flying Saucers, Heavenly Blue, Pearly Gates, Tlitliltzin, Yaxce'lil

Type: Hallucinogen. *See* page 25

Federal Schedule Listing: Unlisted

USA Availability: Nonprescription natural product

Pregnancy Category: None

Uses. Morning glory is a familiar flower. Many varieties exist, and some have drug properties. Although morning glory is an uncontrolled substance, the hallucinogenic varieties contain lysergic acid amide, a Schedule III depressant.

Seeds and roots of the *Ipomoea hederacea* morning glory are used medicinally. The natural product works as a laxative and as a treatment against intestinal worms. Traditional applications include combating flatulence, easing excessive feelings of fullness after a meal, and treating scabies (a skin disease caused by a parasite).

Albert Hofmann, the discoverer of **LSD**, became intrigued by accounts of seed called *ololiuqui* by the Aztecs. Folk medicine used its ointments or potions to treat flatulence, tumors, and venereal disease. Ingesting the seeds allowed Aztecs to commune with their gods, and native peoples still used *ololiuqui* for that purpose during the twentieth century. Hofmann found that the *ololiuqui* seeds of Mexico came from two kinds of morning glory: from *Ipomoea sidaefolia* (also called *Rivea corymbosa*) and from *Ipomoea violacea* (also called *Ipomoea tricolor*, whose seeds are also known as *badoh negro*). Seeds from both plants contained **ergot** chemicals resembling LSD.

Although *Ipomoea violacea* is often viewed in a drug context, the plant has agricultural usage as a natural means of weed control. *Ipomoea purpurea* is sensitive enough to airborne chemicals that researchers use it to measure air pollution.

Drawbacks. Morning glory seeds have been publicized as a substitute for LSD, but no less an authority than Hofmann himself found LSD and morning glory to have different effects. In particular he noted that morning glory emptied thoughts from the mind and made the world seem meaningless, while promoting unease, depression, and a weariness that transformed into sleep. In addition to being a hallucinogen, LSD has powerful stimulant actions, but when morning glory seed was tested on rats, they became less active than normal and, contrary to what would be expected with a hallucinogen, they showed no change in perceptual abilities. A team of researchers who studied reactions of volunteers described morning glory's active chemicals as unlike LSD. Those volunteers nonetheless felt some euphoria; they also had a distorted sense of time and a crossover of senses (in which colors might be smelled or sounds might be seen), but hallucinations or alteration of consciousness did not seem to develop. The research team likened morning glory to the drug ibogalin (which lacks significant psychological effect despite its close relation to **ibogaine**) and to the drug scopolamine found in **belladonna**. A case report about a person being treated for morning glory seed overdose said no hallucinations were present.

Those kinds of observations seem to differ from the effects experienced by the Aztecs and modern native peoples. Indeed, some recreational users (and their medical caregivers) report morning glory experiences quite similar to those of LSD, from hallucinations to philosophical insights—although one short series of case reports about such reactions argued that every instance involved a psychologically abnormal person. Some users describe cold extremities, a possible sign of ergot poisoning. A case report noted other physical reactions: red face and abdominal discomfort eased by "explosive diarrheic bowel movements." The patient also had lowered blood pressure and heart rate, opposite to accounts about LSD.

Morning glory seeds purchased from garden stores are not intended for human consumption and may contain fungicides that could harm a person who ingests them, although one investigator doubts a human stomach can hold enough morning glory seeds to cause fatal poisoning from the fungicide coating. Experimenters have fed uncontaminated seed to rats as various percentages of their diet, from less than 1% up to 8%. After 90 days animals receiving the greatest amount showed a higher death rate than normal, with males more affected than females. Although the animals had less weight gain than would be expected on an ordinary diet, various internal organs enlarged. In addition, liver damage occurred, and blood abnormalities appeared.

Abuse factors. In the 1960s the British government concluded that morning glory seeds were harmless, but American researchers did not reach a consensus about whether danger existed. Some authorities state that *Ipomoea purpurea* morning glory seeds lack psychedelic properties, but other authorities say otherwise.

Drug interactions. Not enough scientific information to report.

Cancer. The Ames test, a laboratory screen used to test substances for cancer-causing potential, reveals that morning glory seeds have that potential.

Pregnancy. Lysergic acid amide has damaged embryo development in mice. Pregnant women are advised to avoid *Ipomoea hederacea* because it is suspected of causing birth defects.

Additional scientific information may be found in:

Blum, O., et al. "Ambient Tropospheric Ozone in the Ukrainian Carpathian Mountains and Kiev Region: Detection with Passive Samplers and Bioindicator Plants." *Environmental Pollution* 98 (1997): 299–304.

Dungan, G.M., and M.R. Gumbmann. "Toxicological Evaluation of Morning Glory Seed: Subchronic 90-Day Feeding Study." *Food and Chemical Toxicology* 28 (1990): 553–60.

Fink, P.J., M.J. Goldman, and I. Lyons. "Morning Glory Seed Psychosis." *Archives of General Psychiatry* 15 (1966): 209–13.

Heim, E., H. Heimann, and G. Lukacs. "Psychotomimetic Effects of the Mexican Drug 'Ololiuqui.' " *Psychopharmacologia* 13 (1968): 35–48.

Hofmann, A. "Teonanacatl and Ololiuqui, Two Ancient Magic Drugs of Mexico." *Bulletin on Narcotics* 23, no. 1 (1971): 3–14.

Ingram, A.L., Jr. "Morning Glory Seed Reaction." *Journal of the American Medical Association* 190 (1964): 1133–34.

"Morning Glory and Hallucinosis." *South African Medical Journal* 40 (1966): 1015–16.

Morphine

Pronunciation: MOR-feen

Chemical Abstracts Service Registry Number: 57-27-2

Formal Names: Astramorph, Duramorph, Infumorph, Kadian, Kapanol Sevredol, Morphine Sulfate, MS Contin, MSIR, MST Continus, MXL, Oramorph, Roxanol

Informal Names: Cube Juice, Dope, Dreamer, Emsel, First Line, God's Drug, Hard Stuff, Hocus, Hows, Lydia, Lydic, M, Miss Emma, Mister Blue, Monkey, Morf, Morph, Morphide, Morphie, Morpho, Mother, MS, Ms. Emma, Mud, New Jack Swing (with **heroin**), Sister, Tab, Unkie, Unkie White, Stuff

Type: Depressant (opiate class). *See* page 22

Federal Schedule Listing: Schedule II (DEA no. 9300)

USA Availability: Prescription

Pregnancy Category: C

Uses. Morphine was identified as **opium**'s main active ingredient in the early 1800s. The body transforms a **heroin** dose into morphine. If stored too long in a water solution, morphine will eventually transform into other chemicals including morphine-N-oxide, a Schedule I controlled substance. Although pharmaceutical supplies of morphine come from opium harvests, mammals produce small amounts of morphine in their bodies. Thus the substance is a natural product in both the plant and animal kingdoms. The drug can also be created entirely in a laboratory.

Morphine's role in medicine did not become prominent until the hypodermic needle was introduced in the 1850s. Injection was long the main means of administration, but other delivery systems (such as absorption by the nasal lining and through rectal suppositories) have since been developed. Oral dosage formats are also available.

Morphine is widely used to sedate people and to ease anxiety. The drug is commonly given to treat acute pain from injury or surgery and chronic pain from assorted afflictions. The hurting does not actually go away, but people become less aware of it. In addition to pain control, morphine also has anti-inflammatory actions and can suppress coughing.

The drug tends to produce better pain relief in women than in men. A small study examined whether Chinese men respond to morphine differently than white men do: Doses lasted longer in the whites, interfered more with their breathing, and produced greater reduction in their blood pressure.

Drawbacks. When used to reduce continual pain in serious disease, too much morphine can increase discomfort rather than relieve it and cause a condition in which a patient experiences pain from activity that should not be uncomfortable.

Morphine can make people drowsy, so they should avoid operating an automobile or other hazardous machinery until they know how the drug affects them. Despite morphine's safety in a medical context, it can be hazardous when injected into fluid circulating through the spinal cord and brain, and if hospital staffs use this technique, they are advised to have resuscitation equipment on hand.

Nausea and vomiting are common unwanted effects from morphine. It promotes constipation and urine retention. Itching and hives can occur. The drug interferes with sexual activity by male rats and lowers **testosterone** levels in human males. Morphine can impede breathing and often is avoided if a person suffers from asthma. Rats dosed with morphine for six weeks developed a weakened immune system. People can experience seizures and accelerated heart activity from a strong dose.

Abuse factors. After several weeks of medical dosage a person can experience noticeable dependence with morphine. Such development should take longer with adulterated street supplies. Medical patients who were surveyed about their experience with morphine claimed to have experienced no difficulty in stopping the drug. Addiction from medical use is almost unheard of. Normally withdrawal symptoms are a mild version of the opiate withdrawal syndrome. Tolerance is normally described as evidence of drug abuse, but morphine tolerance can develop in persons receiving the drug medically for pain relief. Symptoms of such tolerance include a need to take doses more often and at a higher strength in order to produce the same amount of pain relief. This is notable because tolerance to medical effects of a drug tends to be unusual; perhaps the development indicates a substantial psychological component in morphine's pain management. Tolerance is commonly observed among addicts, but they do not continually increase their dosage. At some point they generally reach a level adequate to maintain the sensations they seek. In the 1980s a mice experiment indicated that vitamin C may prevent morphine tolerance and dependence, but judging from subsequent absence of this technique in treating humans, apparently initial hopes for the therapy have not been fulfilled.

One of the main appeals in illicit use of morphine is the drug's ability to induce calmness. People making unauthorized use of the drug for this purpose are not so much using the drug for recreation as for relieving mental suffering. In some people the drug can cause euphoria, a characteristic that can have appeal strictly for recreation but also for self-medication. In these and other respects, morphine and heroin will appeal to the same sorts of people for the same sorts of reasons.

For decades morphine addiction was portrayed as the classic kind of drug abuse. Although the substance was unwelcome in the workplace as the twenty-first century began, a century earlier some workers used the drug to increase productivity in both manual and intellectual tasks by relieving tension that otherwise diminished performance. Other pharmaceuticals later superseded that antianxiety function of morphine. Somewhat surprisingly, given morphine's depressant actions, researchers have found the drug can improve performance on a test of response time in decision making. Other researchers have found no effect on performance in tests of memory, reasoning, muscular coordination, and various additional skills basic to everyday living. Few ill effects seem to come from chronic use of pure morphine (as opposed to adulterated street supplies). Addicts with access to the pure product have lived healthy and productive lives into old age. As drug laws tightened over the past century, use of morphine by ordinary middle-class people declined, shifting the prevalence of nonmedical morphine usage from law-abiding persons into populations with more social deviance. Consequently, illicit use of morphine became more associated with society's outcasts. That association, however, was caused by changes in laws and social attitudes (changes in setting), not by any chemical effect of the drug.

Drug interactions. Animal and human experiments show that more pain relief can come from morphine if **ephedrine** is taken at the same time. **Dextroamphetamine** can improve pain relief provided by morphine. **Alcohol**, tricyclic antidepressants, and monoamine oxidase inhibitors (MAOIs, found in some antidepressants and other medicine) can boost morphine effects. Rat experiments indicate that benzodiazepine class depressants lengthen the effect from a morphine dose. Researchers find that morphine and **nicotine** have cross-tolerance in mice.

Cancer. Morphine is not known to cause cancer. Some laboratory tests and some studies of human users, however, detect cell damage that could lead to cancer. Some people smoke morphine, and the smoke is suspected of causing esophageal cancer. Evidence exists that naturally occurring morphine in lung tissue may constrain development of lung cancer, that nicotine counteracts such protection, and that tobacco smokers have more naturally occurring morphine in their lung tissue than nonsmokers (perhaps because the body increases morphine production when challenged by nicotine). All this evidence, however, involves minute levels of naturally occurring morphine in the body and does not support taking the drug in hopes of avoiding lung cancer.

Pregnancy. When given in amounts exceeding normal human medical doses by hundreds of times, morphine has caused animal birth defects. Malformations involving bones and soft tissues have been observed in animals. Pregnant rats and hamsters dosed on morphine produce male offspring that exhibit feminized behavior. When morphine was routinely given to male adolescent rats, the drug seemed to interfere with sexual maturation. As their offspring reached adulthood, they appeared normal but had hormone abnormalities.

In humans no increase in birth defects has been observed in offspring of women who used morphine during pregnancy. A morphine dose quickly passes from the woman into the fetus, however, and reaches a blood level similar to the woman's. A dose lasts longer in the fetus than elsewhere in a woman's body. The drug reduces fetal motions. A baby born to a chronic morphine user can have dependence on the drug and exhibit withdrawal symptoms after birth. One study found that infants receiving morphine for medical purposes soon after birth show no ill effects five years later in conduct, muscular coordination, or intelligence.

Morphine apparently passes into a mother's milk. One case report described the amount as minimal and found no effect on the nursing infant, but another report tells of an infant receiving so much morphine from milk that dependence developed.

Additional scientific information may be found in:

Hamilton, G.R., and T.F. Baskett. "In the Arms of Morpheus, the Development of Morphine for Postoperative Pain Relief." *Canadian Journal of Anaesthesia* 47 (2000): 367–74.

Hill, J.L., and J.P. Zacny. "Comparing the Subjective, Psychomotor, and Physiological Effects of Intravenous Hydromorphone and Morphine in Healthy Volunteers." *Psychopharmacology* 152 (2000): 31–39.

O'Neill, W.M., et al. "The Cognitive and Psychomotor Effects of Morphine in Healthy Subjects: A Randomized Controlled Trial of Repeated (Four) Oral Doses of Dextropropoxyphene, Morphine, Lorazepam and Placebo." *Pain* 85 (2000): 209–15.

Walker, D.J., and J.P. Zacny. "Subjective, Psychomotor, and Analgesic Effects of Oral Codeine and Morphine in Healthy Volunteers." *Psychopharmacology* 140 (1998): 191–201.

Zacny, J.P., et al. "Comparing the Subjective, Psychomotor and Physiological Effects of Intravenous Pentazocine and Morphine in Normal Volunteers." *Journal of Pharmacology and Experimental Therapeutics* 286 (1998): 1197–207.

Mothballs

Pronunciation: MOTH-ballz
Chemical Abstracts Service Registry Number: None
Formal Names: Naphthalene, Paradichlorobenzene
Type: Inhalant. *See* page 26
Federal Schedule Listing: Unlisted
USA Availability: Generally available nonprescription product
Pregnancy Category: None

Uses. Mothballs typically contain naphthalene or paradichlorobenzene. Neither persons who use mothballs recreationally nor their medical caregivers are always aware of which kind of mothballs have been used. Diaper pail and toilet deodorizers may contain one or the other of those chemicals. Naphthalene varieties look dry, and paradichlorobenzene products appear oily. Normally people inhale fumes, but cases of oral ingestion are known. Naphthalene can also be absorbed through the skin; an infant died from using diapers and blankets contaminated with the substance. Some glues contain naphthalene, but sensations from glue sniffing are normally considered a result of **toluene**.

Drawbacks. Naphthalene may create agitation and tiredness, fever, skin paleness, headache, appetite loss, abdominal discomfort, nausea and vomiting, diarrhea, cataracts, and kidney failure. Blood disorders serious enough to prevent the body from utilizing enough oxygen from the lungs may arise. The kidney failure can create excessive blood potassium levels, which in turn can cause heart failure. Seizures and coma may also occur. Jaundice is a known affliction from naphthalene, and a case report notes fatal liver damage.

A case report tells about difficulty with control of fingers due to inhaling mothball fumes. Paradichlorobenzene is not associated with such an affliction, so the problem is assumed to have come from naphthalene mothballs. Compared to naphthalene, harm from paradichlorobenzene normally takes longer to appear but may include liver and kidney malfunction. A case of anemia is known from eating two paradichlorobenzene toilet freshener blocks per week.

Abuse factors. One person experienced tremors and weariness upon stopping daily oral ingestion of paradichlorobenzene mothballs (which suggests dependence may have developed).

Drug interactions: Not enough scientific information to report.

Cancer. Naphthalene has not been found to cause cancer. Paradichlorobenzene fumes failed to produce cancer in a short animal test. The disease did develop in mice and rats that received oral dosage, and paradichlorobenzene caused cell mutations (a possible indication of cancer-causing potential) in fungi but not in bacteria. Human risk is unknown.

Pregnancy. A normal infant was born to a woman who ate one or two paradichlorobenzene toilet fresheners a week during her pregnancy. A pregnant woman who sniffed naphthalene, however, produced a child with skin color typical of naphthalene poisoning and an enlarged liver and spleen. The organs became normal after treatment.

Additional scientific information may be found in:

Athanasiou, M., et al. "Hemolytic Anemia in a Female Newborn Infant Whose Mother Inhaled Naphthalene Before Delivery." *Journal of Pediatrics* 130 (1997): 680–81.

Santucci, K., and B. Shah. "Association of Naphthalene with Acute Hemolytic Anemia." *Academic Emergency Medicine* 7 (2000): 42–47.

Siegel, E., and S. Wason. "Mothball Toxicity." *Pediatric Clinics of North America* 33 (1986): 369–74.

Weintraub, E., D. Gandhi, and C. Robinson. "Medical Complications Due to Mothball Abuse." *Southern Medical Journal* 93 (2000): 427–29.

Nalbuphine

Pronunciation: nal-BYOO-feen

Chemical Abstracts Service Registry Number: 20594-83-6. (Hydrochloride form 23277-43-2)

Formal Names: Nubain

Type: Depressant (opioid class). *See* page 24

Federal Schedule Listing: Unlisted

USA Availability: Prescription

Pregnancy Category: B

Uses. This opioid is considered about as effective as **morphine** at pain relief and is also used in anesthesia and for sedation. Nalbuphine is used to control substantial pain in conditions ranging from surgery and broken bones to heart attack and sickle cell anemia crisis. Women seem to get more pain relief from the drug than men do. The compound's anesthetic capabilities have been used in military medicine; one scientific report[1] blandly describes nalbuphine usage in cases of "large, multiple gunshot wounds of the trunk and extremities, as well as injuries caused by fragments of projectiles and explosive devices." The drug is also used in dentistry.

Nalbuphine is a narcotic agonist-antagonist, meaning it has opiate properties itself but can counteract other opiates/opioids, a counteraction sometimes strong enough to cause a withdrawal syndrome if someone has dependence on the other opiate/opioid.

The drug's safety for administration to children is considered unproven in the United States, but nalbuphine is given to youngsters in America and elsewhere.

Drawbacks. Unwanted effects include dizziness, perspiration, itching, constipation, nausea, vomiting, and breathing impairment. Hallucinations and euphoria are reported. The drug may interfere with physical and mental abilities needed to operate automobiles or other dangerous devices; tests have demonstrated slower reaction times and impaired decision making among users. The drug can make a person act drunk.

Abuse factors. Research indicates that nalbuphine injections briefly increase blood levels of growth hormone, an increase that may lead some people to think the drug promotes muscle mass. Reports circulating in bodybuilder circles claim the drug can promote muscle mass in another way also, by reducing blood levels of a hormone called cortisol. In the 1990s nalbuphine was popular among bodybuilders using anabolic steroids. These individuals mainly used nalbuphine to reduce pain caused by exercise regimens. Interviews with such users revealed that many were suffering unwanted physical and mental effects from nalbuphine and that many of these persons were abusing other drugs as well. A case report tells of illicit nalbuphine injection causing muscle damage—the opposite of what bodybuilders seek.

In low amounts nalbuphine can produce morphine effects. High doses tend to make users feel nervous and uncomfortable, however, reducing nalbuphine's attractiveness for illicit recreational use. At those higher dosage levels people can experience vision trouble, sleep disturbance, weird dreams, and thoughts running out of control. The drug is generally considered to have a low potential for abuse, lower than **propoxyphene** or **codeine**. Some researchers, however, describe the abuse liability as about equivalent to **pentazocine**, a drug with a notorious reputation for illicit misuse and that has effects similar to those of nalbuphine. Tolerance and dependence may develop if a person uses nalbuphine in amounts higher than normal medical doses. Withdrawal symptoms are described as those of mild opiate withdrawal.

Drug interactions. Not enough scientific information to report.

Cancer. Standard laboratory tests do not indicate the drug has potential for causing cancer. Long-term experiments with rats and mice have failed to produce cancer.

Pregnancy. Animal research using nalbuphine at high doses has not produced birth defects attributable to the drug. It passes from a pregnant woman into the fetus and can build up there; one study found that newborn levels could be six times higher than maternal levels. Due to effects on the newborn's heartbeat and breathing, controversy exists about the drug's appropriateness for easing pain of childbirth. Some researchers believe the substance is risky during childbirth; some believe nalbuphine is safer than combinations of other drugs. Nalbuphine passes into milk of nursing mothers but is not believed to harm breast-feeding infants.

Additional scientific information may be found in:

Jasinski, D.R., and P.A. Mansky. "Evaluation of Nalbuphine for Abuse Potential." *Clinical Pharmacology and Therapeutics* 13 (January–February 1972): 78–90.

Miller, R.R. "Evaluation of Nalbuphine Hydrochloride." *American Journal of Hospital Pharmacy* 37 (1980): 942–49.

Saarialho-Kere, U. "Psychomotor, Respiratory and Neuroendocrinological Effects of Nalbuphine and Haloperidol, Alone and in Combination, in Healthy Subjects." *British Journal of Clinical Pharmacology* 26 (1988): 79–87.

Schmidt, W.K., et al. "Nalbuphine." *Drug and Alcohol Dependence* 14 (1985): 339–62.

Stambaugh, J.E. "Evaluation of Nalbuphine: Efficacy and Safety in the Management of Chronic Pain Associated with Advanced Malignancy." *Current Therapeutic Research: Clinical and Experimental* 31 (1982): 393–401.

Wines, J.D., et al. "Nalbuphine Hydrochloride Dependence in Anabolic Steroid Users." *American Journal on Addictions* 8 (1999): 161–64.

Zacny, J.P., K. Conley, and S. Marks. "Comparing the Subjective, Psychomotor and Physiological Effects of Intravenous Nalbuphine and Morphine in Healthy

Volunteers." *Journal of Pharmacology and Experimental Therapeutics* 280 (1997): 1159–69.

Note

1. Rakaric-Poznanovic, M., Z. Boljevic, and D. Marcec. "Anestezija Nalbufin/Propofol u Kirurskom Zbrinjavanju Ratnih Ozljeda [Nalbuphine/Propofol Anesthesia in the Surgical Treatment of War Injuries]." *Lijecnicki Vjesnik* 115 (1993): 303–305. Abstract in English.

Nandrolone

Pronunciation: NAN-droh-lohn

Chemical Abstracts Service Registry Number: 434-22-0. (Decanoate form 360-70-3; furylpropionate form 7642-64-0; phenpropionate form 62-90-8)

Formal Names: Anabolin LA-100, Androlone D, Deca-Durabolin, Demalon, Dexatopic, Durabolin, Hybolin Decanoate, Nandrolin, Nortestosterone

Type: Anabolic steroid. *See* page 24

Federal Schedule Listing: Schedule III (DEA no. 4000)

USA Availability: Prescription

Pregnancy Category: X

Uses. Nandrolone is used to treat breast cancer and anemia, and the drug has improved asthma and Sjögren's syndrome, a disease that destroys salivary, sweat, and tear glands. Healing action on cornea afflictions has been observed, and rat experiments have explored nandrolone's potential for speeding recovery from tooth extractions. A skin cream containing nandrolone is used against eczema. Human research indicates that the drug can improve osteoporosis, a disease causing brittle bones, although results conflict on how long the improvement lasts. Among some diabetics with a kidney condition called Kimmelstiel-Wilson syndrome, nandrolone has helped both renal and eyesight difficulties. In kidney dialysis, patients' experimental use of nandrolone was able to improve weariness, increase muscle mass, and fight malnutrition. The compound has helped AIDS (acquired immunodeficiency syndrome) patients build up weight, muscles, and strength. The substance has also been given in hopes of stimulating appetite in malnourished cancer patients, although animal cancer research indicates that any weight gain may simply be due to water retention rather than improved nutrition (in contrast to research with healthy animals that produced weight increase associated with protein gain—some livestock raisers illegally dose animals with nandrolone to promote growth). After administration of the drug, improvement occurred in a case of anorexia nervosa, a psychological condition in which people with normal or low weight misperceive themselves as fat.

Drawbacks. Typically, but not always, studies of humans who use nandrolone have measured declines in cholesterol levels (including HDL, the so-called good cholesterol) and elevation of triglycerides (associated with body processes leading to heart attack and stroke). In monkeys, coronary artery damage appeared after long-term administration of nandrolone. After the drug was given for a year or more to female monkeys they showed abnormalities in the uterus. Female reproductive behavior was disrupted in a rat experiment using doses comparable to what humans take. In humans the substance can promote male characteristics in females (such as facial hair and deeper voice), and in men it can enlarge breasts while diminishing sexual organs. Other unwanted effects may include acne, aggressive conduct, urinary difficulty, and fluid retention causing tissues to swell. Nandrolone is supposed to be avoided by males suffering from breast or prostate cancer and by anyone with porphyria, liver disease, heart failure, or kidney failure. The drug may interfere with children's growth and their gender differentiation.

Taking nandrolone without watchful medical supervision can be hazardous. A bodybuilder's use of nandrolone and other steroids is suspected of transforming a routine case of chickenpox into a nearly fatal experience, requiring over a month of hospitalization in an intensive care unit. Daily nandrolone is suspected of leading to kidney and bone marrow disease that paralyzed a 29-year-old bodybuilder, although eventually he recovered enough to walk without help.

Abuse factors. Nandrolone can improve muscle mass, and some athletes use it for that purpose even though sports regulatory agencies forbid use of the compound by competitors. Among athletes tested by the International Olympic Committee in the 1980s nandrolone was the most frequently found illicit anabolic steroid. The sports ban extends beyond human competitions and includes horse racing; however, an experiment testing thoroughbred racing performance found no effect from the drug.

Research demonstrates that consuming boar meat or taking the nonprescription steroid androstenedione can produce false-positive tests for nandrolone. In theory consumption of horse meat might also produce a false positive, as natural body processes in a horse may produce enough nandrolone to be measurable.

Drug interactions. The substance can alter the amount of insulin needed by diabetics. Some experimentation on rats found that nandrolone can boost heart rate acceleration caused by **cocaine**; in other rat work the combination apparently lowered pulse rate. Nandrolone boosts actions of anti–blood clot medicines, putting patients at risk of excessive bleeding.

Cancer. Judging from decades of medical experience, the compound does not seem to cause cancer.

Pregnancy. Due to danger of masculinization of offspring, nandrolone is supposed to be avoided by women who are pregnant or nursing.

Additional scientific information may be found in:

Gerritsma, E.J., et al. "Virilization of the Voice in Post-Menopausal Women Due to the Anabolic Steroid Nandrolone Decanoate (Decadurabolin). The Effects of Medication for One Year." *Clinical Otolaryngology and Allied Sciences* 19 (1994): 79–84.

Gold, J., et al. "Safety and Efficacy of Nandrolone Decanoate for Treatment of Wasting in Patients with HIV Infection." *AIDS* 10 (1996): 745–52.

Johansen, K.L., K. Mulligan, and M. Schambelan. "Anabolic Effects of Nandrolone Decanoate in Patients Receiving Dialysis: A Randomized Controlled Trial." *Journal of the American Medical Association* 281 (1999): 1275–81.

"Nandrolone Decanoate." In *Therapeutic Drugs*, ed. C. Dollery. 2d ed. New York: Churchill Livingstone, 1999. N28–N30.

Radis, C.D., and K.P. Callis. "Systemic Lupus Erythematosus with Membranous Glomerulonephritis and Transverse Myelitis Associated with Anabolic Steroid Use." *Arthritis and Rheumatism* 40 (1997): 1899–1902.

Nicotine

Pronunciation: NIK-uh-teen (also pronounced NIK-uh-tin)

Chemical Abstracts Service Registry Number: 54-11-5

Formal Names: Habitrol, Nicoderm, Niconil, Nicorette, *Nicotiana rustica*, *Nicotiana tabacum*, Nicotrol, Prostrop, Tobacco

Informal Names: Chip (cigarette mixed with **PCP**), Fry Daddy (cigarette mixed with crack **cocaine**)

Type: Stimulant (pyridine alkaloids class). *See* page 18

Federal Schedule Listing: Unlisted

USA Availability: Generally available to adults as a component of tobacco products; nonprescription and prescription in pharmaceutical format

Pregnancy Category: C or D (depending on pharmaceutical format)

Uses. Tobacco's history is mentioned on page 18. Nicotine is the addictive drug component of tobacco and is found in other plants as well. Nicotine is one of the more hazardous drugs, and dosage via tobacco smoke adds still more peril. Although nicotine has medical uses, characteristics of the natural product tobacco fall within the criteria of a Schedule I controlled substance. Nonetheless, federal law explicitly excludes tobacco from such control, making the tobacco industry legal. At the time this book was written debate was under way about limiting adult access to nicotine products, a restrictive effort requiring changes in law.

Traditional medical uses of the drug include treatment of insect bites, skin and intestinal parasites, vomiting, earache, toothache, runny nose, hernia, and heart pain. Although tobacco smoking worsens a gastrointestinal inflammation called Crohn's disease, medical practice uses nicotine skin patches, oral capsules, or suppositories to treat inflammation of the colon and rectum caused by ulcerative colitis. Nicotine chewing gum has been used successfully to treat finger or toe sores deriving from Buerger's disease, an affliction in which blood vessels get blocked off (and which, despite the usefulness of pharmaceutical nicotine, seems to be worsened by smoking). Pharmaceutical nicotine helps some persons suffering from the tics of Tourette's syndrome. Researchers have found cigarette smoking to reduce the likelihood of getting preeclampsia, a potentially serious disease of late pregnancy in which women suffer fluid retention, high blood pressure, and too-high urine protein levels. Cigarette smoking is also associated with a lower probability of getting Parkinson's or Alzheimer's disease. Even though "association" does not demonstrate cause and effect, some experiments using pharmaceutical nicotine to treat those afflictions show positive results. Such results, however, have not yet given nicotine a generally accepted role in treating those diseases. Nicotine reduces hunger pains and raises blood sugar, effects that help users eat less (Native Americans have traditionally chewed tobacco to better endure circumstances involving little food, water, or rest). Nicotine initially raises blood pressure, but continued dosage will lower it.

Drawbacks. Tobacco smoking can lead to lung cancer and heart disease. Many other afflictions are attributed to tobacco smoking: bronchitis, emphysema, cataracts, mouth cancer, pancreas cancer, bone density loss (making broken bones more likely), abdominal aortic aneurysm (a sac ballooning out from the blood vessel wall), brain aneurysm, and gastroesophageal reflux (recurrent backward flow of acid and partially digested food from the stomach to the esophagus, making esophageal cancer more likely). One study noted that smoking tends to produce changes causing women to go through menopause at a younger age than nonsmokers. Laboratory tests imply that smokeless tobacco promotes tooth decay. Still more unwanted actions are known, partly because tobacco has simply been studied so intensively that more is known about it than is known about many other substances. Whether nicotine itself causes afflictions produced by tobacco is uncertain. For example, some investigators suspect that heart disease in smokers comes from carbon monoxide and tar constituents of smoke rather than the nicotine.

In adults 40 mg to 100 mg of pharmaceutical nicotine can produce fatal poisoning; an equivalent dose through cigarettes would require a person to quickly smoke several packs. Smaller dosages can be dangerous for children who play with nicotine patches or gum or who consume tobacco.

Abuse factors. As with many drugs, persons often find nicotine unpleasant at first but learn to ignore bad sensations and focus upon effects that are enjoyed. Experiments examining differences that users perceive in various drugs find that some sensations from nicotine, amphetamine, and cocaine are similar, so similar that in one experiment persons receiving injections of nicotine typically identified it as cocaine. A user can establish a physical dependence with nicotine, causing withdrawal symptoms if dosage stops: nervousness, tenseness, crankiness, lightheadedness, broken sleep, weariness, distractedness, tremors. These symptoms often last a few days, sometimes longer, and can relate to a person's expectations (a psychosomatic component).

Debate exists about how addictive nicotine is. A study published in 1994 noted that about 33% of tobacco smokers become addicted. A study published in 2000 found that 20% to 60% of adolescent smokers are addicted. Many smokers with no interest in quitting can nonetheless substantially reduce their cigarette consumption with little difficulty. In contrast, many smokers wanting to stop find themselves unable to cease, and for them even pharmaceutical nicotine can be an insufficient replacement for tobacco. Among such persons the persistence of a smoking habit suggests that something more than the drug nicotine is involved. Tobacco smoke contains thousands of chemical ingredients besides nicotine; perhaps some of the less-studied ones are important. In addition, the paraphernalia and mechanics of cigarette smoking provide a psychological buffer to users, allowing continual brief respites in interactions with other persons (such as breaking eye contact during a puff). Nicotine itself is a mild stimulant able to release adrenaline and increase pulse rate and blood pressure, with the physiological arousal produced by the drug masking physical arousal provoked by life's tensions, thereby making smokers feel less nervous despite the stimulant effects. Smokers tend to have lower levels of body chemicals that are supplemented by antianxiety and antidepressant drugs. Such pharmaceuticals, unfortunately, seemingly have little ability to help smokers quit their tobacco addiction.

As with any addiction, the power of nicotine and tobacco depends upon needs met by those substances. People do not smoke simply to avoid temporary withdrawal symptoms. If a person's life is filled with situations that smoking eases like nothing else can, breaking the addiction is hard. If a person finds other ways of dealing adequately with those situations, desire for cigarettes can go away and never be bothersome again. Contrary to expectations of researchers, a laboratory test found nicotine to be no more appealing to ex-smokers than to persons who have never smoked—a finding implying that life circumstances, and not just chemistry, determine this drug's appeal.

Alcohol and illicit drug abusers reliably tend to be tobacco cigarette smokers, so reliably that the amount of tobacco use can be used to estimate the amount of cocaine and opiate usage by persons in drug abuse treatment programs. An experiment found that persons smoked less tobacco when they had access to **marijuana**, suggesting that those persons used the two substances for similar purposes. Nonsmokers tend to avoid drug abuse, implying that smokers and nonsmokers use different strategies to cope with life's challenges. Cigarette smoking is more prevalent among schizophrenics, seriously depressed persons, and persons with low-grade psychiatric disturbance that may lack outward symptoms. Almost two thirds of smokers in one research project turned out to have a history of present or past psychiatric abnormality. Among such individuals smoking may be a strategy of self-medication. One study found that withdrawal symptoms can depend on the extent to which the drug is used for self-medication.

Improvement has been measured in alertness, energy, and happiness as cigarette smokers start their day's consumption in the morning. Conversely, cutting off a smoker's supply of cigarettes produces measurable increases in fatigue, irritation, sadness, stress, and disorientation. New users do not get favorable effects sought by experienced users but instead have measurable nausea and general uneasiness. Among new users nicotine reduces job performance skills such as physical coordination and accuracy in memory tasks—the opposite of what happens with experienced users.

Although pharmaceutical nicotine has various medical applications, its main use is for treatment of addiction to tobacco smoking. One authority aptly described nicotine chewing gum as the **methadone** of cigarettes, meaning that such a treatment strategy is intended to switch addicts from tobacco to pharmaceutical nicotine, just as treatment personnel seek to switch **heroin** addicts to methadone. Although such programs may have an official goal of eliminating a person's addiction, in practice simply switching a person from a more harmful drug to a less harmful drug is often considered a success.

Drug interactions. Nicotine interacts with commonly used medical drugs. Antipsychotic drugs and the anti–blood clot medicine heparin flush from the body faster if a person uses nicotine. Nicotine also reduces the sedative effect of benzodiazepines and reduces pain relief from various opioids. Cigarette smoke acts as a monoamine oxidase inhibitor (MAOI), a type of chemical found in some antidepressants and that can have serious adverse effects when used simultaneously with some medicines (though acute danger from cigarette interactions may be small). **Caffeine** seems to make nicotine more pleasurable. Rat studies show that nicotine increases alcohol's appeal and worsens pancreas inflammation caused by both drugs. Birth control pills increase the boost that nicotine gives to pulse rate, and some researchers speculate that such increase is related to the elevated risk of heart disease found among smokers who use birth control pills.

Cancer. Tests indicate that pure nicotine (as opposed to smoke containing nicotine) does not cause cancer.

Pregnancy. Smoking reduces female fertility according to most studies of the topic, and studies of Canadian farm couples and of men in the Netherlands found an apparent reduction in male fertility as well. Pregnant women who smoke tobacco increase the chance of miscarriage, premature birth, smaller full-term infants, and sudden infant death syndrome (SIDS or "crib death"). The children are more likely to have muscle tone abnormalities. Smoking harms male and female gametes, damages chromosomes, and can change DNA in ways linked with childhood cancer. Nicotine usage by a pregnant woman changes movements and heart action of a fetus. One researcher warns that nicotine patches or chewing gum may deliver even more nicotine to a fetus than smoking would. Nicotine enters the milk of nursing mothers. Rat experiments indicate that fetal exposure to nicotine combined with newborn exposure to nicotine in milk increases the risk of offspring developing lung trouble similar to emphysema. Human birth defects have been attributed to tobacco smoking. Although a study of teenage tobacco smokers did not see any increased incidence of birth defects in their infants, research based on animal experimentation and published in 1998 declared that nicotine causes defects in fetal brain development leading to problems in thinking and learning that may not become apparent until years after birth. The children tend to have lower scores on psychological measurements, somewhat reminiscent of "cocaine babies," deficits that continue for years. Some investigators see a link between pregnant smokers and offspring with psychological problems. Investigators tracking mothers and daughters for three decades found that daughters were more likely to take up smoking if their mothers smoked during pregnancy.

Additional information. Scientific studies find that "passive smoking" threatens health of bystanders who inhale smoke from tobacco products and exhalations of smokers. A study of spontaneous abortions found them more likely in pregnant nonsmoking women who inhale environmental smoke *and* use a lot of caffeine or a moderate amount of alcohol. Infants from nonsmoker women who were exposed to tobacco smoke during pregnancy are more likely to have lower birth weight and persistent pulmonary hypertension. Offspring also exhibit the same kinds of lower psychological test scores that are seen in children of active smokers. Inhalation of smoke by infants is suspected of contributing to SIDS. For sure, compared to children in nonsmoking households, infants of smokers are hospitalized more often for pneumonia and bronchitis. The level of environmental smoke necessary for ill effects is often unclear in scientific studies; a person working in a poorly ventilated smokey bar for eight hours a day will have a considerably different exposure than someone in a nonsmoking household who sits outside once a week with a friend who smokes a couple of cigarettes.

Additional scientific information may be found in:

Brown, C. "The Association between Depressive Symptoms and Cigarette Smoking in an Urban Primary Care Sample." *International Journal of Psychiatry in Medicine* 30 (2000): 15–26.

Brown, K.G. "Lung Cancer and Environmental Tobacco Smoke: Occupational Risk to Nonsmokers." *Environmental Health Perspectives* 107 (1999, Suppl. 6): 885–90.

Colby, S.M., et al. "Are Adolescent Smokers Dependent on Nicotine? A Review of the Evidence." *Drug and Alcohol Dependence* 59 (2000, Suppl. 1): S83–S95.

Dursun, S.M., and S. Kutcher. "Smoking, Nicotine and Psychiatric Disorders: Evidence for Therapeutic Role, Controversies and Implications for Future Research." *Medical Hypotheses* 52 (1999): 101–9.

Haustein, K.O. "Cigarette Smoking, Nicotine and Pregnancy." *International Journal of Clinical Pharmacology and Therapeutics* 37 (1999): 417–27.

Parrott, A.C., and F.J. Kaye. "Daily Uplifts, Hassles, Stresses and Cognitive Failures: In Cigarette Smokers, Abstaining Smokers, and Non-smokers." *Behavioural Pharmacology* 10 (1999): 639–46.

Robinson, J.H., and W.S. Pritchard. "The Role of Nicotine in Tobacco Use." *Psychopharmacology* 108 (1992): 397–407.

Stolerman, I.P., and M.J. Jarvis. "The Scientific Case That Nicotine Is Addictive." *Psychopharmacology* 117 (1995): 2–10.

Van Gilder, T.J., P.L. Remington, and M.C. Fiore. "The Direct Effects of Nicotine Use on Human Health." *Wisconsin Medical Journal* 96 (1997): 43–48.

Nitrite

Pronunciation: NIGH-tright

Chemical Abstracts Service Registry Number: 8017-89-8 (amyl nitrite); 542-56-3 (isobutyl nitrite)

Formal Names: Amyl Nitrite, Butyl Nitrite, Cyclohexyl Nitrite, Isoamyl Nitrite, Isobutyl Nitrite, Nitrous Acid

Informal Names: Aimes, Aimies, Ames, Amys, Army, Aroma of Men, Blackjack, Blue Heaven, Bolt, Boppers, Buds, Bullet, Buzz Bomb, Climax, Dixcorama, Hardware, Heart-On, High Ball, Liquid Gold, Liquid Incense, Locker Room, Man Aroma, Oz, Ozone, Pearls, Poppers, Quicksilver, Ram, Rush, Snappers, Thrust, Whiteout

Type: Inhalant. *See* page 26

Federal Schedule Listing: Unlisted, but may be in state schedules

USA Availability: Prescription for some formats; nonprescription for others

Pregnancy Category: X (amyl nitrite, also called isoamyl nitrite)

Uses. Various chemical subvarieties of nitrite inhalants exist. Isobutyl nitrite is popular in some teenager circles and has been called "the cocaine of poor people." Although anyone is physically free to use any drug, authorities find that nitrite sniffing has particular appeal to male homosexuals, especially during sexual activity. Aphrodisiac qualities are claimed for the substance. Amyl nitrite sniffers report euphoria and muscle relaxation. Isobutyl nitrite users report losing their sense of who they are and also becoming calm or, in contrast, becoming prone to wild conduct—differences that may illustrate the impact that someone's personality and surroundings have on drug experiences. Regardless of exact content of a nitrite experience, sensations are brief. Some persons have confused nitrites with nitrates; they have a similar spelling but are different substances.

Drawbacks. Nitrite inhalants have brief action but may incapacitate a person during that time and thus should not be used while engaged in dangerous activity such as driving a car. Unwanted actions of nitrites include feelings of falling and spinning, headache, facial flushing, rapid heartbeat, generalized throbbing feelings, and low blood pressure (low enough to make a person faint). Less common are nausea, vomiting, agitation, sweating, loss of energy and strength, and loss of bladder and rectal control. In mice experiments involving single and multiple exposures, inhaling isobutyl nitrite can cause anemia, harm the immune system, create nose and lung abnormalities, and disturb the spleen. Similar results are seen with rats. Blood and spleen abnormalities developed in a mice experiment using cyclohexyl nitrite. In a human patient, sniffing isobutyl nitrite caused bronchitis severe enough to affect the trachea. Amyl nitrite (which has a long medical history as a heart medicine) and isobutyl nitrite may each cause methemoglobinemia, a sometimes fatal blood disease interfering with the body's use of oxygen; this affliction is particularly likely if a person drinks isobutyl nitrite instead of inhaling the vapor. Isobutyl nitrite interference with the body's ability to use oxygen may be perilous for persons with inadequate oxygen supply to the heart.

In the early days of AIDS (acquired immunodeficiency syndrome) research, scientists noticed that many victims were nitrite sniffers. Because of this association, at one time nitrite sniffing was suspected to be the cause of AIDS, an excellent example of why association of a chemical with a disease cannot be assumed to demonstrate a cause-effect relationship. The substance is still, however, suspected of worsening the progression of AIDS once the disease strikes. In addition, damage to the immune system caused by nitrite inhalation is suspected of making a user more susceptible to AIDS and to a type of cancer called Kaposi's sarcoma.

Abuse factors. Tolerance to amyl nitrite can develop.

Drug interactions. Although amyl nitrite is used as an antidote for cyanide poisoning, isobutyl nitrite can interact with coffee in a way that produces enough cyanide to poison someone who drinks the combination beverage. Using amyl nitrite with **alcohol** can cause heart failure. Nitrites are flammable, making them hazardous around flames or lit cigarettes. Persons with glaucoma are supposed to avoid amyl nitrite. People report burns caused by isobutyl nitrite splashing on skin.

Cancer. Laboratory tests and animal experiments (the latter involving longterm exposure) indicate that isobutyl nitrite liquid and vapor each cause cancer.

Pregnancy. In the body nitrite breaks down into chemicals that may promote birth defects. The lower blood pressure produced by amyl nitrite is believed harmful to a fetus. Whether amyl nitrite passes into the milk of nursing mothers is unknown.

Additional scientific information may be found in:

Bradberry, S.M., et al. "Fatal Methemoglobinemia Due to Inhalation of Isobutyl Nitrite." *Journal of Toxicology: Clinical Toxicology* 32 (1994): 179–84.

Covalla, J.R., C.V. Strimlan, and J.G. Lech. "Severe Tracheobronchitis from Inhalation of an Isobutyl Nitrite Preparation." *Drug Intelligence and Clinical Pharmacy* 15 (1981): 51–52.

Haverkos, H.W., and J. Dougherty. "Health Hazards of Nitrite Inhalants." *American Journal of Medicine* 84 (1988): 479–82.

Haverkos, H.W., et al. "Nitrite Inhalants: History, Epidemiology, and Possible Links to AIDS." *Environmental Health Perspectives* 102 (1994): 858–61.

Israelstam, S., S. Lambert, and G. Oki. "Use of Isobutyl Nitrite as a Recreational Drug." *British Journal of Addiction to Alcohol and Other Drugs* 73 (1978): 319–20.

Lange, W.R., and J. Fralich. "Nitrite Inhalants: Promising and Discouraging News." *British Journal of Addiction* 84 (1989): 121–23.

Soderberg, L.S. "Immunomodulation by Nitrite Inhalants May Predispose Abusers to AIDS and Kaposi's Sarcoma." *Journal of Neuroimmunology* 83 (1998): 157–61.

Nitrous Oxide

Pronunciation: NIGH-truhs OX-eyed

Chemical Abstracts Service Registry Number: 10024-97-2

Formal Names: Dinitrogen Monoxide, Dinitrogen Oxide, Entonox

Informal Names: Fall Down, Gas, Hippie Crack, Hysteria, Laughing Gas, Nitro, Nitrous, Nitrous Acid, Noss, Pan, Shoot the Breeze, Tanks, Thrust, Whippets

Type: Inhalant. *See* page 26

Federal Schedule Listing: Unlisted

USA Availability: Nonprescription, but sales and usage are controlled in some jurisdictions

Uses. This drug has been known since the 1720s. Some authorities describe nitrous oxide as an opioid; some persons even use the gas to counteract effects from stimulants. Nitrous oxide actions and its recreational use are similar to those of other inhalants. Recreational use is illegal in some jurisdictions but has a venerable history. The writer Samuel Taylor Coleridge, thesaurus compiler Peter Mark Roget, and potter Josiah Wedgwood were all eighteenth-century notables who relaxed with nitrous oxide.

Although this substance is a pharmaceutical product, it also occurs naturally. For instance, eating lettuce generates enough nitrous oxide that scientists can measure it in a person's breath. Large quantities are produced by wild prairie grass. Humans do not receive enough nitrous oxide from such natural sources to be affected, however. The substance is also produced by the human body. One study found the amount to increase as oral hygiene declined. As with the amounts produced by grass and lettuce, the level created by the body is too small to have any known effect on a person. From a global environmental perspective, however, nitrous oxide is a gas that promotes the greenhouse effect and ozone layer destruction, and concern exists about medical usage affecting the world's climate. Medical sources are estimated to create 2% of the atmosphere's supply. Such usage may seem insignificant in that regard, but the gas is so durable in the atmosphere that any artificial source has been described as an environmental hazard.

Medically this drug is used as an anesthetic and to relieve pain ranging from dental work to migraine headache and cancer. In a medical context nitrous oxide is considered a reliable sedative. Experimental usage to treat anxiety has been successful, and one authority has noted a therapeutic antidepressant action. The substance has been used to help persons break **pentazocine** addiction. Researchers report success in using the gas to ease **alcohol**, **nicotine**, and opioid withdrawal and to reduce craving for alcohol, tobacco, and **marijuana** among addicts. The latter three substances are so different from one another that nitrous oxide's ability to reduce craving for all of them is remarkable. Some medical practitioners claim that a single dose of the gas actually eliminates craving for those substances, but that claim sounds much like those made for other "miracle cure" addiction treatments over the years but that turned out to be overly optimistic.

In former times, nitrous oxide was used to fight ear afflictions. For many years the substance was believed to make hearing more acute, but tests of hearing ability while using the compound show no improvement—and volunteers in those tests even felt they had lesser ability to detect soft sounds. Nitrous oxide can increase pressure in the middle ear, and a case report tells of treatable hearing loss caused by the drug. Hearing defect has been reported from recreational use as well.

Typical nitrous oxide actions are tingling, numbness, dreaminess, euphoria, dysphoria (the opposite of euphoria), altered sensory perceptions, changed awareness of the body, and different experience of time flow. Although nitrous oxide is not classified as a hallucinogen, some descriptions of experiences are indistinguishable from hallucinations, particularly if a user is talented at creating internal imagery. Some persons claim to achieve mystical insight while under the drug's influence. Intoxication from a dose lasts only a few minutes.

Drawbacks. The substance disrupts learning ability. That action has been exploited medically to promote amnesia of unpleasant procedures. In a typical experiment volunteers who inhaled a low dose of the drug showed worsened reaction time, worsened ability to do arithmetic, and general sedation accompanied by nervous system depression (as opposed to stimulation). Interference with driving ability has been noted one-half hour after a dose. In another experiment volunteers felt stimulated; in still another experiment some individuals were sedated, and others became stimulated. One group became weary, uneasy, and confused. Short-term exposure can cause dizziness, nausea, vomiting, and breathing difficulty. Some recreational users quickly inhale as much nitrous oxide as possible and hold their breath. This technique causes a sudden change of pressure inside the lungs and can rupture small interior structures needed for breathing. Blood pressure can go up or down, depending on dosage. Users can lose consciousness, which may be hazardous in a recreational context due to falls or inability to shut off the gas source. The substance deactivates vitamin B_{12}, an effect that can cause numbness and difficulty in moving arms and legs. Other results can be impotence and involuntary discharge of urine and feces. Nitrous oxide interferes with blood clotting, and long-term exposure has caused blood abnormalities. Persons with chronic industrial exposure have more kidney and liver disease than usual. Nitrous oxide can become very cold when released as a gas from a pressurized container, cold enough to cause frostbite upon meeting skin or throat. Breathing nitrous oxide without an adequate supply of oxygen can be fatal; a little in a closed space or a lot from a face mask can suffocate a user. Although nitrous oxide is called nonflammable, when inhaled it can seep into the ab-dominal cavity and bowels, mixing with body gases to create a flammable combination. If ignited the result would be like setting off an explosive inside the body; the danger is real enough that surgical personnel administering nitrous oxide as an anesthetic have been warned about it.

As with many other drugs, effects of nitrous oxide can be influenced by changes in setting. For example, volunteers who knew what to expect per-formed better on tests than persons who had no information about what ni-trous oxide would do to them.

Abuse factors. In tests of the drug's appeal, people in general chose nitrous oxide no more often than placebo; such lack of preference is a classic sign of low addictive potential. One experiment revealed a catch to such findings, however: Volunteers who enjoyed nitrous oxide effects chose it more often than placebo, and volunteers who disliked the drug actions chose it less often than placebo. Thus, overall in the general population the drug might be no more attractive than placebo, but nonetheless some persons may find it cap-tivating. Such a finding is consistent with drugs having high abuse potential, such as **heroin**; so the fact that persons typically find no attraction in nitrous oxide does not prove low abuse potential for nitrous oxide. Its nickname "hip-pie crack" suggests that users have recognized an abuse potential. Nonethe-less, a medical practitioner who administered the gas as a drug addiction treatment said that in 15,000 cases not a single addict indicated subsequent craving for nitrous oxide; such a patient population would be expected to show particular susceptibility if given a substance with abuse potential. The same practitioner notes that regardless of theoretical possibilities, 200 years of experience demonstrate that nitrous oxide is among the least abused drugs.

Tolerance develops in rats. Human experimentation documents tolerance developing to some effects (such as euphoria and pain relief) but not neces-sarily to all.

Drug interactions. In an experiment comparing light drinkers of alcohol to moderate drinkers, the moderate drinkers found nitrous oxide more appeal-ing. One group of researchers found that alcohol boosts nitrous oxide effects and that the drug combination creates effects produced by neither substance alone. Those researchers concluded, however, that the combination was not potent enough to have more appeal than nitrous oxide alone. That conclusion assumes, of course, that drug abusers base their conduct on rational analysis of scientific findings. In a similar experiment comparing users and nonusers of marijuana, when given a choice neither group preferred nitrous oxide more than a placebo, but nitrous oxide effects felt stronger to marijuana users. In rats **ketamine** boosts effects from nitrous oxide. In a human medical context that combination is routine and appears safe, but the combination causes brain damage in rats. Persons using **morphine** or other opiates can experience mus-cle rigidity when inhaling nitrous oxide, a situation that can interfere with breathing.

Cancer. Studies do not indicate that nitrous oxide causes cancer in animals. Whether the drug causes cancer in humans is unknown. Genetic damage sim-ilar to the amount from daily smoking 10 to 20 cigarettes has been found in health care workers routinely exposed to minuscule amounts of nitrous oxide; such damage might have a potential for causing cancer.

Pregnancy. Fertility is lower in female rats exposed to nitrous oxide than in rats having no exposure. Lower fertility has also been observed among female health care workers with occupational exposure to the gas, and reduced fertility is also reported for males. Offspring of male mice exposed to nitrous oxide have weighed less than normal and have not matured as fast as normal. Birth defects resulted from an experiment exposing pregnant rats to the gas for 24 hours. When given to pregnant women during childbirth the drug builds up in the fetal blood and brain; one authority recommends administering oxygen to any newborn whose mother received nitrous oxide while giving birth. As the twenty-first century began researchers reported that the gas might cause permanent fetal and newborn brain damage, a finding in contrast to previous understanding of the drug. Occupational exposure to nitrous oxide is associated with smaller infants and lower birth weight and may increase likelihood of spontaneous abortion. Pregnant and breast-feeding health workers are advised to avoid rooms where nitrous oxide residues may contaminate the air. Sperm abnormalities and lower fertility have been noted in male rats exposed to nitrous oxide. Wives of men exposed to the gas have shown a higher spontaneous abortion rate, compared to wives of men with no exposure. The compound is not detected in milk of nursing mothers.

Additional information. "Nitrous acid" is an unstable **nitrite** substance. The nickname "nitrous acid" is sometimes used for nitrous oxide, but they are different substances.

Additional scientific information may be found in:

Block, R.I., et al. "Psychedelic Effects of a Subanesthetic Concentration of Nitrous Oxide." *Anesthesia Progress* 37 (1990): 271–76.

Danto, B.L. "A Bag Full of Laughs." *American Journal of Psychiatry* 121 (1964): 612–13.

Dohrn, C.S., et al. "Subjective and Psychomotor Effects of Nitrous Oxide in Healthy Volunteers." *Behavioural Pharmacology* 3 (1992): 19–30.

Linden, C.H. "Volatile Substances of Abuse." *Emergency Medicine Clinics of North America* 8 (1990): 559–78.

Temple, W.A., D.M. Beasley, and D.J. Baker. "Nitrous Oxide Abuse from Whipped Cream Dispenser Chargers." *New Zealand Medical Journal* 110 (1997): 322–23.

Yagiela, J.A. "Health Hazards and Nitrous Oxide: A Time for Reappraisal." *Anesthesia Progress* 38 (1991): 1–11.

Zacny, J.P., et al. "Examining the Subjective, Psychomotor and Reinforcing Effects of Nitrous Oxide in Healthy Volunteers: A Dose-Response Analysis." *Behavioural Pharmacology* 7 (1996): 194–99.

Nutmeg

Pronunciation: NUT-mehg

Chemical Abstracts Service Registry Number: 84082-68-8

Formal Names: Mace, *Myristica fragrans*

Type: Hallucinogen. *See* page 25

Federal Schedule Listing: Unlisted

USA Availability: Nonprescription (food)

Pregnancy Category: None

Uses. Nutmeg is a familiar spice, but when used in larger amounts, it can act as a drug. Nutmeg originated in the Spice Islands of Indonesia. It is a seed coming from an evergreen tree that can reach 45 feet in height. Folk medicine uses nutmeg for treating insomnia, mouth sores, stomach inflammation, gas, diarrhea, and vomiting. Animal research verifies the antiinsomnia and antidiarrhea properties; they have been observed among humans undergoing formal medical care, and recreational users mention sleep-inducing action. The substance is also used as an aphrodisiac, and laboratory tests show that it kills headlice. Nutmeg may be able to help improve dysentery, infections, and rheumatism. In rabbit experiments, nutmeg lowered cholesterol levels and aided in coughing up mucus. Nutmeg, like many other spices, has antimicrobial actions that appear to retard spoilage of unrefrigerated food.

Nutmeg can produce false positives for **marijuana** in a field test that law enforcement officers have used to identify an unknown substance, but of course more sophisticated laboratory examination can correct such an error.

Drawbacks. A nutmeg dose sufficient to produce hallucinations is also sufficient to produce headache, thirst, nausea, constipation, rapid heartbeat, dizziness, and a miserable hangover. Muscular discoordination can be severe enough to mimic multiple sclerosis. Research on cats produced liver destruction. All these results are from dosage quantities much higher than the small amounts used for spicing foods.

Abuse factors. Nutmeg is not considered addictive, although a case report notes a patient hospitalized for nutmeg poisoning, who craved the substance so much that he had a supply smuggled to him during his hospital stay. The report said he was never able to go beyond two weeks without nutmeg.

Some researchers are skeptical that nutmeg possesses hallucinogenic qualities, but for centuries numerous users have said otherwise. Betel chewers sometimes add nutmeg to a quid for extra sensations, and mixing tobacco with nutmeg is a practice reported in Asia. Research indicates that human body chemistry converts part of a nutmeg dose into substances related to amphetamine, affecting mood and sometimes causing hallucinations. The effects from a dose can last three days. Overdose requiring medical intervention is possible, although only one fatality is recorded. Nutmeg has received mixed reviews as a recreational drug. Some people call it incomparable; others resort to it only as an act of desperation when nothing else is available. A favorable description says nutmeg is "capable of removing one completely from the world of reality in a hypnotic trance accompanied by golden dreams and euphoric bliss."[1] In contrast, someone who used nutmeg together with marijuana received emergency hospital treatment for gagging, hot and cold flashes, numbness, blurred vision, double vision, triple vision, and difficulty in controlling movements—among other complaints. Persons who use nutmeg by itself have also reported bad experiences.

Drug interactions. In a mice experiment nutmeg boosted actions of **alcohol** and reduced those of **dextroamphetamine**. One authority describes nutmeg as a weak monoamine oxidase inhibitor (MAOI), and MAOIs interact badly with many drugs described in this book.

Cancer. A laboratory test using a nutmeg extract found evidence that it might cause cancer, and a nutmeg experiment with mice produced DNA changes that might be related to eventual cancer.

Pregnancy. Male mice that received nutmeg in an experiment did not show chromosome damage. A case report notes a normal full-term infant born to a woman who had experienced nutmeg poisoning during pregnancy, but pregnant women are advised to avoid using nutmeg as a drug.

Additional information. As with many other natural products, nutmeg's effects may be produced by the combination of hundreds of chemicals found in the substance. Researchers have identified several chemicals as likely causes of nutmeg's effects: elemicin, eugenol, myristicin, and safrole. Under laboratory conditions myristicin can be chemically converted to **MDMA** and safrole to **MDA**, but this conversion has never been detected in animals or humans. Body chemistry does convert myristicin into substances resembling amphetamine. Myristicin is found not only in nutmeg but in plants related to carrots. An experiment testing myristicin on rats found no poisonous result. Researchers found no evidence of cancer after dosing mice with the substance, but the study did not last long enough to reveal whether cancer would eventually develop. Myristicin's potential for causing birth defects is unknown. Safrole has a faint ability to promote cancer; pregnant women are advised to avoid using it as a drug.

Mace comes from the same seed as nutmeg does, but is a different spice. Folk medicine uses mace to reduce inflammation and pain; research indicates it can protect against some chemically caused cancers. Mace is routinely added to **areca nut** quids.

Additional scientific information may be found in:

Fras, I., and J.J. Friedman. "Hallucinogenic Effects of Nutmeg in Adolescent." *New York State Journal of Medicine* 69 (1969): 463–65.

Lewis, P.W., and D.W. Patterson. "Acute and Chronic Effects of the Voluntary Inhalation of Certain Commercial Volatile Solvents by Juveniles." *Journal of Drug Issues* 4 (1974): 172.

Lewis, W.H., and M.P.F. Elvin-Lewis. *Medical Botany: Plants Affecting Man's Health.* New York: John Wiley & Sons, 1977. 408–10.

Panayotopoulos, D.J., and D.D. Chisholm. "Hallucinogenic Effect of Nutmeg." *British Medical Journal* 1 (1970): 754.

Sjoholm, A., A. Lindberg, and M. Personne. "Acute Nutmeg Intoxication." *Journal of Internal Medicine* 243 (1998): 329–31.

Van Gils, C., and P.A. Cox. "Ethnobotany of Nutmeg in the Spice Islands." *Journal of Ethnopharmacology* 42 (1994): 117–24.

Weiss, G. "Hallucinogenic and Narcotic-Like Effects of Nutmeg." *Psychiatric Quarterly* 34 (1960): 346–56.

Note

1. W.H. Lewis and M.P.F. Elvin-Lewis, *Medical Botany: Plants Affecting Man's Health* (New York: John Wiley & Sons, 1977), 408.

Opium

Pronunciation: OH-pi-uhm

Chemical Abstracts Service Registry Number: 8008-60-4

Formal Names: *Papaver album*, *Papaver somniferum*, Poppy

Informal Names: Ah-pen-yen, Aunti, Aunti Emma, Big O, Black, Blackjack, Black Pill, Black Stuff, Chandoo, Chandu, Chinese, Chinese Molasses, Chinese Tobacco, Chocolate, Cruz, Dopium, Dover, Dover's Deck, Dover's Powder, Dreamer, Dream Gun, Dreams, Dream Stick, Easing Powder, Emma, Fi-Do-Nie, Garden-Poppy, Gee, God's Medicine, Goma, Gondola, Gong, Goric, Great Tobacco, Gum, Guma, Hard Stuff, Hocus, Hop, Indonesian Bud, Joy, Joy Plant, Mawseed, Midnight Oil, Mira, Mud, O, Oil, OJ, OP, Ope, Pen Yan, Pen Yen, PG, Pin Gon, Pin Yen, Plant, PO, Pox, Skee, Tar, Tongs, Tox, Toxy, Toys, When-Shee, Winshee, Yen Shee Suey, Ze, Zero

Type: Depressant (opiate class). *See* page 22

Federal Schedule Listing: Schedule II (DEA no. 9600)

USA Availability: Prescription

Pregnancy Category: C

Uses. Many opium products are discussed elsewhere in this book, but here we are dealing with the substance from which all those products originate. Opium has long been used to relieve pain, fight coughs, cure diarrhea, and control spasms. Traditionally, opium is dried sap harvested from the seed-producing portion of opium poppy plants. At harvest time fields of poppies can have a strong smell, and children in the fields can be overcome by those airborne chemicals. A modern opium variety is "poppy straw," composed of dry or liquid extracts from the plant. The natural product can be used by itself or can be refined to produce various drugs known as "opiates," valued for their medicinal effects.

Archaeologists have found evidence of opium poppy cultivation dating from 15,000 years ago, but examination of historical records has not proven that ancient peoples understood opium's medicinal benefits; the product may have been used traditionally but without understanding how or even whether it worked. Opium may have been used in Roman Empire religious ceremonies, perhaps exploiting the drug's effects to symbolize a process of death and re-incarnation, and even older records imply that ancients may have believed that opium could produce happiness, although evidence of ancient recreational use is nonexistent.

The Opium War from 1840 to 1842 was the first drug war, followed by the second Opium War of 1856 to 1860. These military conflicts were fought against China by England and other European powers in order to force the Chinese government to legalize the opium trade (certainly a goal different from that of the "drug war" familiar to Americans as the twenty-first century began).

Opium and its **morphine** component were widely used to treat wounded soldiers in the American Civil War, and later historians have routinely said that addiction became so common that it was called "the soldier's disease." Such illness may have existed, but an investigator who diligently examined medical writings from that time found none that attributed postwar addictions to war-related medical use. In that era the opium trade was legal, and someone who analyzed opium import statistics found no evidence that consumption rose due to Civil War addictions; a distinguished authority has noted that people of that era called dysentery "the soldier's disease."

Just before World War I an article in the *Journal of the American Medical Association* declared, "If the entire materia medica at our disposal were limited to the choice and use of only one drug, I am sure that a great many, if not the majority, of us would choose opium; and I am convinced that if we were to select, say half a dozen of the most important drugs in the Pharmacopeia, we should all place opium in the first rank."[1] Although many useful drugs have been discovered since then, opium is still the basis for many standard medications. Because opium is a natural product, its morphine content can vary greatly from batch to batch. Opium commercially processed for medical use is adjusted so that 10% of any given amount of medical opium is composed of morphine.

Although medical opinion about opium has changed little, public opinion has changed a lot. Reasons for that shift go beyond the scope of this book, but in the nineteenth century, use of opium and its derivatives had wide social approval in America. **Alcohol** was considered more hazardous to health and home. One of the most telling measures of approval came from the life insurance industry in India, which freely granted policies to known opium users, as mortality statistics showed opium having no effect on life span. A life insurance official reported similar experience in China, although older users in China had higher mortality than older nonusers (probably many users took the drug for diseases that nonusers did not have, with the death rate related more to those diseases than to opium). Some of those statistics would change as the twentieth century progressed because drug laws would change the kinds of people who used opium, thereby associating opium with populations having higher mortality for reasons unrelated to opium's drug properties.

Although identified with China, opium has been grown in the United States. In the late eighteenth century Benjamin Franklin used laudanum (typically wine laced with opium) to treat himself for kidney stones. During the nineteenth century Americans used opium mainly as an ingredient in laudanum and paregoric. Paregoric is a liquid including anise, camphor, and opium.

Paregoric was first produced in the eighteenth century as an asthma medicine. The compound is no longer used for that purpose but can reduce lung congestion by helping people to cough up mucus. Paregoric is a standard diarrhea remedy and is used to help infants suffering from drug withdrawal syndromes. In the 1960s the compound had a flurry of popularity among opiate addicts who would process the product in hopes of isolating the opium, then inject the substance they produced. The outcomes were typical of what happens when oral medications are injected, resulting in lung damage and disfiguring injuries to injection sites.

Less familiar modern opium preparations include home remedy mixtures of the substance with **caffeine**, aspirin, and acetaminophen (Tylenol or other brands). In America opium preparations were once a standard method of quieting noisy infants and children, and that practice is still followed in some parts of the world. One hazard in that custom is the possibility of fatal overdose, as people administering such concoctions do not always understand pediatric dosage.

Drawbacks. Although some opium users have generally unhealthy lifestyles, few ailments have been attributed solely to the drug. Those ailments tend to be in the gastrointestinal tract, such as problems with the small intestine's bile duct. "Cauliflower ear," in which an ear thickens and becomes misshapen, was once associated with opium smoking. The affliction, however, apparently came not from the drug but rather from the habit of lying down for hours in a comatose condition with an ear pressing against a hard surface.

Abuse factors. Recreational use of opium is harder to define than we might think, because even if persons take the drug in a social setting, they can be seeking to reduce mental anxiety or physical pain, which is not the same as using a drug for fun. Some people swallow dry opium or drink tea made with seed or with dried heads of poppy flowers. In the nineteenth century poppy tea was a common medicinal drink, but in the early twenty-first century the habit tends to be limited to opiate addicts. The traditional recreational way to use opium is to inhale its smoke. Heating opium enough to make it smoke can reduce the drug content, and opium is already far weaker than substances refined from it (such as morphine and **heroin**). One authority estimates that the amount of active drug inhaled by someone who smokes a given weight of opium will typically be 300 to 400 times less than the drug content in the same weight of injected heroin. Moreover, while an entire dose of heroin might be ingested in a few seconds, a pipeful of opium is smoked over a much longer period to slowly savor its effects, further reducing the opium's impact. The English poet Samuel Taylor Coleridge started out using opium for medical purposes, as did Thomas De Quincey, and both men produced classic accounts of hallucinations and creative inspiration occurring under opium's influence. Those accounts and later ones may well be true, but for such results people need to be particularly sensitive to the drug and also be prone to such experiences regardless of pharmaceutical encouragement. Arsenic is sometimes added to opium to increase smokers' interest in sexual activity, a practice generating reports of arsenic poisoning among users.

Drug interactions. Not enough scientific information to report about the natural product, although many studies have examined drug interactions with opiates and opioids.

Cancer. Laboratory tests find that opium *smoke* may cause cancer, as may opium dross (waste products, such as scrapings from the inside of an opium pipe, which some persons chew or suck). Opium is suspected of causing esophageal and bladder cancer.

Pregnancy. A pregnant woman using paregoric can give birth to an infant having dependence with opium.

Additional information. Seed from opium poppies is a food product commonly used in breads, cakes, and candies. Consumption of amounts found in a normal meal can cause a false opiate positive in drug screens; controversy exists about whether further analysis of results from such testing can show that poppy seed was the cause. Poppy seed oil is a comparatively unfamiliar product, but animal tests indicate it has good potential for human nutrition. In some parts of the world iodized poppy seed oil has been used instead of iodized salt to treat goiter and has been suggested as a means of preventing nervous endemic cretinism caused by iodine deficiency in the diet of pregnant women. Iodized poppy seed oil is taken up by cancerous portions of a liver, giving the substance clinical usefulness if anticancer drugs are blended into it, as the drugs then concentrate exactly where they are needed in the liver. Results from animal research have led investigators to speculate that consuming normal poppy seed oil may help prevent cancer.

Opium lettuce is not related to opium but can produce mild sensations similar to opium. Sedative and pain relief qualities of opium lettuce have been used for centuries. Lung and urinary tract afflictions have been treated with it. Opium lettuce is smoked for recreational purposes, but results have not caused the practice to gain popularity. A case report tells of individuals who received medical care after injecting a preparation made from the plant. It has other names including Acrid Lettuce, Bitter Lettuce, Compass Plant, Great Lettuce, Green Endive, Lactucarium, *Lactuca virosa*, Poison Lettuce, Prickly Lettuce, Strong-Scented Lettuce, and Wild Lettuce.

Additional scientific information may be found in:

Aurin, M. "Chasing the Dragon: The Cultural Metamorphosis of Opium in the United States, 1825–1935." *Medical Anthropology Quarterly* 14 (2000): 414–41.

Gharagozlou, H., and M.T. Behin. "Frequency of Psychiatric Symptoms among 150 Opium Addicts in Shiraz, Iran." *International Journal of the Addictions* 14 (1979): 1145–49.

Goodhand, J. "From Holy War to Opium War? A Case Study of the Opium Economy in North-Eastern Afghanistan." *Disasters* 24 (2000): 87–102.

Haller, J.S. "Opium Usage in Nineteenth Century Therapeutics." *Bulletin of the New York Academy of Medicine* 65 (1989): 591–607.

Kalant, H. "Opium Revisited: A Brief Review of Its Nature, Composition, Non-Medical Use and Relative Risks." *Addiction* 92 (1997): 267–77.

Lerner, A.M., and F.J. Oerther. "Characteristics and Sequelae of Paregoric Abuse." *Annals of Internal Medicine* 65 (1966): 1019–30.

Quinones, M.A. "Drug Abuse during the Civil War (1861–1865)." *International Journal of the Addictions* 10 (1975): 1007–20.

Strang, J. "Lessons from an English Opium Eater: Thomas De Quincey Reconsidered." *International Journal of the Addictions* 25 (1990): 1455–65.

Note

1. 64 (February 6, 1915): 477.

Oxandrolone

Pronunciation: ok-SAN-droh-lohn

Chemical Abstracts Service Registry Number: 53-39-4

Formal Names: Anatrophill, Anavar, Lipidex, Lonavar, Oxandrin, Provitar, Vasorome

Type: Anabolic steroid. *See* page 24

Federal Schedule Listing: Schedule III (DEA no. 4000)

USA Availability: Prescription

Pregnancy Category: X

Uses. This drug is used to encourage return of adequate heaviness in persons who have lost too much weight from illness, injury, or medical therapy. Experiments with AIDS (acquired immunodeficiency syndrome) patients measured substantial improvement in weight and strength. Oxandrolone may diminish pain from a bone disease called osteoporosis, although the drug has potential for worsening the underlying bone affliction. In rats and in humans the drug has hastened healing of wounds. Experimental therapy using oxandrolone against Duchenne muscular dystrophy has been successful.

Drawbacks. Nausea and diarrhea are among the less serious reports of unwanted effects. The substance can masculinize female users and interfere with menstrual periods. In immature rats oxandrolone has drastically interfered with the male reproductive system, a finding that may be relevant to young athletes using the compound without medical supervision. In humans the substance can promote prostate disease and should be avoided by men with breast cancer and generally by anyone with kidney disease (although doctors sometimes give oxandrolone to dialysis patients). The drug has been used to treat hepatitis in alcoholics despite its ability to interfere with bile flow and to cause jaundice or liver malfunction. Fluid retention can occur and be a serious problem for heart patients. Other unwanted effects may include overall higher cholesterol levels (accompanied by reduction of the HDL "good cholesterol"), although unlike some other drugs of this type, oxandrolone has been seen to reduce levels of triglycerides (which are associated with increased risk of heart attack and stroke), and in some cases oxandrolone reduced overall cholesterol as well. Such effects may, however, depend upon what causes the original levels. Oxandrolone can bring about premature bone maturation in children, preventing attainment of normal adult height. Nonetheless, the compound is used to treat delayed puberty in boys, increasing their height and weight. Turner's syndrome interferes with height and sexual maturation in girls, deficits that have improved with oxandrolone therapy.

Abuse factors. Sports competitors are forbidden to use the substance. Violation of the ban may risk punishment for nothing: Even though oxandrolone can promote muscle mass, a study examining users and nonusers of oxandrolone found no difference between the two groups in muscle mass, strength, and general fitness. Athletes who abuse oxandrolone may suffer bad psychological effects. In one case a person became hyperactive and had racing thoughts. In another case someone abusing this and other steroids became suspicious of other people, rageful, and occasionally suicidal.

An addiction case report mentioned not only psychological craving for oxandrolone and other anabolic steroids but physical dependence as well. When the bodybuilder in question received a dose of a substance that provokes withdrawal symptoms in opiate addiction, he responded with classic opiate withdrawal signs.

Drug interactions. Oxandrolone can alter insulin needs of diabetics and boost actions of anti–blood clot medicines. The steroid can help rats survive an overdose of **meprobamate** or **nicotine**.

Cancer. Potential for causing cancer is unknown. A case report associates oxandrolone with development of colon cancer in a 27-year-old bodybuilder.

Pregnancy. Potential for causing birth defects is unknown. In animal studies testing oxandrolone at nine times the normal human dose, fetal injury has occurred, including introduction of male characteristics into a female fetus. Pregnant women are advised to avoid the drug. Oxandrolone's ability to pass into milk of nursing mothers is unknown.

Additional scientific information may be found in:

Frasier, S.D. "Androgens and Athletes." *American Journal of Diseases of Children* 125 (1973): 479–80.

Freinhar, J.P., and W. Alvarez. "Androgen-Induced Hypomania." *Journal of Clinical Psychiatry* 46 (1985): 354–55.

Levien, T.L., and D.E. Baker. "Reviews of Trimetrexate and Oxandrolone." *Hospital Pharmacy* 29 (1994): 696–702.

Mendenhall, C.L., et al. "Short-Term and Long-Term Survival in Patients with Alcoholic Hepatitis Treated with Oxandrolone and Prednisolone." *New England Journal of Medicine* 311 (1984): 1464–70.

Rosenfeld, R.G., et al. "Six-Year Results of a Randomized, Prospective Trial of Human Growth Hormone and Oxandrolone in Turner Syndrome." *Journal of Pediatrics* 121 (1992): 49–55.

Taiwo, B.O. "HIV-Associated Wasting: Brief Review and Discussion of the Impact of Oxandrolone." *AIDS Patient Care and STDs* 14 (2000): 421–25.

Wilson, D.M., et al. "Oxandrolone Therapy in Constitutionally Delayed Growth and Puberty." *Pediatrics* 96 (1995): 1095–1100.

Oxazepam

Pronunciation: ox-A-zeh-pam (also pronounced ox-AZ-eh-pam)

Chemical Abstracts Service Registry Number: 604-75-1

Formal Names: Anxiolit, Serax, Serenid D

Type: Depressant (benzodiazepine class). *See* page 21

Federal Schedule Listing: Schedule IV (DEA no. 2835)

USA Availability: Prescription

Pregnancy Category: C

Uses. This substance is a metabolite of **diazepam, temazepam, chlordiazepoxide,** and **clorazepate** dipotassium. Oxazepam's primary medical usage is to fight insomnia, hostility, and anxiety. Some researchers have found the drug also works against depression. Studies show oxazepam, diazepam, and **flunitrazepam** to have about the same therapeutic effects, though not the same strengths (oxazepam being the weakest). In the 1990s a survey of pharmacies in Cracow, Poland, illustrated oxazepam's worldwide popularity; around 14% of benzodiazepine prescriptions were for oxazepam, predominantly to women. One advantage of the drug is its safe "therapeutic ratio," meaning that the amount needed to produce a desired medical effect is far below the amount needed to produce a poisonous effect. Thus medical practitioners have considerable flexibility in adjusting dosage to an exact amount needed by a patient.

Experimental use against tinnitus (ringing in the ears) has been promising. Sometimes oxazepam is the preferred antianxiety medicine for alcoholics suffering from cirrhosis, because a fully functioning liver is unnecessary to flush the substance from the body. Oxazepam is used to alleviate **alcohol** withdrawal syndrome and has been used to treat neuroses and schizophrenia. Oxazepam is considered appropriate for short-term treatment of agitation in elderly persons suffering from dementia. Tests indicate the drug can reduce hostility as well as anxiety, an ability that would set oxazepam apart from other benzodiazepines. In a cat experiment, however, the drug increased predator behavior. The drug makes mice more combative. Rats kill more mice when dosed with oxazepam, but researchers interpret that result as illustrating potency of the drug rather than indicating it would promote aggression in humans. Human oxazepam reactions that increase hostility and combativeness are unusual and unexplained, although factors may include size and fre-

quency of dose along with inherent personalities of users. Hostile human reactions are "paradoxical" effects, meaning they are the opposite of what
normally happens after taking an oxazepam dose.

Drawbacks. While under the drug's influence people exhibit memory trouble. Oxazepam lowers body temperature in mice and rats. Case reports tell of
oxazepam causing blisters or other skin eruptions on people. In mice the substance boosts the poisonous action of the cancer medicine ifosfamide. Some
experiments using oxazepam to induce sleep find no hangover effect on persons' performance the next day, but that result is not invariable; size of dose
appears relevant. An experiment testing the drug's effect on vigilance (an
important ability when driving a car) found normal ability while persons were
under the influence of a low dose. Another experiment using a dose four times
greater did find vigilance impairment. Still another experiment showed slower
movements.

Abuse factors. One reviewer of the drug's characteristics reported that it
may have less addictiveness than diazepam. In one study opiate addicts found
oxazepam no more attractive than a placebo. In another study sedative abusers judged the drug less attractive than diazepam and indeed mistakenly identified oxazepam as a placebo one third of the time (a mistake they almost
never made with diazepam) and even considered a placebo more appealing
than oxazepam about one fifth of the time (a preference never occurring with
diazepam). A similar experiment in which drug abusers compared oxazepam,
diazepam, and placebo produced comparable results.

An animal research study found no tolerance produced by the drug. Monkeys, however, exhibit signs of tolerance, dependence, and withdrawal after
taking the drug for a week or two. One human study found tolerance but no
withdrawal symptoms. Nonetheless, melancholy, mood swings, confusion,
anxiousness, panic, and seizures have been observed when doses of the drug
stopped abruptly. Some of those "withdrawal symptoms," however, are also
conditions for which the drug is prescribed; so emergence of those conditions
upon stopping the drug may simply mean the underlying conditions were not
cured. A case report recounts a rare instance of someone having visual hallucinations while undergoing oxazepam withdrawal. Tapering oxazepam does
not necessarily prevent abstinence symptoms, but symptoms have been controlled by substituting another drug. One authority warns that stopping oxazepam can be as touchy as stopping barbiturates. In the 1980s a health official
in Australia portrayed oxazepam dependence as a growing problem. In contrast, another authority reviewing oxazepam's history for a medical journal
found only four accounts of human dependence on the drug and declared
withdrawal symptoms to be unusual upon sudden stoppage. This reviewer
speculated that oxazepam's slow delivery of drug effects and its tendency to
make people dizzy if a lot is consumed help discourage abuse.

Drug interactions. A driving skills test showed that oxazepam worsens impairment induced by alcohol. Cigarette smoking shortens the time span that
an oxazepam dose stays in the body. A mouse study found that animals could
withstand higher doses of **morphine** and **methadone** if oxazepam was also
used.

Cancer. Findings about oxazepam's potential for causing human cancer have been inconclusive. Gene mutations would be a possible sign that cancer might eventually emerge; some laboratory tests show that the drug does not cause gene mutations, but genetic mutations were apparent after a six-month administration of the drug to mice. Oxazepam is described as causing liver cancer in mice. Researchers testing the drug on rats concluded that an unclear potential for causing cancer exists, but their uncertain conclusion was partly based on some dosages so high that apparently they were fatal to various individual animals.

Pregnancy. Experiments have exposed mice to oxazepam during fetal development, and assorted differences in their behavior (compared to mice with no exposure) have been documented, including decreased sociability and decreased interaction with surroundings. What those differences might mean in a human context is unclear. Experimental evidence indicates that prenatal exposure to oxazepam may harm a mouse's learning ability and temporarily slow growth. In humans the drug passes from a pregnant woman into the fetus. A survey of 4,014 instances of birth defects in the Netherlands from 1981 to 1994 found an association between oxazepam and cleft lip. The same association was found in Finland a few years earlier. Mice experiments have also produced head and mouth malformations, but the doses involved were far higher than humans would be expected to take.

Oxazepam is considered to have less impact than other benzodiazepines on a nursing mother's milk supply. Two nursing mothers who had measurable levels of oxazepam in their blood had no evidence of the substance in their milk. A case report tells of a nursing mother whose milk contained about 4.7% of her oxazepam dosage, with no apparent effect on the infant. In other cases, not even 0.001% of the oxazepam dose taken by a mother passed into her milk.

Additional scientific information may be found in:

Ayd, F.J., Jr. "Oxazepam: Update 1989." *International Clinical Psychopharmacology* 5 (1990): 1–15.

Bliding, A. "The Abuse Potential of Benzodiazepines with Special Reference to Oxazepam." *Acta Psychiatrica Scandinavica. Supplementum*, no. 274 (1978): 111–16.

Bucher, J.R., et al. "Toxicity and Carcinogenicity Studies of Oxazepam in the Fischer 344 Rat." *Toxicological Sciences* 42 (1998): 1–12.

Fouks, L., et al. "The Clinical Activity of Oxazepam." *Acta Psychiatrica Scandinavica. Supplementum*, no. 274 (1978): 99–103.

Griffiths, R.R., et al. "Comparison of Diazepam and Oxazepam: Preference, Liking and Extent of Abuse." *Journal of Pharmacology and Experimental Therapeutics* 229 (1984): 501–8.

Mewaldt, S.P., M.M. Ghoneim, and J.V. Hinrichs. "The Behavioral Actions of Diazepam and Oxazepam Are Similar." *Psychopharmacology* 88 (1986): 165–71.

Vaisanen, E., and E. Jalkanen. "A Double-Blind Study of Alprazolam and Oxazepam in the Treatment of Anxiety." *Acta Psychiatrica Scandinavica* 75 (1987): 536–41.

Oxycodone

Pronunciation: ox-i-KOH-dun

Chemical Abstracts Service Registry Number: 76-42-6 (Hydrochloride form 124-90-3)

Formal Names: Endocet, Endocodone, Endodan, M-Oxy, Oxycet, Oxycocet, OxyContin, OxyFast, OxyIR, Percocet, Percodan, Percodan-Demi, Percolone, Roxicet, Roxicodone, Roxilox, Roxiprin, Supeudol, Tylox

Informal Names: Oxicotten, Oxy, Oxycotton, Oxy 80s, Percs

Type: Depressant (opiate class). *See* page 19

Federal Schedule Listing: Schedule II (DEA no. 9143)

USA Availability: Prescription

Pregnancy Category: B

Uses. This drug is considered more addictive than **codeine**, from which oxycodone is derived. Some authorities say oxycodone comes from **thebaine**, which is correct also, because thebaine is the parent chemical that yields codeine. Oxycodone is anywhere from 7 to 12 times stronger than codeine and about 0.3 to 2.2 times the strength of **morphine**, depending on the way the drugs are used. Body chemistry transforms part of an oxycodone dose into **oxymorphone**. Patients have found pain relief from oxycodone to be as satisfactory as relief from **ketamine** and morphine. Oxycodone has been used successfully to reduce pain from dentistry, surgery, cancer, and osteoarthritis (a painful disease of a person's joints). The drug is also used as a sedative and as a cough suppressant. It is sometimes prescribed for "restless leg syndrome," an affliction in which persons keep moving their arms and legs around. The drug has also reduced tics associated with Tourette's syndrome. Oxycodone can relax people and at times even create euphoria. Some researchers speculate that oxycodone's euphoric effects may improve patients' sensation of pain relief, making the substance more effective for that purpose than a drug that lacks euphoric effects. The drug works an antidepressant for some persons.

Blood levels from a given dose of oxycodone tend to be about 25% higher in females than in males. The cause is unknown, but the difference apparently has no impact on medical usage.

Drawbacks. Unwanted effects include nausea, vomiting, constipation, itching, sweating, sleepiness, reduced sex drive, general weakness, impairment of breathing, and momentary low blood pressure when a person stands up. One study found the drug to impair breathing more than various other opiates do, and in another study, doses of oxycodone had to be stopped lest the volunteers be harmed by further breathing difficulty. Normally the drug should be avoided if a person suffers from pancreatitis, enlarged prostate, difficulty with urination, or poorly functioning thyroid or adrenal glands. Experimenters have demonstrated that the drug reduces physical and mental abilities needed for driving automobiles.

Abuse factors. The drug's potential for abuse is considered the same as morphine's, and oxycodone is a sought-after product among opiate abusers. A study that reviewed medical records found no evidence of tolerance developing in a medical context. Regardless of whether people use the drug medically or recreationally, dependence can develop, followed by withdrawal symptoms if dosage stops suddenly. Withdrawal symptoms are described as minor and can be avoided by gradually discontinuing the drug instead of suddenly stopping it or by administering clonidine, a substance normally used to control high blood pressure.

Drug interactions. People should use oxycodone cautiously if they are also taking antihistamines, various antidepressants, or a monoamine oxidase inhibitor (MAOI, found in some antidepressants and other medicine). Combining those sorts of drugs with oxycodone can produce excessive effects. The same is true of **alcohol**. Oxycodone also seems to interact with cyclosporine, a substance used to suppress an individual's immune system (an effect useful in preventing rejection of organs in transplant patients).

Cancer. Oxycodone's potential for causing cancer is unknown.

Pregnancy. Oxycodone is believed to pose a small risk of causing birth defects, but safety for administration during pregnancy has not been determined. An examination of medical records found a slightly higher likelihood of birth defects if pregnant women use oxycodone, but, unlike most drugs associated with malformations, no particular type of birth defect appeared after using oxycodone. That suggests the drug might not be responsible for the observed abnormalities.

Newborns may have dependence on the drug if their mothers have been taking it during pregnancy. Enough of the drug can pass into a woman's milk to cause dependence in a breast-feeding infant.

Combination products. Tylox contains sodium metabisulfite, to which asthmatics and other persons may have a serious allergic reaction, and should be used cautiously if the user is sensitive to sulfites.

Additional scientific information may be found in:

Kalso, E., and A. Vainio. "Morphine and Oxycodone Hydrochloride in the Management of Cancer Pain." *Clinical Pharmacology and Therapeutics* 47 (1990): 639–46.

Saarialho-Kere, U., M.J. Mattila, and T. Seppala. "Psychomotor, Respiratory and Neuroendocrinological Effects of a Mu-Opioid Receptor Agonist (Oxycodone) in Healthy Volunteers." *Pharmacology and Toxicology* 65 (1989): 252–57.

Schick, B., et al. "Preliminary Analysis of First Trimester Exposure to Oxycodone and Hydrocodone." *Reproductive Toxicology* 10 (1996): 162.

Stoll, A.L., and S. Rueter. "Treatment Augmentation with Opiates in Severe and Re-fractory Major Depression." *American Journal of Psychiatry* 156 (1999): 2017.

Walters, A.S., et al. "Successful Treatment of the Idiopathic Restless Legs Syndrome in a Randomized Double-Blind Trial of Oxycodone versus Placebo." *Sleep* 16 (1993): 327–32.

Ytterberg, S.R., M.L. Mahowald, and S.R. Woods. "Codeine and Oxycodone Use in Patients with Chronic Rheumatic Disease Pain." *Arthritis and Rheumatism* 41 (1998): 1603–12.

Oxymetholone

Pronunciation: ok-see-METH-ah-lohn

Chemical Abstracts Service Registry Number: 434-07-1

Formal Names: Adroyd, Anadrol, Anapolon, Anasteron, Oxymethalone

Type: Anabolic steroid. *See* page 24

Federal Schedule Listing: Schedule III (DEA no. 4000)

USA Availability: Prescription

Pregnancy Category: X

Uses. This drug's main medical usage is for treatment of anemia and other blood disorders. The compound has also seen success against hereditary angioedema, a condition involving painful swelling of body tissues. Discouragement of blood clots and encouragement of weight gain are other medical applications. Particular success has been noted in weight gain with HIV/AIDS (human immunodeficiency virus/acquired immunodeficiency syndrome) patients, accompanied by general improvement in quality of life. Cancer patients have also benefitted from the drug's weight-gain property. An experiment indicated that short-term dosage can help persons suffering from heart failure. In another experiment the drug improved bone density in bedridden people. Still another experiment showed that oxymetholone can boost height and weight in boys and girls who are small for their age; such usage requires careful monitoring, as the substance has potential for stopping bone growth and thereby preventing attainment of normal adult height.

Drawbacks. Oxymetholone can produce masculine physical characteristics in women (facial hair, deeper voice) and disrupt the menstrual cycle; some authorities indicate that such masculinization is uncommon. Experimentation with male rats lowered their blood levels of **testosterone** and halted sexual activity. In human males oxymetholone may promote enlargement of the prostate gland. Men with prostate or breast cancer should avoid the drug, as should women who have both breast cancer and signs of a bone-weakening disease called osteoporosis. Oxymetholone can damage the liver and, in unusual circumstances, is associated with fatal harm to the spleen. Cholesterol levels can rise, increasing the risk of conditions leading to heart attack and stroke; kidney dialysis patients are considered to be at special risk for such outcomes. Case reports attribute stroke to oxymetholone. The drug may cause fluid retention, a possible hazard for persons with heart, liver, or kidney disease. Other unwanted effects have included nausea, vomiting, chills, acne, and painful testicles. Case reports have noted severe changes in several persons' ability to handle blood sugar levels. Another case report noted mental confusion that developed in a patient receiving oxymetholone and that continued for weeks after the therapy stopped.

Abuse factors. Some athletes use the compound with the hope it will improve their sports performance. A case report attributed rupture of the triceps tendon to a regimen of oxymetholone, **nandrolone**, and testosterone, although analysts have noted that a nonanabolic steroid called cortisone may have promoted the injury. Another case report told of a 20-year-old athlete developing persistent balance problems after taking oxymetholone and two other steroids; investigators of that case felt that steroids were a likely cause, given their ability to promote brain damage (stroke) and mental difficulties (mood and thinking). A case report notes manic activity in a person using oxymetholone. Another case report notes an even-tempered person who became rageful and violent after beginning a regimen of oxymetholone. Researchers tested one group of athletes who were using that compound and other steroids, a second group composed of former users, and a third group that had never used these drugs. Compared to the other groups, current users perceived themselves as more antagonistic, but investigators found only slight psychological differences among the groups. Chickenpox is a childhood disease that adults can suffer, and a bodybuilder who used oxymetholone and other anabolic steroids came down with a severe case requiring extended hospitalization; the case report did not blame the steroids but considered his drug use important enough to emphasize.

A case report speaks of oxymetholone "dependency" but in the context of persons needing the drug to maintain good health, not dependency in the traditional terminology of drug abuse. Another case report, however, does describe dependence in a bodybuilder who was taking oxymetholone and other anabolic steroids. A noteworthy aspect of this case was the person's sudden development of opiate withdrawal symptoms when he received a drug that provokes opiate withdrawal.

Drug interactions. Not enough scientific information to report, although anabolic steroids as a drug class tend to boost effects from medicines intended to reduce blood clotting.

Cancer. Oxymetholone gives negative results in assorted laboratory tests designed to detect cell mutations that may lead to cancer and gives mixed results in tests involving animals dosed on the substance. Oxymetholone is suspected of causing human cancer, with liver cancer a particular risk. Scientists have been unsure about any connection between the substance and human cancer, but the high level of suspicion is illustrated by numerous published case reports noting development of cancer by patients using oxymetholone.

Pregnancy. The drug may reduce fertility. In rat experiments the substance masculinized female fetuses even more than **methyltestosterone**. Whether oxymetholone passes into human milk is uncertain, but nursing mothers are advised to avoid the substance.

Additional scientific information may be found in:

Alexanian, R., and J. Nadell. "Oxymetholone Treatment for Sickle Cell Anemia." *Blood* 45 (1975): 769–77.

Barker, S. "Oxymethalone and Aggression." *British Journal of Psychiatry* 151 (1987): 564.

Bond, A.J., P.Y. Choi, and H.G. Pope, Jr. "Assessment of Attentional Bias and Mood in Users and Non-Users of Anabolic-Androgenic Steroids." *Drug and Alcohol Dependence* 37 (1995): 241–45.

Hengge, U.R., et al. "Oxymetholone Promotes Weight Gain in Patients with Advanced Human Immunodeficiency Virus (HIV-1) Infection." *British Journal of Nutrition* 75 (1996): 129–38.

Keele, D.K., and J.W. Worley. "Study of an Anabolic Steroid: Certain Effects of Oxymetholone on Small Children." *American Journal of Diseases of Children* 113 (1967): 422–30.

Murchison, L. "Uses and Abuses of Anabolic Steroids." *Prescribers' Journal* 26 (1986): 129–35.

"Oxymetholone." *IARC Monographs on the Evaluation of the Carcinogenic Risk of Chemicals to Man: Some Miscellaneous Pharmaceutical Substances* 13 (1977): 131–39.

Oxymorphone

Pronunciation: ox-i-MOR-fohn

Chemical Abstracts Service Registry Number: 76-41-5. (Hydrochloride form 357-07-3)

Formal Names: Numorphan

Type: Depressant (opioid class). *See* page 24

Federal Schedule Listing: Schedule II (DEA no. 9652)

USA Availability: Prescription

Pregnancy Category: C

Uses. Medically this drug is used to ease pain and assist in anesthesia. It is about 9 to 13 times stronger than **morphine**, with similar actions. Oxymorphone has been likened to **heroin**. Because body chemistry transforms part of an **oxycodone** dose into oxymorphone, scientists wondered if oxycodone's therapeutic actions actually came from oxymorphone; upon investigation, experimenters concluded that oxycodone does produce effects apart from those of oxymorphone. Allowing hospitalized patients to control their own oxymorphone dosage for pain relief has caused no problems. **Hydromorphone** can sometimes be used as a substitute. A case report indicates oxymorphone can have antidepressant actions.

Drawbacks. Unwanted effects of oxymorphone can include nausea, vomiting, and breathing difficulty. Euphoria has been noted in horses that receive the drug.

Abuse factors. Not enough scientific information to report, but the drug is legally classified as highly addictive.

Drug interactions. Other depressants should generally be avoided, and monoamine oxidase inhibitors (MAOIs, found in some antidepressants and other medicine) should also be avoided.

Cancer. Not enough scientific information to report.

Pregnancy. Birth defects appeared after experimenters gave pregnant hamsters 1,500 times the recommended human dose. Effects on human pregnancy are unknown. The drug can influence fetal heartbeat if used in childbirth. Oxymorphone has been found effective for easing pain after caesarean section.

Additional scientific information may be found in:

Heiskanen, T.E., et al. "Morphine or Oxycodone in Cancer Pain?" *Acta Oncologica* (Stockholm, Sweden) 39 (2000): 941–47.

Johnstone, R.E., et al. "Combination of Delta-9-Tetrahydrocannabinol with Oxymorphone or Pentobarbital: Effects on Ventilatory Control and Cardiovascular Dynamics." *Anesthesiology* 42 (1975): 674–84.

Sinatra, R.S., and D.M. Harrison. "Oxymorphone in Patient-Controlled Analgesia." *Clinical Pharmacy* 8 (1989): 541, 544.

Sinatra, R.S., et al. "A Comparison of Morphine, Meperidine, and Oxymorphone as Utilized in Patient-Controlled Analgesia Following Cesarean Delivery." *Anesthesiology* 70 (1989): 585–90.

Stoll, A.L., and S. Rueter. "Treatment Augmentation with Opiates in Severe and Refractory Major Depression." *American Journal of Psychiatry* 156 (1999): 2017.

PCP

Pronunciation: pee-see-pee

Chemical Abstracts Service Registry Number: 77-10-1. (Hydrochloride form 956-90-1)

Formal Names: Phencyclidine

Informal Names: Ace, Ad, Alien Sex Fiend (with **heroin**), Amoeba, Angel, Angel Dust, Angel Hair, Angel Mist, Angel Poke, Animal Trank, Animal Tranq, Animal Tranquilizer, Aurora Borealis, Belladonna, Black Dust, Black Whack, Blotter Acid, Blue Madman, Boat, Bohd, Bush, Busy Bee, Butt Naked, Cadillac, Cannabinol, Cigarrode Cristal, CJ, Clicker, Clickum, Cliffhanger, Columbo, Cozmo's, Crazy Coke, Crazy Eddie, Crystal, Crystal Joint, Crystal T, Cycline, Cyclone, D, Detroit Pink, Devil's Dust, Dipper, DMT, DOA, Do It Jack, Domex, Drink, Dummy Dust, Dust, Dusted Parsley, Elephant, Elephant Trank, Elephant Tranquilizer, Elysion, Embalming Fluid, Energizer, Erth, Fake STP, Flake, Flying Saucer, Fresh, Fuel, Good, Goon, Goon Dust, Gorilla Biscuit, Gorilla Tab, Green, Green Leaves, Green Tea, Happy Sticks, HCP, Heaven & Hell, He-Man, Herms, Hinkley, Hog, Hog Dust, Horse Tracks, Horse Tranquilizer, Ice, Ill, Illy Momo, Jet Fuel, Juice, K, Kap, Kay Jay, K-Blast, Killer, KJ, Kool, Koolly High, Krystal, KW, LBJ, Leaky Bolla, Leaky Leak, Lemon Drop, Lemon 714, Lenos, Lethal Weapon, Little One, Live One, Log, Loveboat, Lovely, Mad Dog, Madman, Magic, Magic Dust, Magic Mist, Mean Green, Mint Dew, Mint Leaf, Mint Weed, Missile, Mist, Monkey Dust, Monkey Tranquilizer, More, New Acid, New Magic, Niebla, Octane (mixed with **gasoline**), Oil, Omen, OPP, Orange Crystal, Ozone, P, Parsley, Paz, PCPA, Peace, PeaCe Pill, Peace Weed, Peep, Peter Pan, Pig Killer, Pikachu (mixed with **MDMA**), Pit, Polvo, Polvo de Angel, Polvo de Estrellas, Puffy, Purple Rain, Red Devil, Rocket Fuel, Scaffle, Scuffle, Selma, Sernyl, Sernylan, Sheets, Sherm, Sherman, Sherm Stick, Skuffle, Smoking, Snort, Soma, Space Base (mixed with crack **cocaine**), Space Cadet (with crack), Space Dust (with crack), Speedboat (with crack and **marijuana**), Spore, Squirrel (with crack and marijuana), Stardust, Stick, STP, Super, Super Grass (with marijuana), Super Joint, Super Kool, Super Weed, Surfer, Synthetic Cocaine, Synthetic THT, TAC, T-Buzz, Tea, Tic, Tic Tac, Tish, Titch, Trank, Wac, Wack, Water, Weed, Wet (alone or with marijuana), Wet Daddy, Whack (with crack or heroin), Whacky Weed, White Devil, White Horizon, White Powder, Wicky Stick (with crack and marijuana), Wobble Weed, Wolf, Wooly (with marijuana), Worm, Yellow Fever, Zimbie, Zombie Dust, Zombie Weed, Zoom

Type: Depressant. *See* page 19

Federal Schedule Listing: Schedule II (DEA no. 7471)

USA Availability: Prescription

Uses. This substance was invented in the 1920s, but not until the 1950s was it introduced as a drug, intended as a human and veterinary anesthetic. Human medical use soon ended because of psychological effects discovered during tests on patients. PCP is related to **ketamine** and, like that substance, has hallucinogenic qualities. Depending on how PCP is used, it can have stimulant, depressant, or hallucinogenic actions. In monkeys PCP is about 10 times stronger than ketamine.

Drawbacks. PCP can make people feel aloof from the world around them, cause numbness, interfere with movement, and distort perception of time. Hallucinations, floating sensations, euphoria, and mania can occur. People may forget what they did while under the drug's influence; such amnesia can last for 24 hours after a dose. Although euphoric effects are well documented, one group of researchers noted bouts of depression brought on by chronic use of the substance, though not by intermittent use. Yet the same researchers also found people successfully using the drug as an antidepressant, and animal studies suggest PCP may have antianxiety properties. The substance reduces appetite in dogs. Rats lost weight when they chronically received PCP.

Law enforcement authorities say the drug can make people hostile and give them extra physical strength, and the same has been experienced by medical personnel dealing with overdose emergencies. Researchers, however, have generally not observed such results from PCP (although one of the very first studies in the 1950s noted violent reactions from about 5% of surgery patients who received the drug as an anesthetic). A study examining PCP cases at a Los Angeles psychiatric hospital emergency room explicitly noted that wild conduct among PCP patients was uncommon. Perhaps police simply have more dealings with hostile individuals; for example, **alcohol** can embolden belligerent persons, but violence is not considered an inherent effect of alcohol. Persons who become violent after taking PCP already have such a history without the substance, and during a police encounter they may well be under the influence of alcohol or other drugs as well. Military research found that PCP hostility did not occur unless persons were under stress, and not all stressed individuals reacted that way. The military study also found that psychotic episodes did not occur with normal persons; someone had to be prone to psychosis in order for such behavior to occur while using the drug (a finding supported by other studies as well). In mice research PCP *reduces* violent behavior. Most species, including monkeys, act more docile after taking the drug. Some violent human episodes are described as coming not from aggression but from a PCP user's panic when police or medical personnel try to restrain the person. One group of addicts spoke of the substance lowering inhibitions, which is not the same as causing violence, although an already enraged person who loses inhibitions may engage in stormy behavior. In addition, users who attract attention from police or emergency medical personnel are not necessarily representative of recreational users in general, either in personality or size of dose or reaction to the dose.

PCP's physical effects include increased salivation, body temperature, pulse rate, and blood pressure. Case reports about humans indicate that PCP can raise blood pressure so high that a medical emergency occurs. The drug can bring on dizziness and double vision, create seizures, and cause muscle discoordination and damage. Numbness caused by PCP can promote injury due to lack of pain signals that ordinarily warn a person to stop doing something. Cases of kidney failure and liver destruction have been associated with the substance.

The higher one rises in the traditional evolutionary scale (for example, from mice to rats to humans), the lower the dose necessary for PCP to create anesthesia. Two observers who noted that trend concluded that human brains are exquisitely sensitive to PCP. Animal experiments reveal brain damage when the substance is used chronically for as little as five days. PCP addicts have complained of memory trouble. A small human study found impaired ability for abstract thinking and for physical movement in response to signals, impairment measured years after the persons said they had stopped using PCP. Moreover, users of the drug may have normal scores on intelligence tests but have emotional disabilities and be crippled in their ability to cope with problems. Those latter defects may be caused by the drug or may instead be reasons why people resort to the drug.

Abuse factors. Initially PCP was a Schedule III drug, but in 1978 government authorities shifted it to Schedule II because of recreational use. At about that time a Los Angeles psychiatric hospital emergency room tested 145 consecutive patients for PCP; 63 were positive (over 40%).

A study of 200 recreational users found differences in effects reported by persons who took a little of the drug once a month and by persons who took a lot every day for years. Heavy users felt more pepped-up, violent, and suicidal. Regular users of PCP are known for self-destruction; one study found that 24% of regular users had tried to commit suicide, and 36% had overdosed on other drugs. A study of PCP users who were treated at a charity hospital found no behavioral difference between black or white males, but black females acted much stranger and more aggressively than white females. The meaning of that finding is unclear—it could be racial, could be cultural, could be a statistical oddity that would disappear after more research.

When monkeys were given a choice between water or PCP, the animals showed no preference; such indifference is a sign of low addictive potential. An experiment measuring rats with prenatal exposure to PCP found the animals were more sensitive to the drug than were rats lacking prenatal exposure—the opposite of tolerance. Dependence has been reported in monkeys that receive PCP. Pigeons that received the drug every day for 215 days did not develop dependence. Human research has found tolerance but not dependence among users, although dependence is suspected.

Various cold remedies contain doxylamine succinate, which can cause a false-positive drug test for PCP.

Drug interactions. In a rat experiment neither alcohol nor PCP affected blood pressure, but blood pressure rose when they were used simultaneously. They also speeded up the heart. One human study found that PCP may be more likely to induce excitability in alcoholics than in nonalcoholics, possibly meaning that alcohol increases the likelihood of a manic reaction. In mice marijuana has reduced hyperactivity caused by PCP.

Cancer. Not enough scientific information to report.

Pregnancy. Two studies published only a few months apart in the 1980s gave different impressions about the prevalence of PCP use among pregnant women. In one study a group of 2,327 pregnant women were tested for PCP use; 19 were taking the drug. Those 19 were typically polydrug abusers. A different study of 200 pregnant women found 24 using PCP, a rate 15 times higher than in the other group.

If a pregnant woman uses PCP, it passes into the fetus. Reports exist of PCP being detected in newborns three months after the mothers claimed to have stopped using the drug during pregnancy, which would mean that the drug remains in a fetus months after a pregnant woman stops taking PCP. Whether the women's claims of abstinence were confirmed by laboratory testing during those months of pregnancy is unclear, however. In mice and pigs PCP builds up in the fetus, reaching levels 7 to 10 times higher than in the female's bloodstream.

The drug is suspected of causing birth defects. At dosage levels high enough to poison the pregnant female, birth defects have been produced in rats and mice. Rats with prenatal exposure to PCP show defective memory and learning ability. The substance is suspected of harming fetal brain development in humans. Pregnant women who use the drug tend to produce infants who are smaller than normal. In a group of 83 infants with prenatal PCP exposure, almost half had a head circumference below the 25th percentile (meaning that 75% of infants in the general population have bigger heads and, by implication, larger brains). Some were below the 10th percentile. Smaller-than-normal infant skulls may interfere with physical growth of the brain. People who abuse one drug tend to abuse others as well; one study of 41 women who used PCP during pregnancy found that most had also been using cocaine. Two studies of women who used PCP during pregnancy found that all were poor; most were unmarried, were in an ethnic minority, and had received inadequate prenatal care. Such factors confound efforts to confirm what effect PCP alone has on pregnancy.

Offspring of mothers who have been using PCP can exhibit symptoms similar to those seen in infants undergoing opiate withdrawal—even though the drug is not an opiate, and research has yet to demonstrate that PCP dependence occurs. Infant distress may be real, but the newborn may be responding to the unpleasant effects of the drug itself rather than responding to sudden absence of the drug.

A year after birth, a group of 57 babies with prenatal PCP exposure showed normal development in mental ability and physical coordination, although almost half were ill-tempered. About 15% had trouble sleeping, and the same percentage lacked normal emotional attachment. Those findings are consistent with other studies. Home environment, of course, may influence behavior as much or more than prenatal drug exposure. Factors noted above (lack of money, absent father, being in a disadvantaged ethnic minority) can weaken home life. Still, the kinds of brain function damage seen in animal studies are the kinds of damage that should interfere with children's abilities to socialize normally—exactly the kind of deficit seen in children who have prenatal exposure to PCP.

In mice PCP not only passes into maternal milk, but milk levels are 10 times higher than maternal blood levels.

Additional information. PCP is related to the Schedule I hallucinogens PCE (CAS RN 2201-15-2), PCPy (2201-39-0), TCP (21500-98-1), and TCPy (22912-13-6). Rat experimentation measured PCPy as about the same strength as PCP. Other laboratory measurement shows TCP as stronger than PCP, and PCE as stronger than TCP. French military experiments found that TCP could protect rats and guinea pigs from the chemical warfare agent soman.

"Cannabinol" is a nickname for PCP and refers to THC, which is the active chemical in marijuana and **dronabinol**, but PCP is not THC. Likewise "**DMT**" and "STP" (**DOM**) are nicknames for PCP, but they are all different drugs.

Additional scientific information may be found in:

Baldridge, E.B., and H.A. Bessen. "Phencyclidine." *Emergency Medicine Clinics of North America* 8 (1990): 541–50.

Brecher, M., et al. "Phencyclidine and Violence: Clinical and Legal Issues." *Journal of Clinical Psychopharmacology* 8 (1988): 397–401.

Giannini, A.J., R.K. Bowman, and J.D. Giannini. "Perception of Nonverbal Facial Cues in Chronic Phencyclidine Abusers." *Perceptual and Motor Skills* 89 (1999): 72–78.

Graeven, D.B., J.G. Sharp, and S. Glatt. "Acute Effects of Phencyclidine (PCP) on Chronic and Recreational Users." *American Journal of Drug and Alcohol Abuse* 8 (1981): 39–50.

Harry, G.J., and J. Howard. "Phencyclidine: Experimental Studies in Animals and Long-term Developmental Effects on Humans." In *Perinatal Substance Abuse: Research Findings and Clinical Implications*, ed. T.B. Sonderegger. Baltimore, MD: Johns Hopkins University Press, 1992. 254–78.

Khajawall, A.M., T.B. Erickson, and G.M. Simpson. "Chronic Phencyclidine Abuse and Physical Assault." *American Journal of Psychiatry* 139 (1982): 1604–6.

Pradhan, S.N. "Phencyclidine (PCP): Some Human Studies." *Neuroscience and Biobehavioral Reviews* 8 (1984): 493–501.

Schuckit, M.A., and E.R. Morrissey. "Propoxyphene and Phencyclidine (PCP) Use in Adolescents." *Journal of Clinical Psychiatry* 39 (1978): 7–13.

Sioris, L.J., and E.P. Krenzelok. "Phencyclidine Intoxication: Literature Review." *American Journal of Hospital Pharmacy* 35 (1978): 1362–67.

Pemoline

Pronunciation: PEM-oh-leen

Chemical Abstracts Service Registry Number: 2152-34-3

Formal Names: Cylert

Informal Names: Popcorn Coke

Type: Stimulant. *See* page 11

Federal Schedule Listing: Schedule IV (DEA no. 1530)

USA Availability: Prescription

Pregnancy Category: B

Uses. In the United States pemoline became available for medical purposes during the 1970s. It is used to treat depression, weariness, and attention deficit hyperactivity disorder (ADHD). The drug's stimulant effects are described as greater than **caffeine** but less than amphetamine. Unlike many scheduled stimulants, pemoline is unrelated to amphetamine.

Studies find pemoline useful in reducing symptoms of depression, and experimental usage of pemoline with monoamine oxidase inhibitor (MAOI) antidepressants has helped depressed persons who obtain insufficient relief with other drugs.

Pemoline has eliminated drowsiness felt by persons taking antihistamines. The drug has been proposed for workplace usage to reduce fatigue but has not been tested extensively for that purpose. Tests have found that the drug improves ability to perform arithmetic when users are tired. In a different but more robust experiment, members of the U.S. Navy Special Warfare group stayed awake 64 hours around the clock while using pemoline. Though their performance appeared to decline as the experiment continued, they not only did better than participants who used placebos, but they also did better than persons using **methylphenidate**. In England, Royal Air Force experimenters concluded that pemoline can help keenness and capabilities during long shifts of duty. A Russian report endorses the drug's usefulness for "urgent increase" of functioning but notes that persons using pemoline cannot maintain initial ability if body temperature rises and oxygen supply declines, nor does the drug help persons push past emotional strain or fulfill complicated task requirements. During the 1980s and 1990s sports officials in Belgium found the drug was frequently used by cyclists seeking a competitive edge. Multiple sclerosis patients using pemoline sometimes report less exhaustion than those using a placebo, but investigators who rigorously reviewed studies about multiple sclerosis fatigue found no evidence of pemoline improving weariness. An instance is known of an elderly man taking pemoline to help him stay awake during lectures, but the regimen seemed to promote prostate trouble. Pemoline has been successfully used against narcolepsy.

Studies find pemoline about as effective as either **dextroamphetamine** or methylphenidate in helping children with ADHD. Pemoline has been used successfully against ADHD in teenagers and adults as well. Growth rates are below normal in some youngsters with ADHD, and pemoline itself can temporarily hold back such development but without long-term harm—youngsters develop normal adult weight and height. Those deficient growth rates may be treated with growth hormone. One study found, however, that pemoline seems to make the hormone treatment less effective in some patients. As the age of ADHD patients grows, so can unwanted effects that they experience from pemoline.

Animal experiments in the 1960s indicated that pemoline boosts learning ability. The lure of a "smart pill" had understandable appeal to suffering students and teachers, but when the drug was tested on college students, no improvement in learning ability occurred. The same dismal outcome occurred when elderly persons received the drug; indeed, some performed worse than elderly persons receiving a placebo. Group results in still another experiment showed either no improvement or worsening of learning scores when people used the drug. In contrast, long-term daily administration of the drug seemed to improve memory in some persons entering senility.

A review covering 10 years of pemoline reports found none attributing euphoria to the drug, a lack that sets it apart from other scheduled stimulants. Unlike some other stimulants, pemoline also seems to have little effect on pulse rate or blood pressure.

Drawbacks. The drug can bring on tics and partial muscle movements, in a particularly severe way if an overdose occurs. An instance is known of muscle damage in an adult misusing pemoline. Pemoline is also known to reduce appetite and salivation, increase crankiness, bring on headaches and stomachaches, cause skin rash, and interfere with sleep. Hallucinations from pemoline have been reported.

In rats and mice pemoline can cause self-harm behavior, and the amount needed to induce such behavior declines when a certain kind of brain damage is present, damage that is often seen in mentally retarded humans. Those findings suggest that such persons receiving pemoline may need monitoring to guard against self-injury. Long-term excessive usage may generate temporary psychotic behavior, but such an outcome appears untypical.

Probably the most serious unwanted results of taking pemoline can be hepatitis and other liver injury, injury so severe as to require a transplant. Damage can continue to worsen after the drug is stopped, and people have died from liver failure induced by pemoline. Victims tend to be children. Such an adverse effect is particularly disquieting because it occurs at therapeutic dosage, rather then being created by reckless abuse. A child can take pemoline for months before harm is apparent, or alarming symptoms can arise after just a week of use. Methylphenidate is suspected of contributing to liver trouble in persons who are also taking pemoline. Debate exists about how dangerous pemoline is to liver function when no other drugs are being taken, but the debate has limited practical significance because many patients taking pemoline receive other drugs as well. Because of concern about liver damage, parents are supposed to sign a written consent form before their children begin pemoline therapy.

Abuse factors. Although pemoline is a scheduled substance, a review of reports covering the first 10 years of its medical availability in the United States found little evidence of addiction or abuse. A Norwegian review of pemoline use boldly described it as "a stimulant which cannot be abused."[1] When given a choice of drugs, animals show no particular interest in pemoline, a sign of low abuse potential. Nonetheless, a case report does exist of a pemoline addict who developed a paranoid psychosis that went away after stopping the drug. A British medical practitioner reported that drug misusers were supplementing their amphetamine habit with pemoline.

An experiment tested pemoline's ability to help reduce **cocaine** usage among persons receiving **methadone** treatment (meaning the persons were addicted to cocaine and **heroin** both). Results were unencouraging. In contrast, favorable response in an ADHD alcoholic caused researchers to predict that pemoline may be useful for treating **alcohol** addiction. Mice experimentation shows that pemoline reduces effects produced by THC, considered the primary drug in **marijuana**.

Drug interactions. Pemoline is suspected of interfering with epilepsy medicines. It can boost mono amine oxidase inhibitor (MAOI) antidepressants and urinary acidifers (the latter action interfering with pemoline's psychostimulant effects).

Cancer. Rat experiments do not indicate any cancer risk from pemoline.

Pregnancy. Experiments with rabbits and rats reveal no harm to fetal development, but influence on human fetal development is unknown.

Additional information. When tested on mentally handicapped workers, magnesium pemoline (CAS RN 18968-99-5) brought on the kinds of temperament modification associated with caffeine but failed to increase either productivity or time worked. Two cocaine addicts who appeared to have mild ADHD were able to reduce their intake of cocaine while receiving magnesium pemoline, a result leading the scientific investigators to wonder if magnesium pemoline might have potential for helping to break cocaine addiction. Animal experiments have shown that both pemoline and magnesium pemoline can provide protection against atomic radiation.

Additional scientific information may be found in:

Bostic, J.Q., et al. "Pemoline Treatment of Adolescents with Attention Deficit Hyperactivity Disorder: A Short-Term Controlled Trial." *Journal of Child and Adolescent Psychopharmacology* 10 (2000): 205–16.

Elizur, A., I. Wintner, and S. Davidson. "The Clinical and Psychological Effects of Pemoline in Depressed Patients—A Controlled Study." *International Pharmacopsychiatry* 14 (1979): 127–34.

Honda, Y., and Y. Hishikawa. "Long Term Treatment of Narcolepsy and Excessive

Daytime Sleepiness with Pemoline (Betanamin)." *Current Therapeutic Research: Clinical and Experimental* 27 (1980): 429–41.

Langer, D.H., et al. "Evidence of Lack of Abuse or Dependence Following Pemoline Treatment: Results of a Retrospective Survey." *Drug and Alcohol Dependence* 17 (1986): 213–27.

Newlands, W.J. "The Effect of Pemoline on Antihistamine-Induced Drowsiness." *The Practitioner* 224 (1980): 1199–1201.

Shevell, M., and R. Schreiber. "Pemoline-Associated Hepatic Failure: A Critical Analysis of the Literature." *Pediatric Neurology* 16 (1997): 14–16.

Sternbach, H. "Pemoline-Induced Mania." *Biological Psychiatry* 16 (1981): 987–89.

Valle-Jones, J.C. "Pemoline in the Treatment of Psychogenic Fatigue in General Practice." *The Practitioner* 221 (1978): 425–27.

Note

1. N. Lie, "Sentralstimuleren Midler ved AD/HD Hos Voksne. Kan De Misbrukes? [Central Stimulants in Adults with AD/HD. Can They Be Abused?]," *Tidsskrift for den Norske Laegeforening* 119 (1999): 82–83. Abstract in English.

Pentazocine

Pronunciation: pen-TAZ-oh-seen

Chemical Abstracts Service Registry Number: 359-83-1. (Hydrochloride form 64024-15-3)

Formal Names: Fortral, Fortralgesic, Fortralin, Fortwin, Liticon, Pentgin, Sosegon, Sosenyl, Talacen, Talwin, Talwin Nx

Informal Names: 4 × 4s, Teacher, Ts, Yellow Footballs. *Combination with **methylphenidate***: Crackers, 1s & 1s, Poor Man's Heroin, Ritz & Ts, Ts & Rits, Ts & Rs, Sets. *Combination with tripelennamine*: Ts & Blues, Ts & Bs

Type: Depressant. *See* page 19

Federal Schedule Listing: Schedule IV (DEA no. 9709)

USA Availability: Prescription

Pregnancy Category: C

Uses. Pentazocine became available in the 1960s. Some authorities classify the drug as an opioid; some do not. Rather than having cross-tolerance with opiates and opioids, pentazocine can provoke a withdrawal syndrome from them. Volunteers who receive pentazocine have been uncertain about what sort of drug it is; some say it is a hallucinogen; some think they are receiving **alcohol**.

Pentazocine has about the same pain relief strength as **codeine**. An experiment using oral surgery patients found pentazocine's pain relief to be the same as aspirin's. After drug abusers began grinding down Talwin tablets and injecting the powder to get **morphine** and **heroin** sensations, the manufacturer introduced Talwin Nx tablets, which include a chemical designed to block those sensations if the substance is injected. Dispute exists about whether the Nx version of Talwin actually prevents effects sought by illicit users.

Research indicates that women surgical patients tend to get better pain relief from pentazocine than male patients. Research also indicates that the drug's surgical pain control is more effective for older patients and less effective for neurotics and for individuals with outgoing personalities. The drug has been routinely used to ease cancer pain and has had success in reducing joint pain caused by various afflictions, including arthritis. After noting that pentazocine does not prolong bleeding times, researchers called it suitable to fight pain from hemophilia, a blood disease that promotes bleeding. The substance has also been given as a treatment for stubborn cases of hiccups.

Investigators have documented that people can briefly experience euphoria after taking the drug. Some users feel more amiable and serene after a dose.

Drawbacks. Unwanted pentazocine actions include rapid heartbeat, blood pressure changes (up or down), fainting, sweating, confusion, sleepiness, blurred vision, nausea, vomiting, and constipation. Studies have found that 1% to 10% of persons receiving the drug (especially an injectable pharmaceutical version) have odd psychological reactions such as hallucinations, delusions, or a sense of unreality about the world. The substance can interfere with decision making and physical movement. Research has shown that driving skills decline when a person uses the drug, and users should avoid operating motor vehicles or other dangerous machinery. Because pentazocine has occasionally been associated with seizures, it should be used cautiously by persons prone to that affliction. The substance should also be used cautiously by people suffering from pancreas malfunction or breathing difficulty. The drug may be particularly hazardous for asthma sufferers who are overly sensitive to aspirin. Pentazocine is associated with skin hardening, which can result in extensive surgical removal of affected areas, to be replaced with skin grafts. Case reports tell of the drug provoking not only skin lesions but internal lesions in the digestive tract. Prolonged use of the substance can also cause muscle destruction that cripples a person's ability to move arms and legs. The compound can dangerously reduce white blood cell levels. Rat experiments indicate the drug may provoke attacks of porphyria, a body chemistry disease that can make people violent and sensitive to light.

One group of researchers documented that pentazocine increased the heart's workload by 22% in cardiac disease patients. Another group found that after a heart attack the drug increases blood pressure and the heart's need for oxygen and concluded that pentazocine is dangerous for heart attack patients. Not all authorities agree with that conclusion, however; some say that such adverse cardiac effects can be avoided through careful dosage, and other opinion says the drug is preferable to morphine for heart attack patients.

Abuse factors. Some abusers inject powder from oral pentazocine tablets. Oral pentazocine tablets contain ingredients not intended for introduction into the bloodstream, and injection can be fatal even though the digestive system can handle the same ingredients without difficulty.

Pentazocine and the antihistamine-anesthetic tripelennamine are a common illicit drug combination called Ts & Blues, sometimes used as a substitute for heroin ("T" standing for Talwin and "Blues" for the antihistamine tablets' color). The combination can create more euphoria than pentazocine alone produces and reduce the discontent caused by some doses of pentazocine. Users report development of memory trouble. Lung damage is a classic consequence of the combination, promoted by injecting oral formats of the drugs. Users have been hospitalized with chest pain, anxiety, spasms, sweating, nausea, and lightheadedness. Fainting and seizures are less common problems. Kidney damage has been noted. Other antihistamines can also be dangerous to use with pentazocine.

Pentazocine tolerance and dependence can occur. After daily doses were given to monkeys for six weeks, mild withdrawal symptoms appeared when the animals received nalorphine, a substance that provokes withdrawal signs if someone has been using opioids. That result supports classifying pentazocine as an opioid, but in humans nalorphine does not cause pentazocine withdrawal—a result consistent with pentazocine not being an opioid. Pentazocine withdrawal is normally likened to a light version of the opiate withdrawal syndrome, although case reports tell of some persons suffering intense physical discomfort for up to two weeks (cramping muscles, painful abdomen and back, nausea, itching, sweating, and general discomposure). Debate exists about whether pentazocine addiction should be treated by substituting other drugs such as **methadone** or whether treatment should avoid substitution altogether. Some authorities have wondered if pentazocine addiction occurs in persons who are not polydrug abusers. Some authorities even question whether pentazocine addiction exists, noting cases in which body fluid testing contradicted drug users' claims to be using the drug (while indicating they were using other substances). German researchers found that addiction reports are at least exaggerated; upon investigation, only 8 of 60 reports turned out to be authentic.

Drug interactions. Persons who smoke or who live in a polluted air environment may need higher doses of pentazocine than persons who breathe clean air. Morphine and pentazocine boost each other's pain-relieving action. Alcohol and possibly monoamine oxidase inhibitors (found in some antidepressants) may react badly with pentazocine.

Cancer. Animal research has not shown pentazocine to cause cancer.

Pregnancy. Normal production of litters has occurred when pentazocine was given to pregnant rats and rabbits, and no birth defects were apparent. The drug is absorbed by the fetus if a pregnant woman takes a dose. Examination of one hospital's records of all pregnant patients who used pentazocine illicitly in a two-year period showed that their infants tended to be premature and undersized, but no malformation was attributed to the drug. Newborns were occasionally dependent. Despite those disadvantages the children seemed to develop normally in their first year of life. When pentazocine was given simply as a pain reliever in childbirth, examination of the infants revealed no difference from children born to women who did not receive a medical dose of the drug during childbirth.

A study found Ts & Blues mothers to have an increased rate of assorted diseases that would not promote healthy fetal development: hepatitis, anemia, gonorrhea, syphilis. Such afflictions indicate a risk-taking lifestyle in which prenatal care is a small concern. A survey of maternity records at one hospital showed that pregnant women who used Ts & Blues tended to produce smaller infants, but no major birth defects were associated with the drug combination. Another study found behavioral abnormalities in newborns that had fetal exposure to Ts & Blues, although the conduct may simply have been a temporary sign of drug withdrawal. Investigators running a rat experiment, however, noted long-term behavioral differences between a group of rats having fetal exposure to the drug combination and another group that was unexposed.

Additional scientific information may be found in:

Brogden, R.N., T.M. Speight, and G.S. Avery. "Pentazocine: A Review of Its Pharmacological Properties, Therapeutic Efficacy and Dependence Liability." *Drugs* 5 (1973): 6–91.

Debooy, V.D., et al. "Intravenous Pentazocine and Methylphenidate Abuse during Pregnancy. Maternal Lifestyle and Infant Outcome." *American Journal of Diseases of Children* 147 (1993): 1062–65.

"Pentazocine." *British Medical Journal* 2 (1970):409–10.

Saarialho-Kere, U., M.J. Mattila, and T. Seppala. "Parenteral Pentazocine: Effects on Psychomotor Skills and Respiration, and Interactions with Amitriptyline." *European Journal of Clinical Pharmacology* 35 (1988): 483–89.

Showalter, C.V. "T's and Blues: Abuse of Pentazocine and Tripelennamine." *Journal of the American Medical Association* 244 (1980): 1224–25.

Zacny, J.P., et al. "Comparing the Subjective, Psychomotor and Physiological Effects of Intravenous Pentazocine and Morphine in Normal Volunteers." *Journal of Pharmacology and Experimental Therapeutics* 286 (1998): 1197–207.

Pentobarbital

Pronunciation: pen-toh-BAR-bi-tal

Chemical Abstracts Service Registry Number: 76-74-4

Formal Names: Cafergot, Nembutal, Pentobarbitone, Phenobarbitone

Informal Names: Nebbies, Nembies, Nemmies, Nimbies, Yellow Bullets, Yellow Dolls, Yellow Jackets, Yellows

Type: Depressant (barbiturate class). *See* page 20

Federal Schedule Listing: Schedule II (oral and parentral, DEA no. 2270), Schedule III for suppositories (DEA no. 2271)

USA Availability: Prescription

Pregnancy Category: D

Uses. This short-acting substance has sedative qualities but is considered ineffective in treating nervous apprehension. Because of the drug's sleep-inducing characteristics, it is used as a preliminary to administering anesthesia and as a short-term treatment for insomnia. Pentobarbital has been observed to lower blood pressure, body temperature, and muscle tone. The compound can be used as an emergency anticonvulsant when a person has seizures, and has been used to treat **alcohol** addicts undergoing withdrawal. Pentobarbital has been found effective in reducing pressure that fluid creates in the brain after severe head injury. Pentobarbital reduces a type of nerve cell death called neuronal apoptosis, and this reduction may help prevent stroke. Animal studies indicate that pentobarbital can help protect brain tissue against radiation, which might have practical application during treatment of brain tumors. Veterinarians use the substance for euthanasia: An unusual demonstration of the drug's strength occurred when a lion was poisoned by eating meat from a horse that had been killed with pentobarbital.

Drawbacks. Although the drug is a sedative, it can cause hyperactivity in children. Sudden stoppage of combined pentobarbital and benzodiazepine therapy in an infant caused temporary chorea (involuntary jerking). A feline experiment showed that tremors reminiscent of Parkinson's disease can occur when pentobarbital is administered with chlorpromazine (also called Thorazine, often used to treat psychotic behavior). Persons with porphyria, a body chemistry affliction that can provoke violence, are supposed to avoid pentobarbital. Examination of epileptic children receiving pentobarbital shows elevated readings for total cholesterol, though levels of high-density lipoprotein (so-called good cholesterol) and triglycerides (associated with heart attack and stroke) seem unaffected.

In a monkey experiment pentobarbital interfered with time perception, ability to learn, short-term memory, attention span, and interest in tasks. The substance impeded task performances in a human experiment, with performance getting worse as the amount of thinking necessary for a chore increased. Such a drug is unlikely to be welcome in the workplace. Although children using the substance apparently have trouble with language skills, a study found language development to be normal two years after the medication ceased.

Abuse factors. In a test, alcohol drinkers who were not alcoholics found pentobarbital less appealing than a placebo and experienced no euphoria from pentobarbital, a finding consistent with other studies of persons who do not abuse drugs. When given choices of assorted substances, monkeys chose pentobarbital less often than water, which indicates the compound has low addictive potential. In contrast, drug abusers participating in an experiment found effects of pentobarbital and **diazepam** to be similar. Those two drugs thus had comparable appeal even though scientists running the experiment found pentobarbital possessing only 10% of diazepam's strength. A study testing various effects on former drug addicts found pentobarbital to be 15 times stronger than **meprobamate**, but **morphine** acted 6 times stronger than pentobarbital. Cross-tolerance among **chlordiazepoxide**, pentobarbital, and alcohol has been observed in rats. A study of sedative drug abusers found alcohol and pentobarbital to deliver similar effects, with pentobarbital possibly having more appeal. A monkey experiment indicates that alcohol increases the attractiveness of pentobarbital. Dependence can develop, and in humans the pentobarbital withdrawal syndrome can duplicate the delirium tremens of alcohol withdrawal. A mice study found that tolerance to pentobarbital developed more rapidly if assorted drugs of abuse were also being administered (morphine, amphetamine, alcohol, or **cocaine**).

Drug interactions. A case report notes that pentobarbital can almost double the speed with which theophylline (commonly used to treat asthma and other breathing difficulties) disappears from the bloodstream, requiring changes in normal theophylline dosage. In a mice experiment alcohol boosted pentobarbital's potency. A human study found that chronic alcohol ingestion reduces the effective length of a pentobarbital dose. Grapefruit juice extends the amount of sleep produced by pentobarbital in rats, and in mice the drug inhibits **caffeine** effects. At one time researchers suspected that taking pentobarbital along with **MDMA** would reduce organic brain damage caused by MDMA, but rat experiments indicate that any apparent benefit comes simply from the lower body temperature produced by pentobarbital. Although cocaine is a stimulant, in a rat experiment it increased the sleep-inducing quality of pentobarbital.

Cancer. In animal experimentation pentobarbital has caused cancer. In humans long-term usage is associated with cancer of the ovaries and bronchi, but that finding is weakened by the patients also smoking cigarettes.

Pregnancy. A large survey of pregnancy outcomes found that pentobarbital does not appear to cause birth defects. Nonetheless pregnant women are supposed to avoid the drug.

Additional information. Some capsule formats of Nembutal (pentobarbital sodium CAS RN 57-33-0) contain FD&C Yellow No. 5 (tartrazine), which can cause asthma attacks or other allergic responses in sensitive persons, particularly if someone has adverse reactions to aspirin. Cafergot PB is a combination of bellafoline, caffeine, and ergotamine tartrate. The combination was tested with and without pentobarbital sodium to determine effect on migraine headache. Presence of pentobarbital not only enhanced reduction of pain but also helped treat anxiety, nausea, vomiting, poor appetite, and low tolerance of light.

Additional scientific information may be found in:

Cole-Harding, S., and H. de Wit. "Self-Administration of Pentobarbital in Light and Moderate Alcohol Drinkers." *Pharmacology, Biochemistry, and Behavior* 43 (1992): 563–69.

Hambly, G., C. Frewin, and B. Dodd. "Effect of Anticonvulsant Medication in the Preschool Years on Later Language Development." *Medical Journal of Australia* 148 (1988): 658, 661–62.

Mintzer, M.Z., et al. "Ethanol and Pentobarbital: Comparison of Behavioral and Subjective Effects in Sedative Drug Abusers." *Experimental and Clinical Psychopharmacology* 5 (1997): 203–15.

Pickworth, W.B., M.S. Rohrer, and R.V. Fant. "Effects of Abused Drugs on Psychomotor Performance." *Experimental and Clinical Psychopharmacology* 5 (1997): 235–41.

Pierce, James I. "Drug-Withdrawal Psychoses." *American Journal of Psychiatry* 119 (1963): 880–81.

Peyote

Pronunciation: pay-OH-tih (also pronounced peh-YOH-teh)

Chemical Abstracts Service Registry Number: 11006-96-5

Formal Names: *Lophophora williamsii*

Informal Names: Bad Seed, Big Chief, Black Button, Britton, Buttons, Cactus, Cactus Head, Challote, Devil's Root, Dry Whiskey, Dumpling Cactus, Half Moon, Hikori, Hikuli, Hyatari, Mescal, Mescal Beans, Mescal Buttons, Mescalito, Mescy, Nubs, P, Pellote, Peyotl, Seni, Shaman, Tops

Type: Hallucinogen. *See* page 25

Federal Schedule Listing: Schedule I (DEA no. 7415)

USA Availability: Illegal to possess

Pregnancy Category: None

Uses. Peyote is part of a cactus plant. Native American folk medicine has used peyote cactus root for doctoring scalp afflictions. In folk medicine peyote has also been used against snake bite, influenza, and arthritis. Scientists have determined that peyote contains substances that might fight infections. Some Native Americans are reported to use light doses of peyote as a stimulant to maintain endurance when engaged in relentless activity permitting little nourishment or water, a practice sounding much like traditional use of **coca**. Spaniards observed such peyote usage in the Aztec empire.

Peyote's main active component is the hallucinogen **mescaline**. Some other varieties of cactus also contain mescaline, although generally in much smaller amounts. Researchers suspect the peyote cactus may additionally contain chemicals similar to those appearing in the brain upon use of **alcohol**.

In addition to causing hallucinations, peyote can change perception of time. Psychic effects can include feeling more peaceful and connected with life; craziness of the everyday world can recede. People can use the experience to work through their concerns and may be more open to suggestions. Physical senses may seem enhanced, and barriers between them may melt, such as allowing sounds to be seen.

Normally a Schedule I substance is illegal to possess except under special permission to do research with it, but for many years members of the Native American Church were allowed to possess and use peyote (but not the pure drug mescaline) for religious purposes. During the 1990s their legal situation became confused, and the issue was a matter of controversy when this book was written.

The religion of Peyotism (of which the Native American Church is but one variety) is a topic beyond the scope of this book, but drug-induced visions are only one part of the practitioners' way of life. Observers have noted that Peyotism can be an effective way of dealing with addiction to alcohol and opiates. Traditional peyote use occurs in a group context, a social gathering of persons sharing and furthering the same beliefs and goals. A solitary user estranged from such a setting is likely to have a far different peyote experience. For instance, one element of a peyote session can be nervousness and fear, emotions that may have different impacts depending on whether a user is alone or is with a group of reassuring and supportive persons. A researcher with the Indian Health Service of the U.S. Public Health Service estimated that traditional peyote usage produced bad psychological experiences once in 70,000 doses, a safety record that the researcher attributed to the social context of traditional use. Physical damage has not been noted from traditional use.

Drawbacks. Chills, muscle tension, nausea, and vomiting are typical unwanted peyote effects.

Abuse factors. A study published in the 1950s concluded that peyote tolerance, dependence, and craving did not occur from traditional usage—a finding supported by other authorities as well. A canine experiment showed that tolerance to the vomiting effect occurred if dogs received daily peyote for a year.

Drug interactions. Not enough scientific information to report.

Cancer. Not enough scientific information to report.

Pregnancy. Peyote has caused birth defects in hamsters. A study comparing peyote users to nonusers from the same Indian group found no increase in chromosome damage among the users.

Additional information. Peyote is sometimes called "mescal," which is also the name of an alcoholic beverage. The two substances are different, and the beverage has no connection with peyote. Likewise "mescal beans" are an alternative peyote name and also the name of a nonhallucinogenic food.

Additional scientific information may be found in:

Bergman, R.L. "Navajo Peyote Use: Its Apparent Safety." *American Journal of Psychiatry* 128 (1971): 695–99.

Boyer, L.B., R.M. Boyer, and H.W. Basehart. "Shamanism and Peyote Use among the Apaches of the Mescalero Indian Reservation." In *Hallucinogens and Shamanism*, ed. M.J. Harner, 53–66. New York: Oxford University Press, 1973.

Bruhn, J.G. "Mescaline Use for 5700 Years." *Lancet* 359 (2002): 1866.

Ellis, H. "Mescal: A New Artificial Paradise." *The Contemporary Review* 71 (1897). Reprinted in Smithsonian Institution's *Annual Report 1897*. Washington, DC: Author, 1898. 537–48.

Huttlinger, K.W., and D. Tanner. "The Peyote Way: Implications for Culture Care Theory." *Journal of Transcultural Nursing* 5, no. 2 (1994): 5–11.

Kapadia, G.J., and M.B.E. Fayez. "Peyote Constituents: Chemistry, Biogenesis, and Biological Effects." *Journal of Pharmaceutical Sciences* 59 (1970): 1699–1727.

La Barre, W. "Peyotl and Mescaline." *Journal of Psychedelic Drugs* 11 (1979): 33–39.

Phendimetrazine

Pronunciation: fen-di-MEH-tra-zeen (also pronounced fen-dye-MEH-trah-zeen)

Chemical Abstracts Service Registry Number: 21784-30-5 (Bontril format); 569-59-5 (Plegine format); 50-58-8 (Prelu-2 format).

Formal Names: Bontril, Plegine, Prelu-2

Informal Names: Pink Hearts

Type: Stimulant (anorectic class). *See* page 15

Federal Schedule Listing: Schedule III (DEA no. 1615)

USA Availability: Prescription

Pregnancy Category: C

Uses. Phendimetrazine is related to **phenmetrazine**. Indeed, the body converts part of a phendimetrazine dose into phenmetrazine, a fact to be remembered if employment drug screening unjustly accuses someone of using phenmetrazine. Short-term weight control is the main medical use of phendimetrazine; one experiment found it 20 more times effective than placebo—an astonishing result for any diet pill. Effectiveness declines as administration continues, and standard practice is then to stop the drug gradually rather than increase the dosage. A derivative of the drug has been found useful for treating pyoderma gangrenosum, a skin affliction involving large sores.

Drawbacks. If dosage suddenly stops, weariness and depression can occur. A small reduction in blood pressure is observed among some users, but generally the drug raises blood pressure and is considered inappropriate for persons with hypertension (high blood pressure). The compound has been linked with hypertension in blood circulation to lungs, a potentially fatal condition causing trouble in breathing. Users have experienced edginess, disturbed sleep, headache, dizziness, lightheadedness, accelerated pulse rate, and feelings of heart tremors. Other muscle tremors can occur. Phendimetrazine can interfere with functioning needed to handle a car or dangerous tools. The compound can dry and even inflame the mouth, upset the stomach, loosen or tighten the bowels, and make urination frequent and painful. Persons should avoid the drug if they suffer from restlessness, glaucoma, excessive thyroid activity, heart disease, hardening of the arteries, or drug abuse. The substance may affect diabetics' insulin needs. Overdose symptoms are similar to those of amphetamine: hyperactivity, fear, aggression, hallucination.

Abuse factors. Phendimetrazine is a chemical relative of amphetamine and is therefore considered addictive. In an experiment using rhesus monkeys to measure phendimetrazine's addictive potential, however, the test animals indicated no interest in it. This same study showed the drug having about 10% to 20% of **dextroamphetamine**'s potency.

Drug interactions. Drinking milk can counteract phendimetrazine's anorectic quality. The drug can dangerously increase blood pressure by interacting with monoamine oxidase inhibitors (MAOIs, found in some antidepressants and other medicine). After highly publicized incidents of adverse effects associated with combination therapy of **phentermine** and **fenfluramine**, medical practitioners became especially alert to any problems associated with diet drugs. Someone taking phendimetrazine two times a day developed heart and lung difficulty that substantially improved when dosage was halted, and a case of temporary skin rash and kidney inflammation is reported from someone who was taking phendimetrazine and phentermine. The latter drug combination is also suspected of responsibility for temporary trouble with blood circulation in the brain (leading to a stroke in at least one instance). Whether these isolated cases can be extrapolated into general principle is questionable, but such reports raise questions worthy of further scientific investigation.

Cancer. Not enough scientific information to report.

Pregnancy. Impact on fetal development is unknown. The drug is not recommended for pregnant women.

Additional scientific information may be found in:

Hadler, A.J. "Sustained-Action Phendimetrazine in Obesity." *Journal of Clinical Pharmacology* 8 (1968): 113–17.

Mazansky, H. "A Review of Obesity and Its Management in 263 Cases." *South African Medical Journal* 49 (1975): 1955–62.

Ressler, C., and S.H. Schneider. "Clinical Evaluation of Phendimetrazine Bitartrate." *Clinical Pharmacology and Therapeutics* 2 (1961): 727–32.

Rostagno, C., et al. "Dilated Cardiomyopathy Associated with Chronic Consumption of Phendimetrazine." *American Heart Journal* 131 (1996): 407–409.

Runyan, J.W. "Observations on the Use of Phendimetrazine, a New Anorexigenic Agent, in Obese Diabetics." *Current Therapeutic Research: Clinical and Experimental* 4 (1962): 270–75.

Sash, S.E. "Anorectic Effects of OBEX LA (D-Phendimetrazine Bitartrate) in the Treatment of Obesity." *Current Therapeutic Research: Clinical and Experimental* 31 (1982): 181–84.

Phenmetrazine

Pronunciation: fen-MET-rah-zeen

Chemical Abstracts Service Registry Number: 134-49-6

Formal Names: Filon, Preludin

Informal Names: Sweeties

Type: Stimulant (anorectic class). *See* page 15

Federal Schedule Listing: Schedule II (DEA no. 1631)

USA Availability: Prescription

Uses. Immediately upon announcement of the drug's discovery in 1954 it was utilized in Germany as an appetite suppressant. A couple years later the same medical use began in the United States with expansive claims about patients obtaining substantial weight loss without having to follow a regimen of dieting, claims that became more modest as experience with the drug spread. One experiment testing the drug's influence on appetite yielded a result relevant to drug experiments in general: The substance worked better when people knew its intended effect. If people knew they were supposed to feel less hungry, they noticed less desire for food and then ate less. Early reports praised phenmetrazine for producing more appetite loss than amphetamine and with fewer unwanted effects. Since then phenmetrazine has fallen into disfavor due to concern about addictive potential even though the drug is described as resembling **caffeine** more than amphetamine.

In dogs phenmetrazine has only one sixth to one tenth the strength of amphetamine. One type of canine experiment showed **dextroamphetamine** to be 250 times stronger than phenmetrazine. In dogs a much higher dose of phenmetrazine is needed for the same weight loss produced by **benzphetamine**, and an experiment with 75 humans had results consistent with that tendency, finding phenmetrazine to be less effective than benzphetamine in promoting weight loss. In contrast, another human weight reduction experiment with 81 persons was unable to demonstrate such a difference. That study did show, however, that users obtain fewer amphetamine effects from phenmetrazine than from dextroamphetamine.

Phenmetrazine has worked as an antidepressant, and for some overweight persons that effect may enhance the drug's appeal (overeating can be a response to depression). The substance shows effectiveness against motion sickness and against symptoms of diabetes insipidus. As a possible cure for bedwetting, the drug produced mixed results. The compound has also been used to treat asthma and Parkinson's disease.

Drawbacks. Intravenous abuse can harm muscles and kidneys. Phenmetrazine can produce standard amphetamine effects such as euphoria, restlessness, jumpiness, insomnia, tics, fatigue reduction, faster breathing, and higher blood pressure. Studies have found phenmetrazine's actions on patients with heart trouble or hypertension (high blood pressure) to be measurable but negligible. Taking the high blood pressure medicine propranolol along with phenmetrazine can relieve cardiac effects without diminishing anorectic effects. Studies with diabetic users find phenmetrazine having little influence on blood sugar levels or on insulin needs.

Fluctuating emotions and even psychosis have been attributed to phenmetrazine abuse. Psychosis can include hallucinations and paranoia. That affliction can stop when drug taking stops, or instead the drug may break down barriers releasing full-fledged and long-lasting schizophrenia. Phenmetrazine interferes with dreaming during sleep, which in itself may cause psychological trouble.

Abuse factors. Tests of drug preference, in which users could choose among several substances, found benzphetamine and phenmetrazine to have about the same amount of appeal even though benzphetamine is a Schedule III substance (a status implying a lower addictive potential than phenmetrazine). In one such test, volunteers found phenmetrazine to be a satisfying substitute for dextroamphetamine but preferred the latter. Abusers of amphetamine and **methamphetamine** have routinely switched to phenmetrazine when their favored drug was unavailable.

Drug interactions. An experiment found that chlorpromazine (Thorazine) interacts with phenmetrazine, hindering phenmetrazine's normal anorectic benefit.

Cancer. In pregnant women phenmetrazine may undergo transformations suspected of promoting childhood tumors.

Pregnancy. Phenmetrazine was formerly prescribed to pregnant women seeking to lose weight. A study of over 10,000 birth and childhood records found the drug having no "severe" impact on fetal development. Other studies have found no birth defects at all, although medical literature from the early 1960s does contain a handful of reports in which the drug is suspected of harming fetuses. Those suspicions were never verified but were strong enough to suspend medical use of the drug in some countries for a while.

Combination products. Filon combines phenmetrazine theoclate (CAS RN 13931-75-4) and phenbutrazate hydrochloride and is promoted as having phenmetrazine's weight loss characteristics while lacking hazard of addiction. Initial clinical trials showed Filon to be an effective anorectic with fewer of phenmetrazine's unwanted qualities, but a later study found the two drugs to have the same unwanted effects. A case of Filon addiction also surfaced, but that single instance hardly proves Filon to have more addictive potential than any other drug considered to have low or zero potential.

Additional scientific information may be found in:

Gilstrap, L.C. III, and B.B. Little, eds. *Drugs and Pregnancy.* New York: Elsevier, 1992.
Martin, W.R., et al. "Physiologic, Subjective, and Behavioral Effects of Amphetamine,

Methamphetamine, Ephedrine, Phenmetrazine, and Methylphenidate in Man." *Clinical Pharmacology and Therapeutics* 12 (1971): 245–58.

Mellar, J., and L.E. Hollister. "Phenmetrazine: An Obsolete Problem Drug." *Clinical Pharmacology and Therapeutics* 32 (1982): 671–75.

Negulici, E., and D. Christodorescu. "Phenmetrazine Psychosis." *British Medical Journal* 3 (1968): 316.

Penick, S.B, and J.R. Hinklele. "The Effect of Expectation on Response to Phenmetrazine." *Psychosomatic Medicine* 26 (1964): 369–73.

Rosen, A., and I.J. Oberman. "Addiction to Phenmetrazine Hydrochloride and Its Psychiatric Implications." *Journal of the American Osteopathic Association* 59 (1960): 722–26.

Spillane, J.P. "The Use of Phenmetrazine." *The Practitioner* 185 (1960): 102–6.

Phenobarbital

Pronunciation: feen-oh-BAR-bi-tall

Chemical Abstracts Service Registry Number: 50-06-6

Formal Names: Arco-Lase Plus, Donnatal, Gardenal, Luminal, Phenobarb, Phenobarbitone, Solfoton

Informal Names: Phennies, Phenos

Type: Depressant (barbiturate class). *See* page 20

Federal Schedule Listing: Schedule IV (DEA no. 2285)

USA Availability: Prescription

Pregnancy Category: D

Uses. This is one of the more familiar pharmaceuticals. For about a century it has been used as an anticonvulsant and was prescribed as a tranquilizer and as a migraine remedy, although all those functions are being superseded by more modern drugs. Phenobarbital is also given to treat cyclic vomiting in children and hyperbilirubinemia (a type of jaundice) in infants. The drug is used against epilepsy and against seizures with other causes, such as fever. The substance has cross-tolerance with **alcohol** and is given temporarily to help relieve withdrawal symptoms from opiates or alcohol. Despite acceptance of phenobarbital for that purpose, scientific proof is lacking for its usefulness in alcohol withdrawal.

Phenobarbital played a walk-on role in the history of drug manufacturing when it was discovered as a contaminant in a batch of the antibiotic sulfathiazole. After that 1941 discovery the U.S. Food and Drug Administration created the system of manufacturing controls that has made the terms "purity" and "American pharmaceuticals" synonymous.

Drawbacks. Experimental use of the drug to treat cerebral malaria in juveniles was disastrous. The treatment halved the seizure rate but doubled the death rate, a rate that climbed even higher when **diazepam** was administered in combination. Some medical personnel have noted that patients taking phenobarbital tend to become more bellicose and uncooperative. A medical curiosity noted as late as the 1960s was that persons could be pronounced dead from a phenobarbital overdose and later be discovered alive.

In some research children receiving the drug for seizures show long-lasting reduction in IQ scores and in scores of other cognitive tests, but different research finds normal results after children have received the drug daily for years. Phenobarbital is known to alter adrenal and thyroid mechanisms. Persons suffering from a body chemistry disorder called porphyria are supposed to avoid the drug. Skin rashes and sores have been attributed to phenobarbital. Scientists suspect the drug causes liver damage in dogs, but an experiment testing a group of dogs for over six months was unable to confirm that suspicion.

Abuse factors. Characteristics are the same as for barbiturate class depressants in general.

Drug interactions. Birth control pills might not work properly while a woman is taking phenobarbital. The drug may interfere with medicines designed to reduce blood clotting. Phenobarbital lowers blood levels of an antischizophrenia medicine called clozapine and thereby affects proper dosage.

Persons taking phenobarbital in a task performance test typed more slowly but more accurately, catching and fixing more errors than when a placebo was used. Taking alcohol at the same time increased both speed and errors, but typists believed they were working as well as ever and were unaware of their worsening inaccuracy. From results in variations of the experiment the researchers concluded that alcohol boosts some effects of phenobarbital.

Cancer. In some mice experiments the drug promotes liver tumors, but complexities in the results have deterred researchers from making conclusions about the drug's ability to do the same in humans. Scientists do find that persons using the drug have higher rates of liver and lung cancer, but a cause-effect relationship has not been demonstrated. In contrast, cigarette smokers who use the drug have lower bladder cancer rates than nonsmokers; as a partial explanation, researchers suspect the drug may reduce the amount of chemicals in tobacco smoke that cause bladder cancer.

Pregnancy. In animal experiments birth defects caused by phenobarbital are described as "profound and prominent." For example, pregnant mice dosed with phenobarbital produce offspring with retarded muscle development, and pregnant rats receiving the drug produce offspring with heart defects.

Debate exists about whether phenobarbital causes human birth defects. Medical records in 151 human pregnancies from the 1970s into the 1990s gave no indication that phenobarbital alone causes malformations, a conclusion supported by another study of 178 pregnancies. In Europe phenobarbital has been classified as safe for using during pregnancy.

Yet a review of almost 20,000 pregnancies found that 4.6% of children born to women who used phenobarbital during early pregnancy had birth defects, almost twice the rate suffered by children from women who used no drugs. An international examination of almost 1,000 birth outcomes in Asia and Europe put the rate of all defects (serious or not) associated with phenobarbital at 5%. Investigations have associated phenobarbital with heart defects, facial deformities, urinary tract malformations, and incomplete development of fingers or toes. One study found that about 20% of pregnant epileptic women taking the drug gave birth to children with serious birth defects, a finding consistent with still more studies. One study compared pregnant epileptic women who used phenobarbital with those who did not and revealed that women using the drug had infants with smaller head size. As children from the phenobarbital group grew older, they had shorter attention spans and more trouble with spelling and math.

Worse deformities have been seen when phenobarbital is used in combination with some other drugs than when used alone. A review of epilepsy medicines published in 1997 said malformations from phenobarbital are no more likely than from carbamazepine, phenytoin, or valproic acid—yet those latter three substances have been found to cause birth defects. A 1994 analysis of outcomes in several hundred pregnancies concluded that birth defects were more likely from phenobarbital than from carbamazepine or phenytoin.

Phenobarbital and other epilepsy drugs may reduce vitamin K levels in a fetus, a reduction that can promote bleeding and cause disfiguring birth defects. Some researchers think that pregnant women using such drugs should ingest extra vitamin K.

Researchers believe that pregnant rats receiving phenobarbital seem to produce male offspring with "feminized behavior" and female offspring with masculine behavior. A group of humans who were prenatally exposed to phenobarbital showed higher rates of homosexual, cross-gender, and transsexual behavior when compared to a matched group that had no prenatal exposure to phenobarbital.

After phenobarbital is given to pregnant rats, their mature progeny act more nervous and uneasy than mature progeny from rats not exposed to the drug during pregnancy and also exhibit defects in reproductive ability. Mice exposed to the drug during fetal development and soon after birth show improper functioning of the hippocampus (a part of the brain affecting memory), and their brains weigh less than normal. Tests of thinking ability in adult humans whose mothers used phenobarbital and phenytoin while pregnant reveal deficiency in perceiving differences among geometrical figures. Other research has found that such adults generally have normal intelligence but are far likelier to have learning difficulties than adults who did not have prenatal exposure to the phenobarbital-phenytoin combination. Two studies have found verbal intelligence scores to be below expectations in men whose mothers took phenobarbital while pregnant, and another study found psychological maturation to be slowed in about 20% of children whose mothers received phenobarbital while pregnant. The director of a National Institutes of Health research center reported contrary findings in which offspring performed better if their mothers had used phenobarbital while pregnant, but analysts have noted methodological aspects in that study that weaken its findings.

The drug is sometimes given to pregnant women having premature labor, to reduce the hazard of infants developing bleeding inside the skull. One follow-through study found that infants born to pregnant women receiving such therapy had better nervous system development than children from mothers who did not receive such therapy, measured both in organic and cognitive factors. Another study measuring two such populations found the phenobarbital children to have lower mental development.

If a pregnant woman uses phenobarbital her infant can be born dependent on the drug; neonatal withdrawal is characterized by peevishness, vomiting, and poor muscle tone. Typically a nursing woman's milk will contain about 45% of the phenobarbital level found in her blood. Breast-feeding by mothers who use phenobarbital is considered marginally acceptable, but infants should be watched for untoward effects.

Combination products. Arco-Lase Plus combines phenobarbital, hyoscyamine sulfate, and atropine sulfate. The product is a remedy for digestive complaints ranging from bloat and cramps to nausea, diarrhea, and ulcers. Arco-Lase Plus can impair vision and is not recommended for persons with glaucoma. The substance increases heart rate and reduces saliva production. The combination product should be avoided by persons suffering from enlarged prostate.

Donnatal combines phenobarbital, hyoscyamine sulfate, atropine sulfate, and scopolamine hydrobromide. The combination product is a treatment for assorted bowel complaints and duodenal ulcers. Normally Donnatal is considered inappropriate for persons with glaucoma or with gastrointestinal or urinary obstruction. The substance may decrease alertness, so a person taking Donnatal should not run dangerous machinery.

Additional scientific information may be found in:

Joyce, C.R., et al. "Potentiation by Phenobarbitone of Effects of Ethyl Alcohol on Human Behaviour." *Journal of Mental Science* 105 (1959): 51–60.

Lerman-Sagie, T., and P. Lerman. "Phenobarbital Still Has a Role in Epilepsy Treatment." *Journal of Child Neurology* 14 (1999): 820–21.

"Phenobarbital." In *Therapeutic Drugs*, ed. C. Dollery. 2d ed. New York: Churchill Livingstone, 1999. P83–P85.

Poindexter, A.R. "Phenobarbital, Propranolol, and Aggression." *Journal of Neuropsychiatry and Clinical Neurosciences* 12 (2000): 413.

Reinisch, J.M., et al. "In Utero Exposure to Phenobarbital and Intelligence Deficits in Adult Men." *Journal of the American Medical Association* 274 (1995): 1518–25.

Rodgers, J.E., and M.A. Crouch. "Phenobarbital for Alcohol Withdrawal Syndrome." *American Journal of Health-System Pharmacy* 56 (1999): 175–78.

Phenoperidine

Pronunciation: fee-noh-PER-i-deen

Chemical Abstracts Service Registry Number: 562-26-5

Formal Names: Operidine

Type: Depressant (opioid class). *See* page 24

Federal Schedule Listing: Schedule I (DEA no. 9641)

USA Availability: Illegal to possess

Pregnancy Category: None

Uses. This drug has no officially approved medical use in the United States. Elsewhere (such as Sweden, France, and Great Britain) the substance is administered for sedation and pain relief, much like **morphine**. For example, phenoperidine is used to calm patients and to cloud unpleasant memory of procedures such as a cataract operation or sticking tubes down passages in the throat or lungs. Phenoperidine is also used in major dental work, such as extraction of wisdom teeth. The substance has been recommended for children in intensive-care units, partly because it normally has modest impact on heart and breathing functions when used in a medical context. Medical practitioners report the drug also has excellent anesthesia results in elderly abdominal surgery patients. Very young and very old populations can be among the most challenging for safe drug treatment, so these favorable results are especially important for evaluating the drug. Phenoperidine takes effect quickly and has a relatively prolonged time of therapeutic action.

One study found phenoperidine, morphine, and **fentanyl** to have about equivalent value for anesthesia, although the drugs are not equivalent in strength. For example, intravenous doses of fentanyl are 6 times stronger than phenoperidine, and phenoperidine is 5 to 10 times stronger than morphine. A study found phenoperidine as effective as **heroin** in relieving pain from cesarean section. Body chemistry transforms a portion of a phenoperidine dose into **meperidine**.

Drawbacks. Unwanted effects can include itching, nausea, vomiting, and breathing trouble. Reports exist of heart and brain damage caused by medical doses.

Abuse factors. Dependence can develop.

Drug interactions. Reports indicate phenoperidine can reduce blood pressure, and the compound is suspected of interacting with propranolol (a drug used to control high blood pressure), thereby producing extremely low blood pressure. Cases of major circulatory collapse are known.

Cancer. Not enough scientific information to report.

Pregnancy. Experimentation with mice has shown birth defects to be less likely from phenoperidine than from other drugs with similar medical uses, but that finding does not mean the substance is safe for use during pregnancy. Clinical observations have detected no fetal or newborn injury when phenoperidine was used as an anesthetic in childbirth.

Additional scientific information may be found in:

Grummitt, R.M., and V.A. Goat. "Intracranial Pressure after Phenoperidine." *Anaesthesia* 39 (1984): 565–67.

Macrae, D.J., et al. "Double-Blind Comparison of the Efficacy of Extradural Diamorphine, Extradural Phenoperidine and I.m. Diamorphine Following Caesarean Section." *British Journal of Anaesthesia* 59 (1987): 354–59.

"Phenoperidine HCl." In *Therapeutic Drugs*, ed. C. Dollery. 2d ed. New York: Churchill Livingstone, 1999. P89–P90.

Werner, D., et al. "A Comparison of Diazepam and Phenoperidine in Premedication for Upper Gastrointestinal Endoscopy: A Randomized Double Blind Controlled Study." *European Journal of Clinical Pharmacology* 22 (1982): 143–45.

Whalley, D.G., et al. "A Comparison of the Incidence of Cardiac Arrhythmia during Two Methods of Anaesthesia for Dental Extractions." *British Journal of Anaesthesia* 48 (1976): 1207–10.

Phentermine

Pronunciation: FEN-ter-meen

Chemical Abstracts Service Registry Number: 122-09-8. (Hydrochloride form 1197-21-3)

Formal Names: Adipex-P, Duromine, Fastin, Ionamin, Obe-Nix 30, Umine

Informal Names: Robin's Eggs

Type: Stimulant (anorectic class). *See* page 15

Federal Schedule Listing: Schedule IV (DEA no. 1640)

USA Availability: Prescription

Pregnancy Category: C

Uses. Phentermine is primarily used on a short-term basis for weight reduction. The compound is related to amphetamine. Effects are similar to but weaker than those of **dextroamphetamine**. For example, phentermine can make users more physically energetic. A study found phentermine more effective than **diethylpropion** for promoting weight loss, a superiority attributed to phentermine's ability to retain therapeutic effectiveness longer before tolerance sets in. Standard medical practice is to stop taking the drug when tolerance develops, instead of increasing the dose.

In one study symptoms of depression improved among overweight people using phentermine. Researchers ascribe that improvement to the drug, but perhaps users simply felt good about shedding pounds. Some research indicates that the drug acts as a monoamine oxidase inhibitor (MAOI), which thereby associates phentermine with a number of antidepressants, but other research has challenged that finding.

Drawbacks. Phentermine may interfere with sleep, cause dry mouth, make bowel movements looser or harder, produce impotence, make people edgy and ill-tempered, or (in contrast) create euphoria. The compound is suspected of involvement with stroke, but reported cases have confounding factors. In one instance the patient had a history of headaches before taking phentermine and a family history of migraine and stroke. In another case the person was also taking **phendimetrazine**, had used birth control pills for 14 years, had smoked cigarettes for two decades, and had a personal history of migraines and a family history of high cholesterol and high blood pressure. Phentermine has also been linked to narrowing of abdominal arteries with a possibility of ruptured aneurysms there. Uncommon accounts exist of phentermine users developing primary pulmonary hypertension, a major and often fatal affliction involving blood circulation through the lungs. The drug is not recommended for persons with heart ailment, serious hardening of the arteries, high blood pressure, glaucoma, or an overactive thyroid gland. The drug may impair ability to operate tools and machinery, such as automobiles.

Someone taking phentermine came down with a psychosis that cleared up after stopping the drug. Initially the affliction was blamed on the drug, but the person later developed paranoid schizophrenia, a development suggesting that the drug promoted but did not cause the initial psychosis. The incident did not demonstrate that phentermine will cause psychosis in healthy people. With someone else, symptoms mimicking schizophrenia appeared when dosage of phentermine increased and stopped after ingestion of phentermine stopped. In another case a user began seeing people appear and vanish, heard things no one else could perceive, and started experiencing paranoia—afflictions attributed to the drug. Such reports became numerous enough that practitioners were advised to limit the drug's use to only a few weeks. Adverse psychological reactions are a known hazard of overdose. Physicians have publicly cautioned against exceeding recommended dosage and against prescribing to persons with personal or family histories of mental illness.

Abuse factors. Research is uncommon on phentermine's specific tolerance, dependence, withdrawal, and addiction potentials, but such factors are probably similar to those of stimulants in general. Animal and human experiments suggest that phentermine may help cocaine addicts decrease their use of the latter drug.

Drug interactions. Because of phentermine's possible MAOI properties it should normally be avoided if a patient is taking some other MAOI, and it may have untoward effect if **alcohol** beverages are consumed.

For years "fen-phen" was a widely prescribed weight reduction combination of phentermine and **fenfluramine**. In 1997 controversy arose about whether the combination caused serious and sometimes fatal heart disease; for details see this book's entry about fenfluramine. Heart disease has been reported following use of phentermine with other drugs as well and, more rarely, without taking any other drugs. In contrast, one practitioner who treated hundreds of patients with phentermine found no evidence of cardiac disease caused by the drug used alone or in combination with the antidepressant fluoxetine (Prozac). That latter "phen-pro" combination has been reported as causing adverse reaction similar to amphetamine overdose, but such reports are uncommon.

Cancer. Not enough scientific information to report.

Pregnancy. Researchers seeking evidence of human birth defects report that standard medical usage in the first trimester found none attributable to the drug.

Additional information. Adipex-P and Fastin are the slightly less potent hydrochloride form of the substance (30 mg of phentermine hydrochloride roughly equals 24 mg of phentermine). The potential for causing cancer or birth defects is unestablished. This form may enter human milk if nursing mothers take the drug.

Additional scientific information may be found in:

Alger, S.A., et al. "Beneficial Effects of Pharmacotherapy on Weight Loss, Depressive Symptoms, and Eating Patterns in Obese Binge Eaters and Non-Binge Eaters." *Obesity Research* 7 (1999): 469–76.

Brauer, L.H., et al. "Evaluation of Phentermine and Fenfluramine, Alone and in Combination, in Normal, Healthy Volunteers." *Neuropsychopharmacology* 14 (1996): 233–41.

Devlin, M.J., et al. "Open Treatment of Overweight Binge Eaters with Phentermine and Fluoxetine as an Adjunct to Cognitive-Behavioral Therapy." *International Journal of Eating Disorders* 28 (2000): 325–32.

Douglas, A. "Plasma Phentermine Levels, Weight Loss and Side-Effects." *International Journal of Obesity* 7 (1983): 591–95.

Griffen, L., and M. Anchors. "The 'Phen-Pro' Diet Drug Combination Is Not Associated with Valvular Heart Disease." *Archives of Internal Medicine* 158 (1998): 1278–79.

Hoffman, B.F. "Diet Pill Psychosis: Follow-up after 6 Years." *Canadian Medical Association Journal* 129 (1983): 1077–78.

Jones, K.L., et al. "Pregnancy Outcomes after First Trimester Exposure to Phentermine/Fenfluramine." *Teratology* 65 (2002): 125–30.

Kokkinos, J., and S.R. Levine. "Possible Association of Ischemic Stroke with Phentermine." *Stroke* 24 (1993): 310–13.

Langlois, K.J., et al. "Double-Blind Clinical Evaluation of the Safety and Efficacy of Phentermine Hydrochloride (Fastin) in the Treatment of Exogenous Obesity." *Current Therapeutic Research: Clinical and Experimental* 16 (1974): 289–96.

Pholcodine

Pronunciation: FAHL-koh-deen

Chemical Abstracts Service Registry Number: 509-67-1

Formal Names: Actuss, Codylin, Dia-Tuss, Duro-Tuss Liquid, Ethnine, Evafol, Galenphol, Hibernyl, Homocodeine, Memine, Neocodine, Pectolin, Pholtrate, Tixylix Night-Time, Tussokon

Type: Depressant (opiate class). *See* page 22

Federal Schedule Listing: Schedule I (DEA no. 9314)

USA Availability: Illegal to possess

Pregnancy Category: None

Uses. This **morphine** derivative has no officially recognized medical use in the United States. Elsewhere, in countries ranging from Germany to Australia, it is used in dozens of cough remedies and has often been given to children for that purpose. Pholcodine is also a component of preparations used to fight colds and influenza, with effects likened to those of **dextromethorphan**. Various species of animals tolerate higher doses of pholcodine than **codeine**, and pholcodine appears safer than codeine in humans. Animal experiments show pholcodine to be an anticonvulsant, unlike morphine, which can worsen convulsions.

The drug has been administered to mice and rats in low daily doses for one to three months without evidence of ill effect. Rats show normal appetite, weight, red and white blood cell counts, and appearance of other body cells.

Drawbacks. Animal studies show pholcodine to depress breathing and heart actions more than codeine does, but impact on those functions has not been noted in humans. Unwanted effects can include sleepiness, nausea, and constipation, but medical doses normally avoid other typical adverse actions associated with opiates. In Scotland accidental poisonings of children who drank a pleasant-tasting cough syrup containing pholcodine became common enough that a call arose to sell the product in child-resistant packaging.

Abuse factors. Pholcodine is one of the few opiates that athletes are allowed to use in Olympic and other sports competitions. The general ban exists not because opiates inherently promote better performance but because their ability to relieve pain can give an athlete an advantage over competitors who are hurting; animal studies show pholcodine to have little value in pain relief.

The substance can still be detected in urine seven weeks after a single dose of cough medicine, a characteristic that can cause positive opiate results for persons undergoing drug screens from employers. Body chemistry slowly breaks down pholcodine into several substances. Some studies find tiny amounts of morphine in breakdown products, but other studies do not. Pholcodine has been described as unable to cause euphoria, a lack that reduces its abuse potential. No tolerance has been observed among patients using the substance every day for months. Experiments looking for dependence find none. Tests for cross-tolerance with morphine produce negative results in humans. One scientific review of pholcodine describes it as having no addiction potential, a view supported by UN drug control authorities. A World Health Organization committee characterizes the drug as having no more addiction potential than codeine. U.S. government officials have ruled that pholcodine is extremely prone to abuse and list the drug as a Schedule I controlled substance.

Drug interactions. Not enough scientific information to report.

Cancer. Not enough scientific information to report.

Pregnancy. Birth defects have not been associated with the substance. A study of women who used pholcodine during pregnancy found no impact on infants. In Europe the drug has been classified as safe for use in pregnancy, but in the United States the drug is not recommended for pregnant women; safety for use during pregnancy has not been established. The substance passes into human milk, and nursing infants are supposed to be watched for signs of drug effects.

Additional scientific information may be found in:

Cahen, R. "The Pharmacology of Pholcodine." *Bulletin on Narcotics* 13 no. 2 (1961): 19–37.

Findlay, J.W. "Pholcodine." *Journal of Clinical Pharmacy and Therapeutics* 13 (1988): 5–17.

"Pholcodine." In *Therapeutic Drugs*, ed. C. Dollery. 2d ed. New York: Churchill Livingstone, 1999. P115–P116.

Piritramide

Pronunciation: pih-RIH-trah-mide

Chemical Abstracts Service Registry Number: 302-41-0

Formal Names: Dipidolor, Dipiritramide, Piridolan

Type: Depressant (opioid class). *See* page 24

Federal Schedule Listing: Schedule I (DEA no. 9642)

USA Availability: Illegal to possess

Pregnancy Category: None

Uses. This drug was developed in the 1960s. It is related to **meperidine** but has no recognized medical use in the United States. Elsewhere (Germany, Belgium, the Netherlands, Eastern Europe) piritramide is used as a long-lasting and powerful pain reliever for adults and children. Its strength is similar to **morphine**'s, though a little less potent. After a wide variety of surgeries (such as facial, heart, urinary system, hip replacement) patients have been allowed to control their own piritramide dosage with satisfactory results. A clinical study found that females received better pain relief, and from smaller amounts of piritramide, than males did. The drug also has a calming action.

The possibility that the drug might protect against ill effects of radiation has been tested in Russian animal research without success. Judging from other articles in the journal reporting that research, the study may have been related to civil defense preparations against nuclear weapons attack during the 1980s.

Drawbacks. Unwanted effects can include perspiration, blood vessel inflammation, localized muscle damage, urine retention, nausea, vomiting, dizziness, and flushing. Breathing difficulty is a possibility but is seldom observed in medical contexts. Human experience and rat experimentation show that habitual intramuscular injection of piritramide can destroy muscle tissue.

Abuse factors. Not enough scientific information to report.

Drug interactions. Not enough scientific information to report.

Cancer. Not enough scientific information to report.

Pregnancy. Not enough scientific information to report.

Additional scientific information may be found in:

Knoche, E., et al. "Clinical Experimental Studies of Postoperative Infusion Analgesia." *Clinical Therapeutics* 5 (1983): 585–94.

Kumar, N., and D.J. Rowbotham. "Piritramide." *British Journal of Anaesthesia* 82 (1999): 3–5.

Lehmann, K.A., B. Tenbuhs, and W. Hoeckle. "Patient-Controlled Analgesia with Piritramid for the Treatment of Postoperative Pain." *Acta Anaesthesiologica Belgica* 37 (1986): 247–57.

Mollmann, M., and U. Auf der Landwehr. "Treatment of Pain in Trauma Patients with Injuries of the Upper Limb." *Injury* 31 (2000, Suppl. 1): 3–10.

Petrat, G., U. Klein, and W. Meissner. "On-Demand Analgesia with Piritramide in Children: A Study on Dosage Specification and Safety." *European Journal of Pediatric Surgery* 7 (1997): 38–41.

Van den Bergh, P.Y., et al. "Focal Myopathy Associated with Chronic Intramuscular Injection of Piritramide." *Muscle and Nerve* 20 (1997): 1598–600.

Prazepam

Pronunciation: PRAY-zee-pam (also pronounced PRAZ-eh-pam)

Chemical Abstracts Service Registry Number: 2955-38-6

Formal Names: Centrax, Demetrin, Verstran

Type: Depressant (benzodiazepine class). *See* page 21

Federal Schedule Listing: Schedule IV (DEA no. 2764)

USA Availability: Prescription

Pregnancy Category: None

Uses. In the human body this long-acting drug converts into desmethyldi-azepam, which is called a metabolite. Desmethyldiazepam is the major metabolite of **diazepam** and also a metabolite of **clorazepate** dipotassium and **chlordiazepoxide**. Some researchers believe this metabolite produces the main drug effects of prazepam and that prazepam should therefore be considered a prodrug (meaning the substance itself has little drug value but that within the body it converts into another substance that is beneficial). Prazepam resembles **oxazepam** both in chemistry and in its effects.

Prazepam is used medically to relieve anxiety and is considered as effective as **alprazolam** and **lorazepam** for that purpose even though they are much stronger drugs than prazepam. One study found prazepam to work better than diazepam for treating anxiety, although diazepam is about twice as potent. A comparison with chlordiazepoxide showed mixed results; chlordiazepoxide produced faster general betterment of anxiety, but prazepam was more effective at improving particular symptoms. Prazepam has also been used successfully for treatment of depression and crankiness. One clinical trial produced weight gain in patients using the drug, but perhaps this was due to better appetite resulting from better mood, rather than an inherent weight-promoting quality of the drug. Some scientists have wondered if the drug improves mood simply by helping patients to get better sleep; researchers investigating that question concluded that the drug does have antianxiety qualities causing the improvement. In evaluating results of a rat experiment, researchers concluded that prazepam may be useful for treating high blood pressure. Animal studies also find the drug to be a muscle relaxant and to reduce convulsions.

The drug has been used to help alcoholics withdraw from **alcohol**. In one study group several patients had experienced delirium tremens when withdrawing from alcohol in the past, but no one suffered the affliction while receiving prazepam. A subsequent study of alcohol withdrawal management rated prazepam as better than placebo but not as good as chlordiazepoxide. The latter study also found that benefits declined with time; after 14 days the placebo, chlordiazepoxide, and prazepam groups of alcoholics were all faring the same. Also during the latter study, in comparison to placebo, about three times as many patients receiving prazepam broke sobriety—a curious and discouraging finding.

Drawbacks. Volunteers taking prazepam showed little sedation and little difference in mental ability tests when compared to performance before taking the drug. Prazepam has been praised for having fewer unwanted effects than diazepam, and for being better absorbed by the body than clorazepate dipotassium. In one experiment a single large dose at night produced less dizziness than taking three divided doses during the day, a factor relevant to the potential of falls (especially among the elderly). Unwanted effects can include dry mouth, weakness, and sleepiness. Tests comparing equivalent-strength oral doses of the drug in liquid and solid formats find the liquid version to be a more potent sedative, a difference ascribed to quicker absorption by the body. In an experiment testing the drug on people of various ages, a dose seemed to last longer in older men, but that change was not seen in older women. An experiment found the drug's effect on movement was similar to that of chlordiazepoxide, suggesting that operating an automobile might be dangerous when using prazepam.

Abuse factors. Not enough scientific information to report about prazepam's specific characteristics, but they should be consistent with general characteristics of the benzodiazepine class of depressants.

Drug interactions. The antacid remedy cimetidine probably slows the body's metabolism of prazepam. Scores on tests of reaction time and mental ability can become worse when alcohol is used along with prazepam.

Cancer. Two experiments, one with rats and one with mice, failed to demonstrate potential for causing cancer. Potential for causing human cancer is unknown.

Pregnancy. A small amount of the drug passes from a nursing mother into her milk.

Additional scientific information may be found in:

Daniel, J.T., and W.W.K. Zung. "Double Blind Clinical Comparison of Prazepam, Lorazepam, Diazepam, and Placebo in the Treatment of Anxiety in a Private Surgical Outpatient Practice." *Current Therapeutic Research: Clinical and Experimental* 30 (1981): 417–26.
Dorman, T. "Multicenter Comparison of Prazepam and Diazepam in the Treatment of Anxiety." *Pharmatherapeutica* 3 (1983): 433–40.
Greenblatt, D.J., and R.I. Shader. "Prazepam and Lorazepam, Two New Benzodiazepines." *New England Journal of Medicine* 299 (1978): 1342–44.
Guelfi, J.D., S. Lancrenon, and V. Millet. "Étude Comparative en Double Insu du Bromazepam versus Prazepam dans l'anxiete Non Psychotique [Comparative Double-Blind Study of Bromazepam versus Prazepam in Non-Psychotic Anxiety]." *L'Encephale* 19 (1993): 547–52. Abstract in English.
Kingstone, E., A. Villeneuve, and I. Kossatz. "Double-Blind Evaluation of Prazepam,

Chlordiazepoxide and Placebo in Non-Psychotic Patients with Anxiety and Tension: Some Methodological Considerations." *Current Therapeutic Research: Clinical and Experimental* 11 (1969): 106–14.

"Prazepam." *IARC Monographs on the Evaluation of the Carcinogenic Risk of Chemicals to Humans* 66 (1996): 143–55.

Shaffer, J.W., et al. "A Comparison of the Effects of Prazepam, Chlordiazepoxide, and Placebo in the Short-Term Treatment of Convalescing Alcoholics." *Journal of Clinical Pharmacology and the Journal of New Drugs* 8 (1968): 392–99.

Zung, W.W.K., et al. "Comparison of the Incidence of Sedation in Anxious Outpatients Treated with Diazepam and Prazepam." *Current Therapeutic Research: Clinical and Experimental* 39 (1986): 480–89.

Propoxyphene

Pronunciation: proh-POX-i-feen

Chemical Abstracts Service Registry Number: 469-62-5. (Hydrochloride form 1639-60-7)

Formal Names: Algaphan, Algodex, Antalvic, Darvocet, Darvon, Depronal, Develin, Dexofen, Distalgesic, Dolene, Dolocap, Doloxene, Doraphen, Erantin, Mardon, Novopropoxyn, Pro-65, Proxagesic, Wygesic

Informal Names: Pink Ladies, Pumpkin Seeds

Type: Depressant (opioid class). *See* page 24

Federal Schedule Listing: Schedule II and Schedule IV controlled substance, depending on amount (large quantities are Schedule II, DEA no. 9273; individual doses are Schedule IV, DEA no. 9278)

USA Availability: Prescription

Pregnancy Category: C

Uses. Propoxyphene has two isomers that are mentioned in drug control matters. Isomers are varieties of a chemical having the same components but different appearances; we might say that a person's right hand is an isomer of the left hand. The levopropoxyphene isomer of propoxyphene may work as a cough suppressant and is not a scheduled substance. The dextropropoxyphene isomer is the controlled substance and for convenience is simply called propoxyphene in this book.

Propoxyphene is a relatively mild pain reliever introduced in the 1950s. As the 1970s began, it was the most commonly prescribed pain reliever in America. One authority describes **codeine** as three times stronger than propoxyphene; another says the two drugs are about equal. Either way, propoxyphene is one of the less potent opioids. A typical use is for easing chronic moderate pain, as in osteoarthritis, rheumatoid arthritis, or other afflictions of the joints. The drug is also given to control early stages discomfort in cancer and has had experimental success in treating headache. In addition to pain reduction, propoxyphene has shown occasional usefulness for treating "restless leg syndrome," a condition in which people have difficulty sleeping and feel a need to frequently move their limbs day and night. Little or no improvement was seen, however, when an experiment used the drug against Tourette's syndrome, an affliction involving tics.

The substance has cross-tolerance with other opiates/opioids and can combat their withdrawal symptoms. Propoxyphene is related to **methadone** so closely that propoxyphene can cause a false positive for methadone in drug screens.

Drawbacks. Normal medical doses of propoxyphene seldom produce unwanted effects, but those can include nausea, vomiting, constipation, sleepiness, and dizziness. Occasional cases of liver damage have been attributed to the drug. Extended use of propoxyphene suppositories can cause ulcerations. Injecting the drug can cause muscle damage at the injection site, and injecting the oral format can cause lung damage. Blood sugar levels can drop when taking propoxyphene, a condition that is easy to treat but that can become serious if ignored (as when an abuser is unconscious). A study of medical records found seizures to be common among abusers who had taken high doses daily for years, but those records did not demonstrate cause and effect. Case reports have attributed deafness and blindness to propoxyphene abuse. Examination of thousands of medical records determined that old people who use propoxyphene are more likely to become unsteady and break their hips in a fall, and this risk increases if the old persons are also taking drugs intended to alter their mental state. Propoxyphene may cause euphoria. That effect is noted in horses as well; the substance also makes them more physically active, perhaps tempting unscrupulous individuals to dose horses before races.

One human experiment found that the substance slowed reaction times and interfered with recognizing pictures, results that may be relevant to driving skills. Another study using the same dosage, however, found the drug to have no significant impact on decision making, picture recognition, or reaction time. Investigators running still another experiment concluded that the normal doses of the drug do not impair driving. Nonetheless, people are supposed to be warned against operating dangerous machinery while using the drug.

Propoxyphene overdose deaths became so common in the 1970s that the U.S. Food and Drug Administration warned that the dangers of this mild drug needed more respect from prescribers and users. Similar concerns were expressed in Great Britain during the 1980s, in Denmark during the 1990s, and in Sweden as the twenty-first century began.

Abuse factors. Despite propoxyphene's relative mildness, tolerance and dependence can occur if a person takes large doses long enough. Case reports tell of individuals who became so addicted that switching the persons to methadone became necessary. Other case reports relate instances of propoxyphene dependence so strong that psychosis developed during withdrawal. Propoxyphene itself has been used as a maintenance drug for addicts being switched from some other opiate/opioid. One study found propoxyphene to be about 80 times weaker than methadone when used for this purpose.

A study noted that a group of adolescents being treated for illicit propoxyphene use had multiproblem lifestyles, and analysis of propoxyphene overdose deaths in Los Angeles revealed that all the persons had led troubled lives involving different drug overdoses, arrests, strife with other persons, mental afflictions, and suicide attempts. That analysis prompted the investigator to ask whether availability of this drug and other opiates/opioids posed a risk to normal persons or just to abnormal people. Other research presented findings relevant to that question: In a group of 37 rheumatic patients using a combination pharmaceutical containing propoxyphene, none were abusing the drug. When a group of 135 hospitalized psychiatric patients received unlimited access to the drug, the level of use roughly correlated with the level of personality disturbance, but all used it for proper medical purposes. Compared to a general population, hospitalized psychiatric patients should be more prone to drug abuse, so their lack of interest in propoxyphene is noteworthy.

Drug interactions. Propoxyphene's actions can be impeded if a person smokes tobacco cigarettes. Propoxyphene can lengthen the time span of effects produced by **alprazolam** and **diazepam**. Studies have found that blood levels from a dose of the epilepsy medicine carbamazepine will be higher if a person also takes propoxyphene, possibly high enough to cause harm. Propoxyphene should be used with particular caution if a person is also using **alcohol**, antidepressants, antihistamines, or tranquilizers. Conceivably the alcohol-propoxyphene combination could seriously impair driving skills, although scientists testing various mental and physical performance effects of the combination found that alcohol had more impact than propoxyphene.

Cancer. The drug has been suspected of promoting a form of cancer called multiple myeloma, but analysis of several hundred sets of medical records failed to link propoxyphene with the disease.

Pregnancy. Rats with prenatal exposure to propoxyphene have seemed physically normal but show some abnormal behavior. Studies with hamsters led an investigator to warn that the drug may cause congenital malformations. A case report discusses birth defects in a child born to a woman who routinely used propoxyphene during pregnancy, but we do not know if those malformations were caused by the drug. Such reports about propoxyphene are rare. A small survey of medical records found no association between propoxyphene and birth defects. The drug passes into a human fetus, and infants born to pregnant women taking propoxyphene can be dependent on the drug. The drug passes into human milk but apparently causes no harm to nursing infants.

Additional information. Propoxyphene napsylate (CAS RN 17140-78-2 or monohydrate form 26570-10-5) is another variety of this drug. Differences between the hydrochloride version and the napsylate version may lead a medical practitioner to choose one over the other for a particular patient, but they are used for the same purposes and have about the same actions. Rat studies found no evidence that the napsylate form caused birth defects.

Additional scientific information may be found in:

"Dangers of Dextropropoxyphene." *British Medical Journal* 1 (1977): 668.

Jonasson, U., B. Jonasson, and T. Saldeen. "Middle-Aged Men—A Risk Category Regarding Fatal Poisoning Due to Dextropropoxyphene and Alcohol in Combination." *Preventive Medicine* 31 (2000): 103–6.

Miller, R.R., A. Feingold, and J. Paxinos. "Propoxyphene Hydrochloride: A Critical Review." *Journal of the American Medical Association* 213 (1970): 996–1006.

Ng, B., and M. Alvear. "Dextropropoxyphene Addiction—A Drug of Primary Abuse." *American Journal of Drug and Alcohol Abuse* 19 (1993): 153–58.

Rosenberg, W.M., et al. "Dextropropoxyphene Induced Hepatotoxicity: A Report of Nine Cases." *Journal of Hepatology* 19 (1993): 470–74.

Saarialho-Kere, U., et al. "Psychomotor Performance of Patients with Rheumatoid Arthritis: Cross-Over Comparison of Dextropropoxyphene, Dextropropoxyphene plus Amitriptyline, Indomethacin, and Placebo." *Pharmacology and Toxicology* 63 (1988): 286–92.

Salter, F.J. "Propoxyphene: Dependence, Abuse and Treatment of Overdosage." *American Journal of Hospital Pharmacy* 28 (1971): 208–10.

Psilocybin

Pronunciation: seye-loh-SEYE-bin (also pronounced seye-loh-SIB-in)

Chemical Abstracts Service Registry Number: 520-52-5

Formal Names: Psilocibin

Informal Names: Blue Caps, Boomer, Buttons, God's Flesh, Hombrecitos, Las Mujercitas, Liberty Caps, Little Smoke, Magic Mushroom, Mexican Mushrooms, Mushies, Mushrooms, Mushroom Soup, Mushroom Tea, Musk, Pizza Toppings, Rooms, Sacred Mushroom, Shrooms, Silly Putty, Simple Simon, Teonanacatl

Type: Hallucinogen. *See* page 25

Federal Schedule Listing: Schedule I (DEA no. 7437)

USA Availability: Illegal to possess

Pregnancy Category: None

Uses. When people speak of hallucinogenic mushrooms they typically refer to various species containing psilocybin, a drug that can also be manufactured in a laboratory and that has some chemical resemblance to **DMT**. Like **peyote** cactus, mushrooms of the *Psilocybe* variety have been part of Native American spiritual experiences for perhaps thousands of years. In the 1500s Spaniards observed use by Aztecs. Such mushrooms grow in North America and elsewhere in the world as well.

For some persons a psilocybin session is a spiritual encounter. Euphoria, self-examination, and meditation about the meaning of life can occur after taking the drug. Along with vivid hallucinations, changes might occur in perception of time and space, and people may feel detached from their bodies or imagine that their bodies are changing shape. As with many other drugs of abuse, scientists find that a user's personality can make a huge difference in what happens with psilocybin; some persons can prevent any hallucinogenic effects at all. Personality may influence physical actions of the drug as well; in one experiment volunteers with less-stable personalities needed less light than usual in order to view reproductions of artwork; volunteers who were more normal needed more light than usual. An experiment found the drug's psychic effects to be stronger on schizophrenics. Experiences can be so extraordinary that some investigators have wondered if the drug can evoke ESP (extrasensory perception) abilities.

One of the most famous scientific studies with psilocybin was conducted by Dr. Timothy Leary before he became a counterculture icon. Leary and his researchers ingested the drug together with state prison inmates to determine whether the experiences would promote life changes motivating inmates to stay out of prison upon release. Leary reported outstanding success, with psilocybin inmates committing far fewer repeat offenses sending them back to prison. Subsequent investigation, however, revealed serious flaws in Leary's research; in reality the percentage of inmates returning to prison for new crime was the same in the psilocybin group as in those who did not receive the drug. Leary's advocacy of widespread hallucinogenic drug use was based partly upon flawed research.

A case report notes successful use of psilocybin mushrooms to ease, though not eliminate, compulsions and obsessions.

Drawbacks. Blood pressure rose in volunteers who received psilocybin; reaction times slowed; hearing became more sensitive; and individuals often felt cold. Dizziness, nausea, and vomiting can occur. Some persons feel nervous and even fearful during a psilocybin experience. After a psilocybin session people may feel worn out for several hours, maybe for more than a day.

Reliable information on mushroom effects is more challenging to obtain than reliable information about psilocybin because mushrooms contain many other chemicals, sometimes including illicit substances that have been added without a user's knowledge. And mushroom eaters may simultaneously use other substances deliberately, further clouding knowledge of what the mushroom itself is doing. With the mushrooms, burning or prickling sensations are routine, as are perspiration, yawning, fatigue, slowed pulse rate, lowered blood pressure and body temperature, and uneasiness. An overdose commonly brings on nausea, vomiting, high blood pressure, and abnormal heartbeat. Heart attack has been reported but seems uncommon.

Abuse factors. An authority who searched scientific reports about 20 drugs considered to have potential for dependence (including **heroin**) found oral psilocybin to have the least. Psilocybin, **LSD**, and **mescaline** all share some cross-tolerance, meaning that they can be at least partially substituted for one another.

Drug interactions. **Alcohol** may cause a flashback of hallucinations up to a week after using psilocybin.

Cancer. A laboratory test found that psilocybin lacked actions expected from chemicals that cause cancer.

Pregnancy. Not enough scientific information to report.

Additional information. Some psilocybin mushroom species contain the Schedule I controlled substance psilocyn (also called psilocin, CAS RN 520-53-6). Mushrooms are not the only source of psilocyn; laboratories can manufacture it artificially, and reportedly human body chemistry transforms psilocybin into psilocyn. A case report notes someone who successfully used psilocyn to reduce obsessions and compulsions. The chemical can reduce appetite in dogs. Researchers report that tolerance develops in mice. Experimentation with mice found no evidence that psilocyn causes birth defects.

Additional scientific information may be found in:

Doblin, R. "Dr. Leary's Concord Prison Experiment: A 34-Year Follow-up Study." *Journal of Psychoactive Drugs* 30 (1998): 419–26.

Hofmann, A. "The Mexican Relatives of LSD." In *LSD, My Problem Child*. Trans. J. Ott. New York: McGraw-Hill, 1980. Ch. 6.

McDonald, A. "Mushrooms and Madness: Hallucinogenic Mushrooms and Some Psychopharmacological Implications." *Canadian Journal of Psychiatry* 25 (1980): 586–94.

Parashos, A.J. "The Psilocybin-Induced 'State of Drunkenness' in Normal Volunteers and Schizophrenics." *Behavioral Neuropsychiatry* 8 (1976–1977): 83–86.

Peden, N.R., S.D. Pringle, and J. Crooks. "The Problem of Psilocybin Mushroom Abuse." *Human Toxicology* 1 (1982): 417–24.

Rynearson, R.R., M.R. Wilson, and R.G. Bickford. "Psilocybin-Induced Changes in Psychologic Function, Electroencephalogram, and Light-Evoked Potentials in Human Subjects." *Mayo Clinic Proceedings* 43 (1968): 191–204.

Stein, S.I., G.L. Closs, and N.W. Gabel. "Observations on Psychoneurophysiologically Significant Mushrooms. I. Clinical Details Pertaining to the Ingestion of *Panaeolus venenosus* and *Psilocybe caerulescens* Mushrooms." *Mycopathologia et Mycologia Applicata* 11 (1959): 205–16.

Thatcher, K. "Personality Trait Dependent Performance under Psilocybin. II." *Diseases of the Nervous System* 31 (1970): 181–92.

Quazepam

Pronunciation: KWAY-ze-pam (also pronounced KWA-ze-pam)

Chemical Abstracts Service Registry Number: 36735-22-5

Formal Names: Doral, Dormalin

Type: Depressant (benzodiazepine class). *See* page 21

Federal Schedule Listing: Schedule IV (DEA no. 2881)

USA Availability: Prescription

Pregnancy Category: X

Uses. Insomnia is one of the main medical conditions treated by this drug, which also has anticonvulsant properties. The compound has been found useful to counteract insomnia actions of some psychiatric medicines. Although one insomnia study showed doses losing some effectiveness over time, patients continued to sleep better for 15 nights after dosage stopped, an improvement not observed when people stop taking some other antiinsomnia drugs. Similar findings have come from other experimentation. Antiinsomnia drugs commonly have "rebound" effects in which insomnia temporarily becomes worse than ever when dosage stops. Little or no rebound is observed with quazepam, perhaps because it is eliminated rather slowly from the body. A study noted that quazepam not only reduced anxiety among insomniacs but that the decline in anxiety continued for 15 days after dosage stopped.

The drug has been tested against other substances used against insomnia: **triazolam, temazepam,** and **flurazepam.** In some respects triazolam was six times stronger than quazepam, but researchers judged quazepam as superior to triazolam and temazepam in aiding sleep. In animals quazepam produced brainwave measurements that resembled normal sleep more than flurazepam did. Flurazepam leaves people groggier than quazepam the day after bedtime use. In contrast to flurazepam, quazepam slows mice without making them physically discoordinated. Still another advantage of quazepam is its relative safety; in one experiment a particular dose of flurazepam killed animals, but four times that amount of quazepam left animals apparently unharmed—and still larger doses caused sickness but not death. One group of experimenters was unable to find the LD50 (lethal dose 50) of quazepam. "LD50" is the amount of drug that will kill half the animals receiving it; the researchers could not find a dose producing fatal poisoning in more than 10% of the animals. Other experimenters, however, report success at achieving LD50. Animal studies find quazepam to have little influence on blood pressure, heartbeat, and breathing. A human study found no change in daytime attentiveness or muscular coordination after awakening from a nighttime dose. In one study researchers were surprised to discover improvement in ability to move limbs quickly and precisely the day after taking a normal bedtime dose of quazepam.

Drawbacks. Depending on size of doses, people might feel drowsy and slow-moving during the daytime after taking quazepam the night before, but some researchers describe that effect as minor. Various attempts to measure other adverse effects of the drug have found none, but an experiment using a dosage six times stronger than a recommended therapeutic dose made people dizzy and sleepy and lowered their ability to function normally. In humans an impairment of eye movement and eye-hand coordination can be measured, but the practical significance of those deficits is unclear. Animal studies with the drug produce abnormalities in the liver and in male gonads.

Abuse factors. Tolerance and dependence can develop. Sudden stoppage of quazepam after a full year of dosing produces withdrawal symptoms in animals: restless moving around, easy agitation, convulsions.

Drug interactions. In mice quazepam boosts **alcohol**'s effects, but in humans a test of skill in movement found the combination to have the same effect as alcohol plus placebo.

Cancer. Oral dosage in mice and hamsters did not produce cancer.

Pregnancy. Research is scanty about quazepam's potential for causing birth defects, but the drug is considered a producer of fetal malformations. In mice a substantial amount of a quazepam dose passes into a fetus. Human testing has shown that about 0.1% of a quazepam dose (and its metabolites) passes into the milk of nursing mothers.

Additional scientific information may be found in:

Ankier, S.I., and K.L. Goa. "Quazepam: A Preliminary Review of Its Pharmacodynamic and Pharmacokinetic Properties, and Therapeutic Efficacy in Insomnia." *Drugs* 35 (1988): 42–62.

Kales, A. "Quazepam: Hypnotic Efficacy and Side Effects." *Pharmacotherapy* 10 (1990): 1–10.

"Quazepam: New Hypnotic." *Medical Letter on Drugs and Therapeutics* 32 (1990): 39–40.

Rush, C.R., and J.A. Ali. "A Follow-up Study of the Acute Behavioral Effects of Benzodiazepine-Receptor Ligands in Humans: Comparison of Quazepam and Triazolam." *Experimental and Clinical Psychopharmacology* 7 (1999): 257–65.

Remifentanil

Pronunciation: rehm-ih-FEHN-tuh-nill

Chemical Abstracts Service Registry Number: 132875-61-7. (Hydrochloride form 132539-07-2)

Formal Names: Ultiva

Type: Depressant (opioid class). *See* page 24

Federal Schedule Listing: Schedule II (DEA no. 9739)

USA Availability: Prescription

Pregnancy Category: C

Uses. This drug is related to **fentanyl** and became available for medical purposes in the United States during the 1990s. Remifentanil is used for pain relief and to help induce anesthesia. Depending on the type of measurement used, studies of the drug's potency find it to be 15 to 70 times stronger than alfentanil (described in this book's fentanyl listing), which means remifentanil is strong indeed. Remifentanil is fast acting but is generally not considered long lasting. An experiment, however, challenged standard belief that the drug's actions last only a few minutes, with investigators finding that the substance still impeded physical movement an hour after taking a dose (although volunteers using the drug felt normal at that point). Researchers have suggested the substance might have a specialized use in treating certain eye injuries because the drug can reduce pressure that may otherwise build up inside the eyeball and cause the contents to leak out. Some investigators have found that women need a larger remifentanil dose than men for an equivalent relief from pain.

Drawbacks. Unwanted actions from remifentanil can include muscle tenseness and trouble with breathing and heartbeat. These conditions can become so dangerous that the drug is not supposed to be used unless emergency resuscitation equipment is on hand and the medical practitioner administering the substance is an expert. Less serious unwanted effects can include perspiration, itching, nausea, vomiting, and lightheadedness.

Abuse factors. An experiment in a medical setting found that remifentanil appears to create tolerance to other opioids given for pain control, but another medical study did not find that effect. A group of recreational opioid users testing remifentanil declared it to have stronger effects than fentanyl, but researchers running the experiment noted that remifentanil's brief action meant that it might appeal only to abusers seeking short spurts of sensation. Although the researchers implied that limited access to necessary safe dosage equipment might deter illicit use of remifentanil, safety concerns are not universal among drug abusers.

Drug interactions. Not enough scientific information to report.

Cancer. The drug's ability to cause cancer is uncertain. Most laboratory tests reveal no potential for cancer from remifentanil, although one type of laboratory test using mouse cells does give positive results.

Pregnancy. Decline in fertility was observed among male rats that received remifentanil daily for over two months at doses 40 times the recommended human level. No birth defects were attributed to the drug when pregnant rabbits received 125 times the recommended human dose. The same negative result occurred when rats received 400 times the maximum human dose. In both species the drug passed into the fetus. Those offspring, in turn, developed and reproduced normally. Effects on human pregnancy are unknown. One study observed no ill effect in infants when women received remifentanil during childbirth, but another study found the drug to have such a negative impact on women giving birth (itching, vomiting, low oxygen level in blood, and insufficient pain relief) that the experiment was abandoned. The drug passes into the milk of rats, but whether it passes into human milk is unknown.

Additional scientific information may be found in:

Baylon, G.J., et al. "Comparative Abuse Liability of Intravenously Administered Remifentanil and Fentanyl." *Journal of Clinical Psychopharmacology* 20 (2000): 597–606.

Black, M.L., J.L. Hill, J.P. Zacny. "Behavioral and Physiological Effects of Remifentanil and Alfentanil in Healthy Volunteers." *Anesthesiology* 90 (1999): 718–26.

Ferguson, C.N., and R.M. Jones. "Remifentanil—Introduction and Preclinical Studies." *Drugs Today* 33 (1997): 603–9.

Guignard, B., et al. "Acute Opioid Tolerance: Intraoperative Remifentanil Increases Postoperative Pain and Morphine Requirement." *Anesthesiology* 93 (2000): 409–17.

Patel, S.S., and C.M. Spencer. "Remifentanil." *Drugs* 52 (1996): 417–27.

Puckett, S.D., and J.J. Andrews. "AANA Journal Course: Update for Nurse Anesthetists—A Comprehensive Review of Remifentanil: The Next Generation Opioid." *AANA Journal* 66 (1998): 125–36.

Sibutramine

Pronunciation: sih-BYOO-tra-meen

Chemical Abstracts Service Registry Number: 106650-56-0. (Hydrochloride anhydrous form 84485-00-7; Hydrochloride monohydrate form 125494-59-9)

Formal Names: Meridia, Reductil

Type: Stimulant (anorectic class). *See* page 15

Federal Schedule Listing: Schedule IV (DEA no. 1675)

USA Availability: Prescription

Pregnancy Category: C

Uses. This weight control medicine appears to work by making people feel more full while eating a meal, thereby reducing appetite. People using sibutramine eat less regardless of whether they are trying to lose weight. In rats the drug increases the rate at which the body consumes stored energy, burning off calories. A similar action has been measured in humans. Sibutramine has also been used for treating nerve pain caused by diabetes. One research study found that the drug improved attention and muscular coordination.

A given dose of the drug tends to produce higher drug levels in women than in men, but the difference is not considered significant enough to affect calculation of dosage. Blood levels from a given dose also tend to be higher in blacks than in whites, but again the difference is considered insignificant.

Drawbacks. The drug elevates heart rate and blood pressure. Headache, insomnia, dry mouth, and constipation are typical unwanted effects. The medicine may promote bleeding. Sibutramine is not recommended for persons suffering from narrow-angle glaucoma or for persons who have had seizures.

Abuse factors. Although chemical details are highly technical, sibutramine operates in ways fundamentally different from the weight-loss drugs **fenfluramine** and **dextroamphetamine**, differences that may make abuse of sibutramine less likely. Volunteers with a history of drug abuse were paid to participate in a study. They found sibutramine unpleasant (causing confusion, unease, and loss of energy), so unpleasant that in order to avoid a high dose they were willing to accept reduction in the fee. In another study, examining how recreational stimulant users react to sibutramine, researchers concluded the drug had no more appeal than a placebo.

Drug interactions. Sibutramine should normally be avoided if a person is taking a monoamine oxidase inhibitor (MAOI—found in some antidepressants and other medicine). The drug is a "serotonin reuptake inhibitor," meaning it can interact with various medicines (including **dextromethorphan**, **fentanyl**, **meperidine**, and **pentazocine**) to cause "serotonin syndrome," a serious condition that can involve hyperactivity, confusion, and influenzalike symptoms. Sibutramine should be used cautiously if a person is taking **ephedrine**, contained in some cold and allergy remedies.

Cancer. Mice experiments involving blood plasma levels similar to normal human dosage found no evidence that sibutramine causes cancer. In experimentation producing levels of sibutramine metabolites (breakdown products) many times higher than those seen in humans, female rats showed no evidence of cancer; but male rats developed tumors that are commonly caused by hormone changes. Typical laboratory tests used to measure a chemical's cancer potential show none for sibutramine, though its breakdown products produced ambiguous results in one test.

Pregnancy. Rat studies involving doses strong enough to produce metabolite blood levels 43 times higher than normal human levels yielded no observable birth defects. Some rabbit studies involving doses high enough to be poisonous have produced birth defects, but other testing at a poisonous dosage level has not. Sibutramine's potential for causing human congenital abnormalities is unknown, and pregnant women are advised to avoid the drug. Its potential for transfer into milk is unknown, so nursing mothers are advised to avoid the drug.

Additional information. The hydrochloride anhydrous form of sibutramine was tested as an antidepressant in the 1980s, but medical literature has reported little about this form of the drug since then. The hydrochloride monohydrate form became available in the 1990s to help people lose weight.

Additional scientific information may be found in:

Cole, J.O., et al. "Sibutramine: A New Weight Loss Agent without Evidence of the Abuse Potential Associated with Amphetamines." *Journal of Clinical Psychopharmacology* 18 (1998): 231–36.

James, W.P., et al. "Effect of Sibutramine on Weight Maintenance after Weight Loss: A Randomised Trial." *Lancet* 356 (2000): 2119–25.

Lean, M.E. "Sibutramine—A Review of Clinical Efficacy." *International Journal of Obesity and Related Metabolic Disorders* 21 (1997, Suppl. 1): S30–S36.

Luque, C.A., and J.A. Rey. "Sibutramine: A Serotonin-Norepinephrine Reuptake-Inhibitor for the Treatment of Obesity." *Annals of Pharmacotherapy* 33 (1999): 968–78.

Schuh, L.M., et al. "Abuse Liability Assessment of Sibutramine, a Novel Weight Control Agent." *Psychopharmacology* 147 (2000): 339–46.

"Sibutramine for Obesity." *Medical Letter on Drugs and Therapeutics* 40 (1998): 32.

Stanozolol

Pronunciation: stan-OH-zoh-lahl (also pronounced stan-OH-zoh-lohl)
Chemical Abstracts Service Registry Number: 10418-03-8
Formal Names: Stromba, Strombaject, Stromba Winject, Winstroid, Winstrol
Type: Anabolic steroid. *See* page 24
Federal Schedule Listing: Schedule III (DEA no. 4000)
USA Availability: Prescription
Pregnancy Category: X

Uses. This synthetic drug is related to **testosterone**. Stanozolol is used to combat hereditary angioedema, a disease causing body tissues to swell. The substance is also used to reduce weight loss from cancer or AIDS (acquired immunodeficiency syndrome) and has been used experimentally to improve physical activity of elderly persons and to enhance nutrition of surgery patients (a case report warns, however, that the substance may cause iron deficiency). Raynaud's disease, in which persons experience painful spasms of fingers and toes, has been combated with stanozolol, and the drug can improve a skin affliction called pityriasis rubra pilaris. Other skin conditions responsive to stanozolol treatment include hives and cryofibrinogenemia (a blood vessel blockage disorder that can also involve the heart and lungs). Using the drug to treat a very serious blood disease called aplastic anemia has yielded uncertain results. Itching from liver cirrhosis has been relieved with stanozolol. Dentists give the drug to ease tooth-pulling. In a clinical experiment the drug increased muscle mass. Some cattle raisers have used stanozolol to boost meat production, but the practice is banned in assorted jurisdictions.

Drawbacks. Unwanted effects from stanozolol may include weariness, cramps, fluid retention, and migraine headaches. While taking stanozolol a person's high-density lipoproteins (so-called good cholesterol) may decline, while low-density lipoproteins (bad cholesterol) increase. This effect might worsen risk of artery blockage leading to heart attack or stroke, but the changes in lipoprotein levels normally disappear after dosage stops. Uncommon case reports indicate that stanozolol may increase blood pressure in the brain and cause a stroke. A case report raises the possibility that the compound may worsen tics suffered by persons having Tourette's syndrome. Stanozolol should be avoided by men with cancer of the breast or prostate and by women with breast cancer accompanied by high blood levels of calcium—stanozolol may weaken bones in such women. The drug is not recommended for persons with serious kidney inflammation. In young persons stanozolol has the potential for stunting attainment of adult height, a special concern if the drug is used by growing athletes without medical supervision. Any use by athletes, however, violates rules governing sports competitions. The drug can masculinize women (losing hair from the top of the head, gaining hair elsewhere, coarsened voice). A clinical experiment noted disruption of menstrual periods among women using stanozolol.

Reports of liver damage among persons using the compound are numerous; however, most scientists stop short of asserting a cause-and-effect relationship. Researchers have noted liver damage in rat experiments that point further suspicion in the drug's direction.

Stanozolol appears to interfere with blood clotting. In some medical conditions, however, anticlotting action can be useful; for example, stanozolol has benefited persons suffering from conditions like thrombophlebitis, a painful blockage of veins caused by the buildup of clotlike material.

Researchers running a mice experiment looked for evidence that the drug promoted aggression but found none.

Abuse factors. Not enough scientific information to report about tolerance, dependence, withdrawal, or addiction.

Drug interactions. Medical observers have noted instances in which the drug interacts badly with the anti–blood clot medicine warfarin, with patients experiencing too much anticlotting action.

Cancer. The drug is suspected of causing human liver cancer. Tests of liver function are recommended for patients receiving this drug, lest they develop cancer or other serious problems that are difficult to treat after overt symptoms appear.

Pregnancy. The drug is suspected of reducing fertility. Stanozolol has masculinized female rat fetuses and is believed to harm human fetal development.

Additional scientific information may be found in:

Helfman, T., and V. Falanga. "Stanozolol as a Novel Therapeutic Agent in Dermatology." *Journal of the American Academy of Dermatology* 33 (1995): 254–58.

Hosegood, J.L., and A.J. Franks. "Response of Human Skeletal Muscle to the Anabolic Steroid Stanozolol." *British Medical Journal* 297 (1988): 1028–29.

Lye, M.D., and A.E. Ritch. "A Double-Blind Trial of an Anabolic Steroid (Stanozolol) in the Disabled Elderly." *Rheumatology and Rehabilitation* 16 (1977): 62–69.

"Stanozolol." In *Therapeutic Drugs*, ed. C. Dollery. 2d ed. New York: Churchill Livingstone, 1999. S91–S93.

Yoshida, E.M., et al. "At What Price, Glory? Severe Cholestasis and Acute Renal Failure in an Athlete Abusing Stanozolol." *Canadian Medical Association Journal* 151 (1994): 791–93.

TCE

Pronunciation: tee-see-ee

Chemical Abstracts Service Registry Number: 71-55-6

Formal Names: Chloroethene, Chlorotene, Chlorothene, Ethane, Methyl Chloroform, Methylchloroform, Methyltrichloromethane, 1,1,1-Trichloroethane

Type: Inhalant. *See* page 26

Federal Schedule Listing: Unscheduled

USA Availability: Generally available as a chemical, or as a component in various
products

Pregnancy Category: None

Uses. TCE is a solvent with many industrial functions, ranging from manufacturing of ink and textiles to cleaning wigs and motion picture film. The
substance has been an ingredient in "liquid paper" correction fluids used to
cover blemishes on documents and photocopies. Small amounts of TCE can
be driven into food that is microwaved in paper and plastic containers fur-
nished for microwave cooking, but this exposure is considered safe. A standard medical use of the substance is for removing adhesive tape from a
patient's skin.

In animal experiments TCE has depressant actions similar to those of **ether**,
such as reducing coordination in movement and lessening muscle strength.
Rats exhibit brain chemistry changes comparable to changes produced by benzodiazepines. Mice act as if TCE provides some effects similar to those of
pentobarbital, diazepam, ether, and **alcohol**, but those reactions in highly
technical experiments do not mean that TCE would provide humans with any
therapeutic benefits or recreational sensations produced by those four drugs.
TCE has, however, altered sensory perception and caused hallucinations in
humans.

Drawbacks. Caregivers have been cautioned to take steps to avoid accumulation of vapor inside incubators if TCE is used to remove adhesive tape
from infants. Nonprescription aerosol cold remedies have contained TCE as a
solvent component, and deaths have been attributed to the TCE in those products.

Recreational usage of TCE is intended to produce euphoria. Depending on
amount of inhalation, TCE can make mice more active or less active. In humans the substance tends to excite persons at first, then make them lethargic.

Typical instances requiring medical assistance involve patients who were so stimulated that they began running vigorously until they collapsed. An intoxicating dose may produce dizziness and difficulty in moving arms and legs. Inhaling low levels of TCE can irritate a person's nose, and presumably higher amounts would be worse. The vapor may cause eyes to water. Although experiments exposing volunteers to fumes showed little or no adverse effect on several tests of mental sharpness (and even improvement in some measures, depending on dosage), persons with industrial exposure to fumes have become peevish and moody, showed trouble maintaining their balance, and exhibited problems with concentration and short-term memory. Numbness, tingling, or other sensory defects can occur, as can headache, nausea, and low blood pressure. Brain, liver, kidney, lung, and heart disease have been observed. Respiratory arrest is recorded, as are stroke and coma. Fatal changes in cardiac rhythm can occur. Heart attack can result from an overdose, but that is uncommon. A case report tells of chronic exposure causing fatal damage to blood, skin, and internal organs. Autopsy in another instance revealed liver, kidney, and lung damage in a teenager who died from a TCE overdose. In addition to sniffing, the chemical can also be absorbed through the skin, posing a hazard to persons touched by the liquid.

Because TCE liquid will not burn, the substance is often treated as nonflammable. The vapor will burn, however. TCE is used to clean the interior of space shuttle solid fuel booster casings for relaunch, and a worker was killed at a cleaning facility when the TCE vapor ignited.

Abuse factors. Tolerance is reported. Dependence can develop in mice. Withdrawal symptoms in mice can be reduced by dosing them with alcohol, pentobarbital, or **midazolam**. Such cross-tolerance suggests that TCE operates as a depressant, and humans have experienced depressant actions from it.

Drug interactions. In animal experiments TCE causes fatal cardiac rhythm trouble that is worsened by alcohol.

Cancer. Laboratory tests indicate TCE might cause cancer, but the compound's ability to produce the disease in animals and humans is unclear.

Pregnancy. Industrial exposure is suspected of causing fetal abnormality and spontaneous abortion. One group of experimenters found that chronic fetal exposure caused heart defects in rats, but another group of researchers found no effect. Other rodent work has produced birth defects involving bones. In mice, fetal exposure experiments simulating recreational abuse patterns cause low birth weight along with slower maturation in brains and in behavior of offspring.

Additional information. Scientific writings occasionally use the abbreviation "TCE" for trichloroethylene, also called trichlorethylene (CAS RN 79-01-6). That compound and 1,1,1-trichloroethane are sometimes found in the same product, but they are different chemicals. Trichloroethylene is not considered a substance of abuse.

Additional scientific information may be found in:

"Aerosols for Colds." *Medical Letter on Drugs and Therapeutics* 15 (1973): 86–88.
D'Costa, D.F., and N.P. Gunasekera. "Fatal Cerebral Oedema Following Trichloroethane Abuse." *Journal of the Royal Society of Medicine* 83 (1990): 533–34.

Kelafant, G.A., R.A. Berg, and R. Schleenbaker. "Toxic Encephalopathy Due to 1,1,1-Trichloroethane Exposure." *American Journal of Industrial Medicine* 25 (1994): 439–46.

King, G.S., J.E. Smialek, and W.G. Troutman. "Sudden Death in Adolescents Resulting from the Inhalation of Typewriter Correction Fluid." *Journal of the American Medical Association* 253 (1985): 1604–6.

"1,1,1-Trichloroethane." *IARC Monographs on the Evaluation of Carcinogenic Risks to Humans*, pt.2, 71 (1999): 881–903.

Pointer, J. "Typewriter Correction Fluid Inhalation: A New Substance of Abuse." *Journal of Toxicology: Clinical Toxicology* 19 (1982): 493–99.

Temazepam

Pronunciation: teh-MAZ-eh-pam (also pronounced tem-AZ-eh-pam)

Chemical Abstracts Service Registry Number: 846-50-4

Formal Names: Euhypnos, Levanxol, Normison, Planum, Restoril, Temazepam Gelthix

Informal Names: Eggs, Temazies, Temmies

Type: Depressant (benzodiazepine class). *See* page 21

Federal Schedule Listing: Schedule IV (DEA no. 2925)

USA Availability: Prescription

Pregnancy Category: X

Uses. This metabolite of **diazepam** is used to fight anxiety and insomnia. Those medicinal characteristics give sedative properties to the drug. Temazepam has had experimental success in treating posttraumatic stress disorder, a condition that may be aggravated by poor sleep. In one study the substance reduced depression, although in another study some people said it made them melancholy. The drug has been used in veterinary large-animal anesthesia.

Laboratory tests indicate the drug can help rotating-shift workers turn their sleep schedule around and perform better at night work; those tests did not detect a hangover problem. Researchers report that aspect of the drug may be particularly useful for emergency changes of sleep schedule imposed upon combat pilots. The drug's usefulness for that purpose was studied in Operation Desert Storm during the Gulf War of 1991; in one unit about half the pilots using the drug reported it useful for shifting their sleep schedule. The drug has official U.S. Air Force approval for combat support. The substance has also been used to treat jet lag, which is fatigue caused when air travelers cross too many time zones without being able to adjust their sleep schedule. Military researchers concerned about effects of jet lag and other sleep disturbances on parachute troops concluded that temazepam could help parachutists get proper rest before making an assault. Elite athletes have used the drug to promote proper rest, with no adverse effect noted on performance.

During mountain climbing in the Himalayas at altitudes well over 4,000 meters (13,123 feet) the compound improved quality of sleep, but researchers were unsure about whether it interfered with breathing at such heights, where atmospheric oxygen begins to become inadequate. Diminished oxygen pressure was measured in the blood of mountain climbers who took temazepam at an altitude of 3,000 meters (9,843 feet); the change did not occur at 171 meters (561 feet) with the drug, nor at either altitude with placebo. Judging from those results, avoiding the drug might be a good idea if a person must engage in physical exertion at high altitude. A British Mt. Everest expedition, however, found no change in oxygen saturation when temazepam was used at 5,300 meters (17,388 feet); the mountaineers reported more restful sleep as well.

Drawbacks. In a test of driving ability 12 hours after taking a dose, operators of a test vehicle showed increased carelessness and decreased ability to avoid colliding with objects. Researchers concluded that temazepam users would be dangerous if they drove a car. In another experiment, however, little effect on reaction time was observed in volunteers who received a dose almost three times stronger than those received by the drivers. In still another test the day after a nighttime dose, in which temazepam users drove a car on a test course and in actual traffic, observers thought control of the vehicle was better than normal. No effect at all was seen in one more test, in which temazepam users drove a car in traffic for over 50 miles the day after a bedtime dose.

Various experiments have sought to determine whether the drug affects thinking and judgment. Unsurprisingly, results generally show the impact to depend upon size of dose and how much time has elapsed since taking it. The more important practical results are those from the morning after taking a normal bedtime dose, a typical situation for persons using the drug medically. Some of those experiments have documented impaired reaction time and trouble in observing short events, but other tests have been unable to measure differences from normal performance. One study indicated that healthy volunteers do worse than insomniacs who use the drug; perhaps the latter group is more rested and alert after a good night's sleep, in contrast to healthy volunteers who get no extra sleep benefit and are a little groggy from the drug. An experiment with elderly persons the morning after a dose found vigilance and speed of movement to be unchanged or sometimes better. That finding is particularly striking because effects of such drugs are often stronger on elderly persons than on others. The drug is characterized as short acting, meaning it should have fewer hangover effects (tiredness, lightheadedness, impaired eye-hand coordination) than other benzodiazepine class substances, an expectation supported by some experiments and refuted by others. The drug tends to build up in the bloodstream after repeated dosing.

In studies involving thousands of patients, about 6% reported unwanted effects. The most frequent complaint was drug hangover; less common were headache, nausea, and dizziness. Temazepam can also reduce blood pressure, accelerate heartbeat, and produce tingling. An unusual case report notes a person who experienced hallucinations of music while taking the drug along with **lorazepam**, but the individual was already hearing things before the drug regimen began. Temazepam can produce amnesia about things that occur while a person is under the drug's influence, more so than **flurazepam** in one experiment. Volunteers who took temazepam have reported it causes otherworldly feelings. Blisters have occurred after overdose. Injecting the drug into an arm or leg artery can cause dire injury resulting in amputation. Arterial injection can also cause skin rash, swelling from fluid buildup, muscle damage, and kidney failure. Intravenous injection of oral temazepam can be fatal due to tablet ingredients not intended to circulate in the bloodstream. Some abusers inject the oral gel format into the groin; this practice can form leg blood clots that may dislodge and travel to the lung, where they can halt breathing.

Abuse factors. Investigators found no "significant" dependence after giving temazepam to persons for three months. Examination of patients on long-term temazepam dosage revealed no tolerance, and in one study temazepam retained its antiinsomnia effectiveness when given to a group of volunteers each night for over a month; they did not develop tolerance. A study involving a second group did show tolerance developing, findings supported in still more experimentation as well. The first group did not experience rebound when dosage stopped (insomnia did not come back), but experimenters working with a third group were sometimes able to provoke a rebound, which they interpreted as evidence that temazepam is addictive—although not everyone would agree that return of an ailment upon stoppage of medication means that the medicine is addictive. Nonetheless, a case of addiction is reported in which someone regularly used temazepam before drinking **alcohol** and also to reduce tremors.

A report published in 1990 noted that in northwest England about 25% of persons engaged in AIDS (acquired immunodeficiency syndrome) risk conduct were using temazepam. This does not mean the drug promotes such conduct, but it does mean the drug was popular among reckless persons. Such popularity may have been due to pharmaceutical effects, or due to availability, or due simply to fashionability, or perhaps a combination of all. In Scotland as the twenty-first century began, researchers found temazepam abuse to be the third-largest cause (after alcohol and **heroin**) of muscle damage leading to kidney failure and limb amputation.

Drug interactions. Researchers have seen that a dose of temazepam lasts longer in women than in men. Birth control pills may reduce the amount of time that temazepam stays in the body. Disulfiram, a drug used to treat alcoholism, can turn a medicinal dose of temazepam into a poisonous one.

Cancer. Tests on animals do not reveal potential for causing cancer.

Pregnancy. High-enough dosage during pregnancy has caused rib malformations in offspring of rats and rabbits. Temazepam is believed to pass from a pregnant woman into the fetus. Taking the drug together with diphenhydramine hydrochloride (found in many cold and allergy remedies) is followed by a stillbirth and newborn death rate of 80% in rabbits, and a human case is reported. The drug passes into the milk of nursing mothers. A case report noted no effect on a nursing infant.

Additional scientific information may be found in:

Ferrer, C.F., Jr., R.U. Bisson, and J. French. "Circadian Rhythm Desynchronosis in Military Deployments: A Review of Current Strategies." *Aviation, Space, and Environmental Medicine* 66 (1995): 571–78.

Fox, R., et al. "Misuse of Temazepam: 1." *British Medical Journal* 305 (1992): 253.

Fraschini, F., and B. Stankov. "Temazepam: Pharmacological Profile of a Benzodiazepine and New Trends in Its Clinical Application." *Pharmacological Research* 27 (1993): 97–113.

Heel, R.C., et al. "Temazepam: A Review of Its Pharmacological Properties and Therapeutic Efficacy as an Hypnotic." *Drugs* 21 (1981): 321–40.

Kunsman, G.W., et al. "The Use of Microcomputer-Based Psychomotor Tests for the Evaluation of Benzodiazepine Effects on Human Performance: A Review with Emphasis on Temazepam." *British Journal of Clinical Pharmacology* 34 (1992): 289–301.

McElnay, J.C., M.E. Jones, and B. Alexander. "Temazepam (Restoril, Sandoz Pharmaceuticals)." *Drug Intelligence and Clinical Pharmacy* 16 (1982): 650–56.

Testolactone

Pronunciation: tes-toh-LACK-tohn

Chemical Abstracts Service Registry Number: 968-93-4

Formal Names: Teslac, Testololactone

Type: Anabolic steroid. See page 24

Federal Schedule Listing: Schedule III (DEA no. 4000)

USA Availability: Prescription

Pregnancy Category: C

Uses. Experiments have shown that testolactone can produce substantial reductions in size of tumors, although such results are not invariable. Medical practitioners mainly use this drug to ease suffering from breast cancer in older female patients and in younger women who no longer have functioning ovaries. The drug may permanently reduce the amount of estrogen hormones in a woman's body; such hormones affect pregnancy and female physical characteristics. Unlike other anabolic steroids, testolactone seems to have no masculinizing effect on women. Clinical experimentation using testolactone as part of the regimen against a juvenile adrenal gland disorder found no adverse effect on children's bone growth, in contrast to most anabolic steroids' ability to prematurely halt bone growth in young people. Testolactone has had success in treating premature male puberty, in restoring normal growth characteristics, and in improving young men's mood—all without harming bone development. The substance has also reduced abnormal enlargement of breasts that some males experience during adolescence. Although the drug is not recommended for women who have yet to pass through menopause, testolactone has seen experimental success in controlling premature puberty among girls suffering from McCune-Albright syndrome (a disease also involving bone and skin abnormalities). In rat experiments the drug had no apparent effect on fertility, but in humans the substance has been used to improve male fertility with mixed success. Testolactone has also been given to counteract human male sexual dysfunction caused by some epilepsy therapy. Experimental use against enlarged prostate has had promising results.

Drawbacks. Unwanted effects are described as uncommon but can include headache, skin rash, tingling, nausea, constipation or diarrhea, and abdominal discomfort. By elevating amounts of calcium in the blood, the drug can make a person become confused. Temporary hair loss was reported with two patients who were also taking a corticosteroid.

Abuse factors. Not enough scientific information to report about tolerance, dependence, withdrawal, or addiction.

Drug interactions. Testolactone may promote bleeding if a person is also taking anti–blood clot medicine.

Cancer. Testolactone's potential for causing cancer is unknown.

Pregnancy. In rat experiments at doses far higher than humans normally receive, the drug increased the amount of fetal malformations and deaths. No birth defects were found when pregnant rabbits received over seven times the normal human dose. The drug is not designed for pregnant women, and impact on human pregnancy is unknown. Whether the drug passes into human milk is unknown.

Additional scientific information may be found in:

Goldenberg, I.S., et al. "Combined Androgen and Antimetabolite Therapy of Advanced Female Breast Cancer." *Cancer* 36 (1975): 308–10.

Howards, S.S. "Treatment of Male Infertility." *New England Journal of Medicine* 332 (1995): 312–17.

Laue, L., et al. "Treatment of Familial Male Precocious Puberty with Spironolactone and Testolactone." *New England Journal of Medicine* 320 (1989): 496–502.

"Testolactone Aqueous Suspension (Teslac)." *Clinical Pharmacology and Therapeutics* 11 (1970): 302–6.

Testosterone

Pronunciation: tes-TOS-tuh-rohn

Chemical Abstracts Service Registry Number: 58-22-0

Formal Names: Androderm, Andronaq, Delatestryl, Depo-Testosterone, Hydro-test, Malogen, Oreton, Percutacrine Androgénique Forte, Primotoston, Testo-derm, Testoral Sublings, Testoviron

Type: Anabolic steroid. *See* page 24

Federal Schedule Listing: Schedule III (DEA no. 4000)

USA Availability: Prescription

Pregnancy Category: X

Uses. Testosterone was discovered in the 1930s. It is primarily a male hormone but is found in females as well. Various forms of testosterone exist, and body chemistry can transform them into still other substances. They play major roles in maintaining male physical characteristics: genitals and prostate, beard and other body hair, voice quality, and body build. Testosterone is suspected of influencing thinking abilities and definitely can influence behavior, such as encouraging mania and aggression. One study found high testosterone amounts in criminals with personality disorder, with repeat offenders having the highest amounts. Experimenters documented that giving high doses to mares resulted in "markedly vicious stallion-like" conduct. Low testosterone levels in men can make them tired and depressed, reduce their interest in sexual activity, and cause male physical characteristics to diminish. In contrast to high and low amounts, one study found that normal levels of testosterone in men promoted normal behavior and feelings, such as geniality and contentment.

Doses of the drug can supplement the body's natural supply of male hormones if the supply is abnormally low. Testosterone is a treatment for male sexual dysfunction. Experimental use of the drug to alleviate depression and weight loss in HIV/AIDS (human immunodeficiency virus/acquired immunodeficiency syndrome) patients has been successful. The drug has also improved liver cirrhosis and a blood disease called aplastic anemia and is used against a bone affliction called myelosclerosis. In experiments testosterone improved the condition of heart patients suffering from angina (pain caused by insufficient cardiac oxygen supply), and an experiment showed benefit for coronary artery disease patients. A case report tells of success in treating

Felty's syndrome, an affliction involving rheumatoid arthritis accompanied by abnormalities in the blood and spleen. In men testosterone is used to combat osteoporosis, a disease causing brittleness in bones. Ordinarily the drug is not given to women but is sometimes appropriate in cases of hormonal imbalance or sexual dysfunction.

Examination of fluid circulating in the human brain shows higher-than-normal levels of testosterone in smokers addicted to **nicotine** and lower-than-normal levels in persons suffering from posttraumatic stress disorder. Blood studies find that female smokers and overweight women have higher testosterone levels than nonsmokers or lean persons. Such discoveries have led investigators to speculate that testosterone affects those conditions. Heightened testosterone levels have also been seen in women experiencing major depression. Among men with low body levels of testosterone, supplemental doses may help reduce depression. The drug's ability to affect depression was under investigation when this book was written.

Drawbacks. Unwanted effects of testosterone dosage may include acne, headache, higher blood pressure and cholesterol levels, gastrointestinal bleeding, promotion of baldness, and enlargement of prostate and male breasts. The drug should be avoided by men with breast or prostate cancer. Liver damage is suspected. Breathing interruptions during sleep can occur. The substance may cause fluid to build up in body tissues, which can be a serious problem for persons with heart, liver, or kidney disease. A case report associated a stroke with high levels of testosterone in a 21-year-old man who was injecting himself. When administered in a skin patch the compound can cause rashes, burning sensations, and even blisters.

Normally women are supposed to avoid taking the substance. It can cause their voices to deepen, promote hair growth on various parts of the body, induce irregular menstrual periods, and bring about genital changes. Sometimes women inadvertently receive doses from residual amounts on the skin of men who are using testosterone creams or skin patches. Such inadvertent dosage can be enough to bring on some male physical characteristics in a woman (such as development of facial hair). A case study notes premature puberty that began in a child who received the same type of exposure. Another inadvertent source of testosterone is meat from livestock that has been illegally dosed. Agricultural sources of the drug are not necessarily illicit; for example, chicken litter is used for cattle feed, and chicken manure may contain testosterone excreted by the birds, thereby dosing the cattle. Even some feeds used in salmon farming contain testosterone. Human consumption of such food animals may well be safe, but they are possible dosage routes for the drug in humans if regulations about agricultural use of the substance are disregarded.

Abuse factors. If used properly testosterone can stimulate muscle development, which tempts some athletes to try the drug regardless of whether a doctor is willing to prescribe it. Such unauthorized use can have bad consequences. One bodybuilder injected the substance into his right leg, which resulted in severe muscle damage making the right leg 40% weaker than his left one. Illicit testosterone use is also suspected of reducing male fertility; indeed, the drug has been investigated as a possible male contraceptive. Taking the compound without medical supervision can be particularly risky for adolescents, as testosterone can first make a young person taller but then prematurely halt further bone growth, thereby preventing attainment of normal adult height. Still another bad consequence of an athlete's illicit usage of testosterone may occur if sports regulatory authorities discover that an athlete is using it; the drug is banned from competitions.

Drug interactions. An experiment found that eating licorice reduces testosterone levels in men, enough that the candy may contribute to problems of male sexual function. Adolescent hamsters that drink **alcohol** show elevated testosterone levels, and a human study showed high levels among some alcoholics. Testosterone impairs blood clotting, which may dangerously boost actions from medicines given to reduce blood clots.

Cancer. Although testosterone is a naturally occurring substance in mammals, additional doses of testosterone have caused cancer of the breast, uterus, and cervix in mice and are suspected of promoting liver cancer in mice and rats. An experiment using both testosterone and estrogen produced cancer in hamsters. Testosterone is not proven to produce cancer in humans but is under suspicion. The drug may help bring about human prostate cancer but is not necessarily a direct cause. A case of kidney cancer has been ascribed to lengthy dosage, and in other case reports, testosterone was suspected of causing liver cancer. Paradoxically the drug has been used to help treat cancer.

Pregnancy. In animal tests the drug has caused pregnancy failure and has masculinized female offspring. Human fetal harm is a suspected consequence if pregnant women take doses of testosterone. A case report said that using the drug during pregnancy caused ambiguous gender appearance in a child, an appearance so ambiguous that the child was misidentified as male for several years even though she was female (as demonstrated by assorted medical tests and by the fact that as an adult she gave birth to a child). Testosterone has been investigated as a potential drug for stopping a woman's milk production. Regarding pregnancy and nursing, one manufacturer of the drug bluntly states that the product "must not be used in women."

Additional information. In addition to testosterone itself other pharmaceutical varieties (called "esters") are testosterone cypionate, testosterone decanoate, testosterone enanthate, testosterone isocaproate, testosterone propionate, and testosterone undecanoate. These are used for the same purposes that testosterone is used, and they basically have the same effects.

Additional scientific information may be found in:

Dabbs, J.M., and M.F. Hargrove. "Age, Testosterone, and Behavior among Female Prison Inmates." *Psychosomatic Medicine* 59 (1997): 477–80.

Freeman, E.R., D.A. Bloom, and E.J. McGuire. "A Brief History of Testosterone." *Journal of Urology* 165 (2001): 371–73.

Gambineri, A., and R. Pasquali. "Testosterone Therapy in Men: Clinical and Pharmacological Perspectives." *Journal of Endocrinological Investigation* 23 (2000): 196–214.

Giorgi, A., R.P. Weatherby, and P.W. Murphy. "Muscular Strength, Body Composition and Health Responses to the Use of Testosterone Enanthate: A Double Blind Study." *Journal of Science and Medicine in Sport* 2 (1999): 341–55.

Hayes, F.J. "Testosterone—Fountain of Youth or Drug of Abuse?" *Journal of Clinical Endocrinology and Metabolism* 85 (2000): 3020–23.

Killinger, D.W. "Testosterone." *Canadian Medical Association Journal* 103 (1970): 733–35.

Mazur, A., and A. Booth. "Testosterone and Dominance in Men." *Behavioral and Brain Sciences* 21 (1998): 353–63.

Pope, H.G., E.M. Kouri, and J.I. Hudson. "Effects of Supraphysiologic Doses of Testosterone on Mood and Aggression in Normal Men: A Randomized Controlled Trial." *Archives of General Psychiatry* 57 (2000): 133–40.

Rolf, C., and E. Nieschlag. "Potential Adverse Effects of Long-term Testosterone Therapy." *Bailliere's Clinical Endocrinology and Metabolism* 12 (1998): 521–34.

Thebaine

Pronunciation: THEE-buh-een (also pronounced thi-BAY-in)
Chemical Abstracts Service Registry Number: 115-37-7
Formal Names: Paramorphine
Type: Depressant (opiate class). *See* page 22
Federal Schedule Listing: Schedule II (DEA no. 9333)
USA Availability: Prescription
Pregnancy Category: None

Uses. Although thebaine is listed as a depressant in this book because the substance is an opiate, the substance is an unusual opiate lacking many effects seen in drugs of that class—and indeed sometimes seems more like a stimulant. Thebaine is one of the chemicals found in **opium** and in a poppy plant called *Papaver bracteatum*. Trace amounts are manufactured in brains of cows and presumably in brains of other mammals, and scientists suspect that mammals transform thebaine into **morphine**. Animal studies show that thebaine possesses mild ability to relieve pain and can lower pulse rate and blood pressure, but the drug has no medical use. Instead, its value is that other drugs can be produced from it: **buprenorphine, codeine, etorphine, hydrocodone, nalbuphine, oxycodone,** and **oxymorphone**. Opiate manufacturing creates waste products from which thebaine can be reclaimed, thereby allowing fuller use of an opium harvest. Thebaine in urine is considered evidence that a person testing positive for opiates has ingested a poppy seed food instead of an illicit drug.

Drawbacks. Tests with a variety of animal species, including human beings, show that thebaine can produce convulsions. That effect is so typical that two researchers have described thebaine as more a poison than a medicine. Compared to morphine, a much smaller dose of thebaine can be fatal.

Abuse factors. Experiments with monkeys indicate that thebaine has less addiction potential than codeine, but results were inconclusive about whether thebaine produces dependence. A World Health Organization advisory committee concluded that high doses of thebaine do produce dependence in monkeys, but the committee doubted that drug abusers could take high-enough doses to produce dependence. Only faint evidence of dependence developed in a canine study, and rat research produced no dependence at all. Some researchers have expressed uncertainty about whether dependence develops with thebaine itself or with breakdown products formed from thebaine through body chemistry. The same researchers declared that thebaine's ability to cause dependence is less than codeine's. One dog experiment yielded unclear evidence of tolerance, evidence that has not been supported by other work. Cross-tolerance with morphine has not been found in monkeys.

Drug interactions. In rats thebaine boosts **caffeine**'s effects.

Cancer. Not enough scientific information to report.

Pregnancy. After pregnant hamsters received thebaine their offspring had more birth defects than normal, and such defects did not appear if the hamsters first received various drugs known to reduce opiate effects. A thebaine dose sufficient to cause birth defects in hamsters tended to kill the pregnant females, so not much has been determined about the drug's potential to cause hamster malformations.

Additional scientific information may be found in:

Halbach, H., et al. "The Dependence Potential of Thebaine." *Bulletin on Narcotics* 32, no. 1 (1980): 45–54.

Waclawski, E.R., and R. Aldridge. "Occupational Dermatitis from Thebaine and Codeine." *Contact Dermatitis* 33 (1995): 51.

Woods, J.H., C.R. Schuster, and C.R. Hartel. "Behavioral Effects of Thebaine in the Rhesus Monkey." *Pharmacology, Biochemistry, and Behavior* 14 (1981): 805–9.

Yanagita, T., et al. "Dependence Potential of Drotebanol, Codeine and Thebaine Tested in Rhesus Monkeys." *Bulletin on Narcotics* 29, no. 1 (1977): 33–46.

Toluene

Pronunciation: TAHL-yoo-een

Chemical Abstracts Service Registry Number: 108-88-3

Formal Names: Methylbenzene

Informal Names: Glue, Tolly

Types: Inhalant. *See* page 26

Federal Schedule Listing: Unlisted

USA Availability: Found in assorted products; sales of the pure chemical are restricted because it can be used to manufacture controlled substances

Pregnancy Category: None

Uses. Toluene is a common component in **gasoline**, glues, and paint products (including nail polish). The chemical is used to manufacture the explosive TNT and may be found in DDT insecticides. Drinking toluene would be unhealthy, although experimental animals have survived oral dosage of the pure chemical. Many recreational users have no access to the pure chemical, and most (if not all) products containing it are poisonous.

Recreational use is by inhaling vapor from toluene, often in a group setting. Toluene intoxication lasts longer than intoxication from assorted other inhalants. Some actions of toluene are comparable to **alcohol**. Toluene can relax users, cheer them up, and produce hallucinations. Mood may change and become unpleasant, however, often in response to content of hallucinations. People may have delusions of nonexistent abilities to fly or swim or that they must obey commands from some entity. Real-world scenes may seem more brightly lit than normal. Time may be perceived as passing faster. People may feel confused and dizzy and experience difficulty with balance and with controlling their limbs. Mice react to toluene, **pentobarbital**, and **PCP** in some of the same ways. Rats respond to toluene, pentobarbital, and **ether** in similar manners. At a smaller dosage toluene stimulates rats to scurry about, but at larger doses the animals move around less—reminiscent of alcohol. Although some persons use toluene recreationally, others may use it to blunt psychological pain.

Drawbacks. Volunteers who inhaled toluene fumes experienced headache, eye discomfort, and lower performance on tests of thinking ability. Recreational users have reported slowness in thinking, and they have scored lower in intelligence testing than nonusers do. Dementia can be a consequence of the habit. Recreational users may have trouble remembering what they did while intoxicated, and persons with occupational exposure have shown memory damage. Sniffers may also experience nausea, appetite loss, tremors, speech difficulty, double vision, and ringing in the ears. Permanent hearing damage occurs in rats. Industrial exposure may harm a person's ability to move around; such problems may be unnoticeable in everyday life but can be detected with scientific tests. In contrast to such occupational exposure, daily abuse for several years may cause significant problems in mobility; those symptoms may mimic beriberi.

Brain, lung, eye, and liver injury can occur in recreational users. Investigators find that some physical damage may improve if exposure to toluene stops, although brain damage may be permanent. High blood pressure is reported in blood circulating through the lungs. Controversy exists about whether cardiac injury occurs, although a case report notes a heart attack suffered after a teenager sniffed toluene. Another case report tells about a previously healthy toluene sniffer, hospitalized with an extremely slow pulse rate that could result in heart stoppage. Anemia and other changes in blood composition may develop, changes affecting males and females in different ways. For example, in one study of persons chronically exposed to the substance, women had higher blood cholesterol levels than normal, and men had lower levels than normal. Chronic abuse can deplete a person's potassium levels; such depletion can damage muscles and produce irregular heartbeat. Although researchers concluded from one experiment that moderate exposure causes no kidney damage, stronger exposure may result in such harm. The chemical may produce a kidney malfunction called renal tubular acidosis, which might lead to rickets. Renal tubular acidosis can have fatal complications, but case reports indicate the condition can clear up if a victim stops toluene sniffing.

Regular exposure can be dangerous enough, but an overdose can create a medical emergency. In humans an overdose can dangerously speed up the heart, cause seizures and convulsions, and produce coma. Fatalities occur. An unusual hazard comes from the chemical's ability to increase salivation; in one case, a semiconscious person nearly drowned in his own saliva as it flowed into his lungs.

The liquid can be absorbed through skin and may cause skin irritation. Toluene is flammable, thus hazardous around flames or burning cigarettes.

Abuse factors. Monkeys have exhibited as much interest in toluene as in opiates and amphetamines. Tolerance has developed in rats and humans. Dependence is reported in humans, with a withdrawal syndrome including queasiness, perspiring, facial tics and abdominal cramps, peevishness, and difficulty with sleep. Symptoms last for several days. One reviewer of scientific studies, however, has questioned whether either tolerance or dependence has really been seen. Two experiments with monkeys found that they would self-administer toluene, behavior that is a classic indication of addictive potential, but circumstances in those tests did not simulate conditions of human recreational use. Animals that are strapped down with tubes shoved into a body orifice might well find a drug that reduces discomfort to be more attractive than a placebo, a choice having little to do with the drug's appeal in other circumstances.

Drug interactions. Not enough scientific information to report.

Cancer. Most, but not all, laboratory tests indicate toluene has no potential for causing cancer. Animal experiments have not produced cancer. Whether toluene causes cancer in humans is unknown.

Pregnancy. Toluene passes from a pregnant female into the fetus. Animal experiments designed to duplicate toluene abuse patterns have produced low birth weight and slow maturation of offspring; intermittent birth defects are also observed but without enough evidence to be sure they are caused by toluene, particularly since dosages tend to be so high as to sicken the pregnant females. Chronic exposure to the substance caused pregnancy failure in rabbits. In a mice experiment the death rate of offspring with prenatal exposure was nearly twice the rate of nonexposed offspring. Industrial exposure to toluene has been associated with human fetal deformity and spontaneous abortion, but toluene's exact role is uncertain because the women were exposed to other chemicals as well. Association has been noted with birth defects of the heart and of the digestive and urogenital systems. Such association does not prove cause and effect, but it does indicate areas needing further research. A study of 18 infants with prenatal exposure to toluene found that 39% were premature births, with 9% dying soon afterward. Over half were smaller than normal and had trouble catching up to usual size in ensuing months. Fully 67% had smaller-than-normal heads, implying smaller-than-normal brains. Almost all had classic head and facial characteristics of fetal alcohol syndrome. Similar findings came from a study of 30 infants born to 11 toluene abusers and from a study of another 21 infants. Case reports are consistent with those findings. Most, if not all, toluene abusers also abuse other drugs, so firm conclusions about fetal effects of toluene cannot be reached from these studies and cases. Indeed, one group of researchers concluded that some effects blamed on toluene were actually caused by alcohol abuse during pregnancy.

Additional scientific information may be found in:

Aydin, K., et al. "Cranial MR Findings in Chronic Toluene Abuse by Inhalation." *AJNR. American Journal of Neuroradiology* 23 (2002): 1173–79.

Devathasan, G., et al. "Complications of Chronic Glue (Toluene) Abuse in Adolescents." *Australian and New Zealand Journal of Medicine* 14 (1984): 39–43.

Evans, A.C., and D. Raistrick. "Phenomenology of Intoxication with Toluene-Based Adhesives and Butane Gas." *British Journal of Psychiatry* 150 (1987): 769–73.

Filley, C., R.K. Heaton, and N.L. Rosenberg. "White Matter Dementia in Chronic Toluene Abuse." *Neurology* 40 (1990): 532–34.

Glaser, H.H., and O.N. Massengale. "Glue-Sniffing in Children: Deliberate Inhalation of Vaporized Plastic Cements." *Journal of the American Medical Association* 181 (1962): 300–304.

Goodwin, T.M. "Toluene Abuse and Renal Tubular Acidosis in Pregnancy." *Obstetrics and Gynecology* 71 (1988): 715–18.

Kamiyoshi, S., et al. "[Generalized Muscle Weakness Mimicking Periodic Paralysis in a Patient with Toluene Abuse.]" *No To Shinkei* [*Brain and Nerve*] 54 (2002): 427–30. Abstract in English.

King, P.J., J.G. Morris, and J.D. Pollard. "Glue Sniffing Neuropathy." *Australian and New Zealand Journal of Medicine* 15 (1985): 293–99.

Lurie, J.B. "Acute Toluene Poisoning." *South African Medical Journal* 23 (1949): 233–36.

Marjot, R., and A.A. McLeod. "Chronic Non-Neurological Toxicity from Volatile Substance Abuse." *Human Toxicology* 8 (1989): 301–6.

Massengale, O.N., et al. "Physical and Psychologic Factors in Glue Sniffing." *New England Journal of Medicine* 269 (1963): 1340–44.

Trenbolone

Pronunciation: TREN-boh-lohn

Chemical Abstracts Service Registry Number: 10161-33-8. (Acetate form 10161-34-9)

Formal Names: Fina, Finaject, Finajet, Finaplix, Parabolan

Informal Names: Tren

Type: Anabolic steroid. See page 24

Federal Schedule Listing: Schedule III (DEA no. 4000)

USA Availability: Prescription

Uses. Trenbolone is a familiar agricultural drug used for encouraging growth in meat animals. Human bodybuilders have used the substance in hopes of gaining competitive advantage.

Drawbacks. The drug can promote masculine characteristics in females. Research on the drug's effects in pigs noted that testes decreased in size; research on cows noted disruption of ovarian cycles. Reports exist of human users complaining about headache, high blood pressure, nosebleeds, acne, fever, loss of appetite, queasy stomach, darkened urine, and aggressive conduct while taking the substance.

Abuse factors. Muscle mass has increased in steers receiving a growth treatment that included the drug. Some bodybuilders and weight lifters use various forms of trenbolone, making little distinction among them. The drug, however, is banned from sports competitions (including horse racing).

Drug interactions. Not enough scientific information to report.

Cancer. Laboratory tests generally have not revealed trenbolone to have a cancer-causing potential, but the substance has nonetheless been associated with cancer in mice and rats. Some researchers believe tumors probably result from hormonal effects of trenbolone dosage rather than a direct chemical action (the practical consequence may be the same for an animal either way, but the difference is important for scientists seeking better understanding of the drug).

Pregnancy. Animal experiments do not indicate that the drug causes birth defects, but women are routinely advised to avoid drugs of this type during pregnancy.

Additional scientific information may be found in:

Johnson, B.J., et al. "Effect of a Combined Trenbolone Acetate and Estradiol Implant on Feedlot Performance, Carcass Characteristics, and Carcass Composition of Feedlot Steers." *Journal of Animal Science* 74 (1996): 363–71.

Peters, A.R. "Effect of Trenbolone Acetate on Ovarian Function in Culled Dairy Cows." *Veterinary Record* 120 (1987): 413–16.

Richold, M. "The Genotoxicity of Trenbolone, a Synthetic Steroid." *Archives of Toxicology* 61 (1988): 249–58.

Van Leeuwen, F.X. "The Approach Taken and Conclusions Reached by the Joint FAO-WHO Expert Committee on Food Additives." *Annales de Recherches Veterinaires—Annals of Veterinary Research* 22 (1991): 253–56.

Triazolam

Pronunciation: try-Ā-zoh-lam

Chemical Abstracts Service Registry Number: 28911-01-5

Formal Names: Halcion

Type: Depressant (benzodiazepine class). *See* page 21

Federal Schedule Listing: Schedule IV (DEA no. 2887)

USA Availability: Prescription

Pregnancy Category: X

Uses. Triazolam became available for medical use in the United States during the 1980s. The substance is supposed to be used for treating insomnia on a short-term basis (typically one or two weeks), but sometimes prescribers tell patients to take the medicine for months. A brief insomnia rebound can occur when people stop taking the drug, meaning that for a night or two they have more trouble sleeping than before they used the drug. Another medical application of the drug is to make patients less nervous as they await dental work.

Experiments indicate the substance can help workers change their sleep schedules. In a simulated transportation of troops into combat, however, triazolam was unhelpful in shifting the sleep schedule of soldiers; and in a military exercise flying soldiers from the United States to the Middle East, the drug failed to produce adequate sleep. In still another experiment, the U.S. Army noted that the drug can induce sleep under adverse conditions but that soldiers will not do as well as normal if forced to perform while under triazolam's influence. A military experiment tested whether the drug could affect ability to engage in cold temperature operations, with ambiguous results.

Murders have been committed using triazolam in a beverage to make victims defenseless against attack. The substance is 4 to 34 times stronger than **diazepam**, 40 times stronger than **zolpidem**, and 1,000 times stronger than **chloral hydrate**; and it is normally considered about 60 times stronger than **flurazepam** and **temazepam**, but that normal assumption has been questioned by researchers examining those drugs' potencies. For some effects, such as memory impairment and control of body appendages, triazolam is hundreds of times stronger than **pentobarbital**. Despite triazolam's inherent strength, experiments show its effects as no greater than other benzodiazepine class depressants if doses are adjusted to compensate for strength differences.

Drawbacks. Triazolam has been likened to **flunitrazepam** in ability to cause amnesia. Memory trouble has been scientifically demonstrated after triazolam dosage, and an experiment measured continued memory impairment a week after taking the compound. Triazolam is associated with "traveler's amnesia" when people on the go (such as airline passengers) take the drug for a quick sleep and rouse themselves for activity before the substance has worn off; they forget things they did while under the drug's influence. That condition is sometimes associated with simultaneously ingesting **alcohol**, an unwise practice with any benzodiazepine class substance. The amnesia can be startling. Physicians have taken triazolam to promote a good night's sleep, attended to professional duties the next day (including carrying out medical procedures), and suddenly realized they have no memory of anything they have done in that time period. Colleagues and patients observed nothing amiss; by coincidence one doctor was videotaped during the "blackout" period, and the videotape showed him acting normally. Such an effect can happen without drugs; some car drivers suddenly realize they have gone for several blocks or miles with no recollection of stoplights or turnoffs. Under triazolam amnesia people function normally and do not do anything they would not ordinarily do but simply fail to acquire memory of what they did. Flumazenil is a drug that counteracts benzodiazepine effects, and U.S. Army research has determined that administering flumazenil with triazolam prevents the memory trouble.

Triazolam may promote extraverted behavior, mania, aggression, hallucinations (visual, auditory, tactile), confusion, and difficulty in communicating. These responses are mostly limited to users who are elderly or who have a prior history of psychiatric difficulties. A study of psychiatric patients receiving high dosage of triazolam documented that they engaged in alarming conduct (ranging from self-induced vomiting to panic attacks and suicide attempts) with no memory of the activity after the drug wore off. Persons who commit violent acts after taking triazolam seem to be persons who are already psychologically abnormal. In the general population such effects are unusual: Examination of results from clinical trials testing the drug on over 5,400 persons revealed no reports of psychotic reaction. Nonetheless, in the early 1990s unwanted psychological effects prompted a ban against triazolam by governments around the world (although not by the United States). After further consideration, most of those countries restored access to the drug. Two authorities have suggested that the most sensible approach is simply to avoid prescribing the drug to persons who are elderly or mentally ill.

A study in Finland concluded that despite occasional bizarre behavior prompted by the drug, triazolam was not associated with violent death; indeed, in fatalities the drug was detected less often than would be expected by chance. A comparison of psychiatric patient records found that triazolam is no more prone to lower someone's inhibitions than temazepam, and an experiment testing adverse effects in normal volunteers found little difference between those two drugs in comparable dosing.

A reviewer who examined dozens of scientific studies involving thousands of triazolam users found unwanted sedation to be the only adverse effect reliably associated with medical doses of the substance, although a reviewer of studies sponsored by the manufacturer noted occasional complaints of headache, dizziness, incoordination, and nervousness. Hangover from the drug is common after awakening, although some studies show hangover to be lighter with triazolam than with flurazepam or barbiturates. Triazolam can produce double vision, and hours after taking a dose people can still have difficulty controlling their movements—a particular problem for elderly persons who already have trouble avoiding falls.

Alarmingly, people are not necessarily aware of how much they are affected by a triazolam dose. While under the drug's influence, users should avoid operating dangerous machinery such as automobiles. A U.S. Army experiment found that people could perform normally on computerized tests six hours after taking a triazolam dose, but not everyone is as physically fit as combat-ready soldiers (physical condition can make a difference on how fast a drug is flushed from the body). For example, Swiss military and airline pilots showed impaired performance when tested seven hours after taking the same dose used in the U.S. Army study.

An unusual case report tells of vision damage in two persons who looked at a television camera's brilliant light while using triazolam. Another case report notes the drug can interfere with male fertility. Triazolam is not recommended for use by children, although experiments have revealed no ill effects in juveniles who receive the drug.

Abuse factors. Experimentation indicates that the greater a person's history of sedative abuse, the more appealing triazolam will be. Persons who did not abuse drugs and who took triazolam in an experiment did not like it, and compared to other benzodiazepines, the drug is considered to have average or below-average potential for abuse. A published review of research on triazolam concluded that its potential for abuse is less than pentobarbital's. Research finds little evidence of triazolam tolerance, but cases are reported of the drug's sleep-inducing and antianxiety properties declining in some persons, who respond by taking more and more triazolam. Dependence can develop, causing a withdrawal syndrome if the drug is cut off. Withdrawal symptoms may be trivial but can include psychosis, delirium, and seizures. Indeed, some psychological problems once attributed to the drug have later been attributed partly to withdrawal. Typically someone experiencing dependence on triazolam has already had trouble with drug abuse or is suffering from anxiety or panic attacks.

Drug interactions. Normally people using triazolam should avoid the antidepressant drug nefazodone due to its tendency to prolong effects of a triazolam dose. The female hormone supplement progesterone makes the body more sensitive to triazolam. The blood pressure medicine diltiazem, the human immunodeficiency virus AIDS (acquired immunodeficiency syndrome) medicine ritonavir, and the antifungus drugs itraconazole and ketoconazole not only extend the length of a triazolam dose but increase its effects. The antacid cimetidine (Tagamet) is suspected of doing the same. Grapefruit juice may increase the amount of triazolam accessible to the body after a dose, but results have been inconsistent in experiments testing whether the combination increases drug actions. Drugs that lessen effects of a triazolam dose include **caffeine**, the tuberculosis medicine rifampin, and the anticonvulsant medicines carbamazepine and phenytoin. The antibiotics roxithromycin and erythromycin interfere with the body's use of triazolam. In rat experiments alcohol increased triazolam levels in the brain even though blood levels were virtually unaffected. In human experiments some researchers have concluded that alcohol boosts some triazolam effects, but other researchers feel that the lengthening and deepening of triazolam actions after drinking alcohol simply mean that both substances have similar effects, not that the two drugs are interacting. Regardless, combining the two can be fatal.

Cancer. A two-year triazolam experiment with mice using up to 4,000 times the normal human dose yielded no sign that the drug causes cancer.

Pregnancy. Triazolam is not recommended for pregnant women. A case report tells of a full-term pregnant woman who took 100 times the normal dose of triazolam plus alcohol, arrived at a hospital unconscious, and delivered a normal-seeming infant—an exceptional case, however, as lighter triazolam amounts have proved fatal.

In rat studies triazolam passes into milk of nursing rodents. The drug's level in rat milk is about 70% of levels in the maternal rat's blood.

Additional scientific information may be found in:

Ghaeli, P., R.L. Dufresne, and C.A. Stoukides. "Triazolam Treatment Controversy." *Annals of Pharmacotherapy* 28 (1994): 1038–40.

Griffiths, R.R., et al. "Relative Abuse Liability of Triazolam: Experimental Assessment in Animals and Humans." *Neuroscience and Biobehavioral Reviews* 9 (1985): 133–51.

Klett, C.J. "Review of Triazolam Data." *Journal of Clinical Psychiatry* 53 (1992, Suppl.): 61–67.

Pakes, G.E., et al. "Triazolam: A Review of Its Pharmacological Properties and Therapeutic Efficacy in Patients with Insomnia." *Drugs* 22 (1981): 81–110.

Perry, P.J., and D.A. Smith. "Triazolam—Never-Ending Story." *DICP: The Annals of Pharmacotherapy* 25 (1991): 1263–64.

Rothschild, A.J. "Disinhibition, Amnestic Reactions, and Other Adverse Reactions Secondary to Triazolam: A Review of the Literature." *Journal of Clinical Psychiatry* 53 (1992, Suppl.): 69–79.

Rush, C.R., et al. "Acute Effects of Triazolam and Lorazepam on Human Learning, Performance and Subject Ratings." *Journal of Pharmacology and Experimental Therapeutics* 264 (1993): 1218–26.

Schneider, P.J., and P.J. Perry. "Triazolam—An 'Abused Drug' by the Lay Press?" *DICP: The Annals of Pharmacotherapy* 24 (1990): 389–92.

Spinweber, C.L., and L.C. Johnson. "Effects of Triazolam (0.5 Mg) on Sleep, Performance, Memory, and Arousal Threshold." *Psychopharmacology* 76 (1982): 5–12.

Trimeperidine

Pronunciation: treye-meh-PER-i-deen

Chemical Abstracts Service Registry Number: 64-39-1

Formal Names: Isopromedol, Promedol

Type: Depressant (opioid class). *See* page 24

Federal Schedule Listing: Schedule I (DEA no. 9646)

USA Availability: Illegal to possess

Pregnancy Category: None

Uses. This drug is somewhat like **meperidine** but has no officially sanctioned medical use in the United States. Elsewhere it is used as a pain reliever. Australian work has examined using trimeperidine, meperidine, and **methadone** together for pain control. In Russia trimeperidine is given to adults and children both and has been used to treat shock (low blood pressure and heartbeat abnormality) as well as pain. A report from a Moscow surgery facility indicated that trimeperidine is used routinely there and implied that patients are allowed to select whatever dosage is effective for them. Another report from Russia judged the substance to be an excellent choice for anesthesia in abdominal cancer operations, although an additional study described the drug as less effective than **fentanyl** in anesthesia. Trimeperidine has been used to ease childbirth, but a clinical report from Bulgaria says that other drugs work better. Russian military medicine used trimeperidine for treating combat casualties evacuated from the Afghanistan and Chechnya wars but found it less effective than other pharmaceuticals. In the 1980s Russian research studied possible uses for the drug in treating combined burn and radiation injuries, a direction of research suggesting preparation for nuclear war.

Drawbacks. The drug has been known to halt breathing.

Abuse factors. A rat study demonstrated that dependence can develop with trimeperidine.

Drug interactions. Not enough scientific information to report.

Cancer. Not enough scientific information to report.

Pregnancy. Not enough scientific information to report.

Additional information. Trimeperidine and the Schedule I substances alphameprodine (CAS RN 468-51-9), betameprodine (468-50-8), and proheptazine (77-14-5) all have the same molecular formula, but they are different drugs.

Additional scientific information may be found in:

Alderman, C. "Trimeprazine as a Component of Pain Cocktails." *Australian Journal of Hospital Pharmacy* 19 (1989): 205–6.

Bazarevich, G.I., et al. "Sravnitel'naia otsenka protivoshokovogo deistviia nekotorykh otechestvennykh farmakologicheskikh preparatov" (Comparative evaluation of antishock activity of various Soviet pharmacological agents) (In Russian). *Vestnik Khirurgii Imeni I. I. Grekova* 130, no. 6 (1983): 73–77.

Il'iuchenok, T.Iu., I.A. Matveeva, and R.O. Budagov. "Changes in the Pharmacodynamic Properties of Promedol, Droperidol and Dimedrol in Burn Shock and Combined Radiation-Thermal Injury" (in Russian). *Farmakologiia i Toksikologiia* 50 (1987): 71–74.

Kichin, V.V., and M.Iu. Buldakov. "Anesthesiological Accompaniment for the Wounded during Transport" (in Russian). *Voenno-Meditsinskii Zhurnal* 320 (1999): 23–26, 96.

Malinovskii, N.N., R.N. Lebedeva, and V.V. Nikoda. "The Problem of Acute Pain in Postoperative Period" (in Russian). *Khirurgiia (Mosk)*, no. 5 (1996): 30–35.

Radev, R. "Postoperative Analgesia in Cesarean Section" (in Bulgarian). *Khirurgiia (Sofiia)* 49 (1996): 33–36.

Shcherbakov, I.V., et al. "The Choice of a Method of General Anesthesia for Patients with Cancer of the Abdominal Cavity" (in Russian). *Anesteziologiia i Reanimatologiia*, nos. 5–6 (1992): 48–50.

Note: English summaries of all the above articles are available through the PubMed Web site: http://www.ncbi.nlm.nih.gov/entrez/query.fcgi

2C-B

Pronunciation: too-see-bee

Chemical Abstracts Service Registry Number: 66142-81-2

Formal Names: Alpha-Desmethyl DOB, 4-Bromo-2,5-Dimethoxyphenethylam-ine, 2-CB

Informal Names: BDMPEA, Bees, Bromo, Bromo-Mescaline, Erox, Eve, Herox, Honey Flip (with **MDMA**), Illusion, MFT, Nexus, Performax, Spectrum, Synergy, Venus, Zenith

Type: Hallucinogen. *See* page 25

Federal Schedule Listing: Schedule I (DEA no. 7392)

USA Availability: Illegal to possess

Pregnancy Category: None

Uses. This drug was created in the 1970s and is related to amphetamine, **DOB**, and **mescaline**.

Reports about alleged effects are plentiful, but 2C-B's Schedule I status means that most persons who think they are using 2C-B have acquired their product from an illegal drug dealer. Therefore, they do not really know what substance they are taking, and their accounts have no value. The drug's inventor Alexander Shulgin portrays the chemical as facilitating psychological insights that improve mental health, a quality that gained 2C-B a role in psychotherapy—both alone and in combination with MDMA, a combination that promoted empathy between users and other persons. Reports conflict about how much empathy is promoted by 2C-B itself. Intense emotions can occur, ranging from euphoria to fear. Physical senses can become more acute after the drug is administered. Research reported by a World Health Organization agency indicates 2C-B can make the senses of smell, taste, and touch more acute. This and other research describes 2C-B as a possible aphrodisiac. The substance is also a hallucinogen that can alter visual perceptions. The U.S. Drug Enforcement Administration made 2C-B a Schedule I substance in 1994.

Drawbacks. The drug is reported to have general stimulant actions that increase pulse rate and blood pressure and may be hazardous to epileptics and diabetics. Headache, chills, sweating, nausea, cramps, tremors, and reddened complexion are reported. Although sense of touch may be enhanced, sensitivity to pain may paradoxically be reduced, making a person less aware of injury—thereby increasing risk of harm. One authority warns against using the drug along with monoamine oxidase inhibitors (MAOIs), found in some antidepressants, lest the combination make a 2C-B dose too strong.

Abuse factors. Not enough scientific information to report.

Drug interactions. Not enough scientific information to report.

Cancer. Not enough scientific information to report.

Pregnancy. Not enough scientific information to report.

Additional scientific information may be found in:

De Boer, D., et al. "More Data about the New Psychoactive Drug 2C-B." *Journal of Analytical Toxicology* 23 (1999): 227–28.

Giroud, C., et al. "2C-B: A New Psychoactive Phenylethylamine Recently Discovered in Ecstasy Tablets Sold on the Swiss Black Market." *Journal of Analytical Toxicology* 22 (1998): 345–54.

"Schedules of Controlled Substances; Placement of 4-Bromo-2,5-Dimethoxyphenethylamine into Schedule I." *Federal Register* 55 (1996): 28718–719.

Who Expert Committee on Drug Dependence. "Thirty-Second Report." *WHO Technical Report Series* 903 (2001): 6–8.

Yage

Pronunciation: YAH-hay

Chemical Abstracts Service Registry Number: None

Formal Names: Ayahuasca, *Banisteriopsis caapi*, Yaje

Informal Names: Caapi, Daime, Huasca, La Purga, Vine, Vine of Death, Vine of the Soul, Visionary Vine

Type: Hallucinogen. *See* page 25

Federal Schedule Listing: Unlisted

USA Availability: Nonprescription natural product

Pregnancy Category: None

Uses. This powerful plant comes from the Amazon jungle. "Ayahuasca" is a name both for the plant and for a potion composed of yage and other ingredients (often including plants containing **DMT**). Disagreement exists about whether a particular name is properly applied to the plant, to the potion, or to both. Small doses of yage produce euphoria; larger ones produce hallucinations (blue is reportedly a predominant color in the visual images). Sexual imagery has been noted, but debate exists on whether ayahuasca preparations are aphrodisiacal. An account from recreational users says yage itself has barely any hallucinogenic actions but describes yage as enhancing such effects from DMT. Sedative properties appear as the drug experience proceeds.

Among native peoples of the Amazon, the ayahuasca potion is used in contexts of healing and religion. Healing may be psychological; in some regions yage is called "vine of death," a name that one authority interprets as referring to liberation from a troubled life and being born again into a better life after using yage. Evidence exists that the ayahuasca potion may have antidepressant actions. In its traditional Amazon setting drinkers of the preparation claim to experience ESP (extrasensory perception) and sensations of flying.

Drawbacks. Unwanted yage effects include nausea, vomiting, and ringing or other noise in the ears. Users of ayahuasca drinks report an urgent need to defecate; other reactions may include tremors, perspiration, and tingling in hands or feet.

Abuse factors. Not enough scientific information to report about tolerance, dependence, withdrawal, or addiction.

Drug interactions. Not enough scientific information to report about the natural product, but see below for information about interactions with chemicals in yage.

Cancer. Not enough scientific information to report.

Pregnancy. Not enough scientific information to report.

Additional information. Harmine, harmaline, and tetrahydroharmine are chemicals found in yage. Harmaline users have noted vision distortions when looking at real objects, accompanied by loss of sensitivity in other physical senses. Unwanted effects may include dizziness, pressure in chest, nausea, vomiting, and weariness. Feelings of anxiety may arise. One investigator gave harmaline to urban residents and was intrigued that they hallucinated jungle animal imagery; according to some reports, dosage must be almost poisonous for such effects; otherwise, actions are more sedative than psychedelic. Some authorities declare that harmaline aids psychotherapy; others dispute that assertion. Harmine has been tested as a treatment for Parkinson's disease, with mixed results. Harmine can slow heartbeat, lower blood pressure, produce tingling and dizziness, and make hands and feet cold. Hallucinations and a feeling of floating have been reported.

The harmine, harmaline, and tetrahydroharmine in yage are all monoamine oxidase inhibitors (MAOIs). Yage might cause overdose effects if a person is taking other MAOI drugs (found in some antidepressants and other medicine), and yage could cause problems if a person is also using drugs that interact badly with an MAOI.

Additional scientific information may be found in:

Freedland, C.S., and R.S. Mansbach. "Behavioral Profile of Constituents in Ayahuasca, an Amazonian Psychoactive Plant Mixture." *Drug and Alcohol Dependence* 54 (1999): 183–94.

Grob, C.S., et al. "Human Psychopharmacology of Hoasca: A Plant Hallucinogen Used in Ritual Context in Brazil." *Journal of Nervous and Mental Disorders* 184 (1996): 86–94.

Harner, M.J., ed. *Hallucinogens and Shamanism.* New York: Oxford University Press, 1973.

Naranjo, C. "Ayahuasca, Caapi, Yage. Psychotropic Properties of the Harmala Alkaloids." *Psychopharmacology Bulletin* 4, no. 3 (1967): 16–17.

Riba, J., and M.J. Barbanoj. "A Pharmacological Study of Ayahuasca in Healthy Volunteers." *Bulletin of the Multidisciplinary Association for Psychedelic Studies* 8 (Autumn 1998): 12–15.

Shulgin, A.T. "Profiles of Psychedelic Drugs: 4. Harmaline." *Journal of Psychedelic Drugs* 9 (1977): 79–80.

Yohimbe

Pronunciation: yoh-HIM-bee

Chemical Abstracts Service Registry Number: None

Formal Names: Actibine, Aphrodine, Aphrodyne, Baron-X, *Corynanthe yohimbe*, Corynine, Dayto Himbin, Hydroaergotocin, *Pausinystalia yohimbe*, Procomil, Prohim, Quebrachine, Thybine, Testomar, Yocon, Yohimar, Yohimex, Yohydrol, Yoman, Yomax, Yovital

Informal Names: Yo-Yo

Type: Stimulant. *See* page 11

Federal Schedule Listing: Unlisted

USA Availability: Nonprescription natural product

Pregnancy Category: None

Uses. Yohimbe is an evergreen tree found in African jungles. The bark contains the prescription drug yohimbine (CAS RN 146-48-5), which is also commercially produced in a hydrochloride form (CAS RN 65-19-0).

In folk medicine yohimbe bark is a treatment for fever, coughs, weariness, pain, and leprosy and is considered an aphrodisiac. Preparations including the natural product have been marketed as a bodybuilding aid, although the U.S. Food and Drug Administration (FDA) has shown skepticism about that claim. Theoretical reasons exist to suspect that yohimbine might have antidepressant capability, but documentation of such benefit has eluded investigators. Yohimbine has also been marketed as an appetite suppressant, but scientific research has found it to have no such action. In an experiment using patients on a controlled diet, however, those who received yohimbine achieved more weight loss, perhaps through enhancement of energy expenditure. Human experiments have failed to show that the drug promotes loss of fat, although that effect has been measured in canines.

Veterinarians have used yohimbine to speed awakening of anesthetized animals ranging from foxes and finches to buffaloes and budgerigars.

Research indicates the drug can increase male sexual drive and performance; a case report indicates similar effects in females also, but formal experimentation has not shown such benefit for females. Experimenters administered capsules of yohimbine to male crocodiles (by tossing food morsels in which the capsules had been hidden). The males did not copulate more frequently, despite showing more sexual desire, but the fertility rate increased among eggs laid by females that were mated by the treated crocodiles.

Normal sensations returned to legs of diabetics after they received yohimbine in an experiment. Another experiment showed that yohimbine can help persons fight the sleepiness of narcolepsy. The substance can be used to improve salivation in individuals troubled by dry mouth and can dilate the eye's pupil. The drug increases blood pressure of normal persons, and in persons prone to fainting, yohimbine can improve that affliction by increasing blood pressure. A branch of the FDA, however, has declared yohimbine to be a substance that lowers blood pressure. Experimental use of yohimbine shows that it can help bring forth repressed memories and help people deal with them. Research also reveals that yohimbine can improve performance on some kinds of reaction-time tests.

Drawbacks. Unwanted effects from yohimbine include headache, tremors, cramps, mental tenseness, confusion, insomnia, chills, perspiration, dizziness, indigestion, nausea, vomiting, diarrhea, skin eruptions or flushed appearance, impaired hearing, accelerated heartbeat, and decreased urine production. Daily usage may cause breathing difficulty and symptoms reminiscent of lupus. Persons should avoid operating dangerous machinery if the substance is making them dizzy. People are advised to avoid yohimbine if they suffer from diabetes or diseases of the heart, liver, or kidney. Case reports attribute kidney failure and heart difficulty to yohimbine; an experiment documented that yohimbine reduces the heart's efficiency while a person is resting and makes the heart work harder while a person is exercising. Persons with kidney or liver malfunction are advised to avoid the natural product yohimbe as well. Claims exist about the natural product yohimbe causing hallucinations, but scientific information is nil about that subject. Hallucinations are not included among unwanted effects listed by the manufacturer of the Aphrodyne brand of yohimbine.

Yohimbine may increase anxiety and panic; research has shown the substance to worsen symptoms experienced by persons suffering from posttraumatic stress disorder—experimentation demonstrates that yohimbine facilitates recall of emotionally charged memories, and such recall is not always a good thing. Instances of manic behavior following yohimbine administration are known, as is lesser stimulation involving mere restlessness.

Abuse factors. Not enough scientific information to report about tolerance, dependence, withdrawal, or addiction.

Drug interactions. Although yohimbine can improve pain relief provided by **morphine**, yohimbine can interfere with clonidine, a pain reliever and sedative that is also used to fight high blood pressure and migraine. Yohimbine may also interfere with other drugs used against high blood pressure; indeed, it has worked as an antidote for overdose from clonidine. Yohimbine's ability to increase blood pressure can be boosted by tricyclic antidepressants. Phenothiazine tranquilizers may raise the chance of yohimbine poisoning. In a dog experiment yohimbine increased **cocaine**'s adverse actions on the heart. Yohimbine's unwanted effects may be promoted by **ephedrine** and by naltrexone, a drug given to treat **alcohol** and **heroin** addiction. At a high-enough dose yohimbine acts as a monoamine oxidase inhibitor (MAOI), and various drugs described in this book react badly with MAOIs.

Cancer. Not enough scientific information to report.

Pregnancy. Women are supposed to avoid yohimbine during pregnancy and if they are nursing an infant.

Additional information. Although yohimbine may help treat sexual dysfunction, and sexual dysfunction is a topic of robust interest to sufferers and caregivers alike, someone who reviewed scientific studies about yohimbine noted comparatively little investigation of the substance and attributed this apathy to yohimbine's status as an "orphan drug." An orphan drug is one that is ignored because it has little potential for commercial profitability. Yohimbine is such an old drug that it can no longer be patented; no pharmaceutical company can gain a monopoly on it and thereby force patients to pay a premium price. Consequently, scientists can obtain little financial or institutional support for exploring yohimbine's potential.

Additional scientific information may be found in:

Albus, M., T.P. Zahn, and A. Breier. "Anxiogenic Properties of Yohimbine. I. Behavioral, Physiological and Biochemical Measures." *European Archives of Psychiatry and Clinical Neuroscience* 241 (1992): 337–44.

Biaggioni, I., R.M. Robertson, and D. Robertson. "Manipulation of Norepinephrine Metabolism with Yohimbine in the Treatment of Autonomic Failure." *Journal of Clinical Pharmacology* 34 (1994): 418–23.

De Smet, P.A., and O.S. Smeets. "Potential Risks of Health Food Products Containing Yohimbe Extracts." *BMJ* 309 (1994): 958.

Linden, C.H., W.P. Vellman, and B. Rumack. "Yohimbine: A New Street Drug." *Annals of Emergency Medicine* 14 (1985): 1002–4.

Morpurgo, B., I. Rozenboim, and B. Robinzon. "Effect of Yohimbine on the Reproductive Behavior of the Male Nile Crocodile *Crocodylus niloticus*." *Pharmacology, Biochemistry, and Behavior* 43 (1992): 449–52.

Southwick, S.M., et al. "Yohimbine Use in a Natural Setting: Effects on Posttraumatic Stress Disorder." *Biological Psychiatry* 46 (1999): 442–44.

"Yohimbine for Male Sexual Dysfunction." *Medical Letter on Drugs and Therapeutics* 36 (1994): 115–16.

Zaleplon

Pronunciation: ZAH-leh-plon

Chemical Abstracts Service Registry Number: 151319-34-5

Formal Names: Sonata

Type: Depressant. *See* page 19

Federal Schedule Listing: Schedule IV (DEA no. 2781)

USA Availability: Prescription

Pregnancy Category: C

Uses. This substance is a sleep inducer that also has anticonvulsant properties. Zaleplon is neither an opiate nor a barbiturate nor a benzodiazepine depressant.

The drug's sleep-inducing effects wear off so quickly that zaleplon seems suitable for use in the middle of the night without risk of hangover drowsiness after waking up. The substance has been approved for NASA (National Aeronautics and Space Administration) space shuttle crews and has been carried on flights, an environment where immediate alertness is required upon awakening. Despite lack of grogginess after people rouse themselves, they should nonetheless avoid dangerous activity (such as driving a car) right after taking a drug intended to induce sleep. Researchers testing zaleplon when it was active, rather than after its effects should have worn off, found that it interfered with people's actions to about the same extent as **triazolam** but less than **lorazepam** or **zolpidem**. Sleep medicines with short action sometimes make people nervous after extended use, and nervousness has been reported by some persons using zaleplon, but that unwanted effect was not observed in formal tests with the drug. Experiments with rats and mice find zaleplon to have an antianxiety property. Results of human research conflict on whether zaleplon has a brief rebound insomnia effect, but the trend is to find no rebound. "Rebound" is when people have trouble sleeping for a night or two after dosage stops.

One study found doses to be more potent among Japanese than among Americans. The reason is unclear; it may be related to average body weights or to some ethnic factor.

Drawbacks. Zaleplon can cause people to forget what happens for a couple of hours after a dose, and some persons still have amnesia trouble the day after a dose. One experiment found the intensity of that effect to be comparable to lorazepam's but shorter in duration. Because of possible memory difficulty, an individual using zaleplon may want to avoid situations involving important decisions. Other unwanted effects may include skin rash, muscle tightness, pain in chest and back, migraine headache, constipation, difficulty in concentrating, and emotional depression. Euphoria is a less common effect.

Abuse factors. Studies indicate zaleplon has about the same potential for abuse as benzodiazepine class depressants do. Researchers using volunteers who had previously abused drugs concluded that zaleplon and triazolam have the same abuse potential. No tolerance emerged in studies where people took zaleplon for weeks and months. No dependence developed either, but that finding is not considered conclusive. In animal studies dependence has occurred, severe enough that some animals died when the drug was cut off. Researchers conducting a baboon experiment found zaleplon to have about the same dependence potential as triazolam.

Drug interactions. **Alcohol** should be avoided when taking zaleplon. Tests have demonstrated that zaleplon boosts the effects of alcohol and also boosts some action of the psychiatric medication thioridazine.

Cancer. Cancer emerged in some mice that received 6 to 49 times the maximum human dose of zaleplon for two years, but cancer did not develop in rats that received 5 to 10 times the maximum human dose. Likewise, laboratory tests of the drug's cancer-causing potential have had mixed results.

Pregnancy. The drug has not caused birth defects in rats and rabbits receiving almost 50 times the maximum human dose. Rat offspring had impaired growth, however. The drug passes into maternal milk of rats at levels high enough to affect offspring; keep in mind, however, that these milk levels result from doses exceeding the maximum recommended for humans. In humans the drug passes into milk of nursing mothers; impact on the infants is unknown but is presumed to be harmless. At its peak the amount of zaleplon in milk is less than 0.02% (two one-hundredths of one percent) of the mother's dose, and that amount declines rapidly an hour after a mother takes zaleplon.

Additional information. Sonata tablets contain FD&C Yellow No. 5 (tartrazine), to which some persons seem allergic, particularly if they have an aspirin sensitivity.

Additional scientific information may be found in:

Chagan, L., and L.A. Cicero. "Zaleplon: Possible Advance in the Treatment of Insomnia." *P&T: A Peer-Reviewed Journal for Formulary Management* 24 (1999): 590.
Heydorn, W.E. "Zaleplon—A Review of a Novel Sedative Hypnotic Used in the Treatment of Insomnia." *Expert Opinion on Investigational Drugs* 9 (2000): 841–58.
Mangano, R.M. "Efficacy and Safety of Zaleplon at Peak Plasma Levels." *International Journal of Clinical Practice: Supplement* 79, no. 116 (2001): 9–13.
Rush, C.R., J.M. Frey, and R.R. Griffiths. "Zaleplon and Triazolam in Humans: Acute Behavioral Effects and Abuse Potential." *Psychopharmacology* 145 (1999): 39–51.
Troy, S., and M. Darwish. "Maximal Effects and Residual Effects: Zaleplon vs. Zolpidem and Triazolam." *American Society of Hospital Pharmacists Annual Meeting* 56 (June 1999): 59.
Troy, S., et al. "Comparison of the Effects of Zaleplon, Zolpidem, and Triazolam on Memory, Learning, and Psychomotor Performance." *Journal of Clinical Psychopharmacology* 20 (2000): 328–37.
"Zaleplon for Insomnia." *Medical Letter on Drugs and Therapeutics* 41 (1999): 93–94.

Zolpidem

Pronunciation: zohl-PIH-dem

Chemical Abstracts Service Registry Number: 82626-48-0. (Tartrate form 99294-93-6)

Formal Names: Ambien, Stilnoct, Stilnox

Type: Depressant. *See* page 19

Federal Schedule Listing: Schedule IV (DEA no. 2783)

USA Availability: Prescription

Pregnancy Category: B

Uses. Zolpidem became available for medical purposes in the United States during the 1990s, after already being used in Europe. The substance can be used to relax people shortly before they undergo surgery. Zolpidem promotes sleep and has both sedative and anticonvulsant properties. Generally insomnia patients are not supposed to take the drug for much more than a week. They are also not supposed to take the drug until they are ready for sleep; the substance is fast acting, and a person could doze off while in the middle of doing something. Elderly nursing home residents have been known to fall after taking zolpidem. People may forget things they do while under the drug's influence; a U.S. Army test found that the amnesia can be prevented if the drug flumazenil is taken soon enough after a zolpidem dose (flumazenil is used to counteract benzodiazepine depressants).

Scientific studies of zolpidem generally find no hangover drug effects, but people should be careful about what they do after waking up from a dose until they know they are functioning normally. No problem in that regard surfaced when the drug was tested on French military pilots and ground crews to determine if zolpidem could improve rest during prolonged military activity, nor did Swiss researchers find any reduction in performance if athletes used zolpidem to get a good night's sleep before a sporting competition. Not everyone, of course, has the same vigor as those populations. Experimenters running the French military test concluded that the drug is suitable for active military duty, and the substance also has U.S. Air Force approval for aircrew use.

The drug has been used to counteract jet lag, allowing travelers to compensate for changes in their sleep/wake cycles and to function effectively while crossing many time zones. During a simulation of such conditions for long-distance troop transport the U.S. Army found that zolpidem worked for promoting sleep but had no advantage over **triazolam**. Another U.S. Army experiment tested human performance during at least 38 hours of continual wakefulness, with ambiguous results about whether short naps induced by zolpidem would be useful in combat circumstances. French researchers found the drug to be useful for improving quality of sleep in low air pressures found at high altitude (4,000 meters or 13,123 feet) while producing no breathing difficulty, a finding relevant not only to mountaineers but to aviators and astronauts.

Many insomnia medicines produce a rebound effect, meaning that the insomnia comes back worse than ever for a few days after people stop taking the medication. Rebound is seldom observed with zolpidem, however. An experiment with the drug produced temporary improvement in Parkinson's disease symptoms, and zolpidem has helped clear up catatonia. A case report tells of the drug being given to treat anorexia nervosa, a condition in which thin people do not eat much because they imagine they are overweight, but results were unsatisfactory.

Animal experiments show that various chemicals related to zolpidem relieve pain, reduce inflammation and body temperature, and protect against gastric ulcers. Chemically these substances differ from barbiturates and benzodiazepines, but have effects similar to them and operate in some ways similar to benzodiazepines. Monkeys responded in ways indicating that zolpidem shares similarities with benzodiazepines but few or none with barbiturates. Despite those resemblances to benzodiazepines, rats trained to distinguish differences in drug effects acted as if zolpidem was unlike the benzodiazepine **chlordiazepoxide**. Various other differences have been documented. To take one example, **caffeine** typically counteracts some benzodiazepine actions, but counteraction does not necessarily happen when caffeine is administered with zolpidem. In animal experimentation chemicals related to zolpidem can produce sedation at doses low enough to avoid unwanted effects that occur with benzodiazepine sedation. Substances like zolpidem are generally believed to accomplish some of the same therapeutic actions as benzodiazepines, with less abuse potential.

Drawbacks. Caution is recommended if a depressed person takes zolpidem, as the drug can deepen despondency and even promote suicidal thinking. Less serious occasional unwanted effects include dry mouth, headache, hiccups, nausea, and diarrhea. Hallucinations and other psychotic reactions (ranging from delirium to euphoria) are even less common but documented nonetheless.

Abuse factors. Drug abusers report mental pleasure from zolpidem and say that higher doses feel similar to **diazepam**. Human experience indicates that tolerance does not occur with zolpidem, although two or three disputed case reports exist. Typically, animals who have been dosed with zolpidem for months show no tolerance, dependence, or withdrawal symptoms. Diligent experimenters, however, have been able to produce dependence and withdrawal in baboons. Those effects have seldom been observed in humans, but case reports exist. Someone took 30 to 40 times the normal daily medical dosage on his own accord for months and developed dependence. This person showed enough cross-tolerance with **clorazepate** dipotassium that this chemical could help control withdrawal symptoms caused by zolpidem dependence, indicating that zolpidem shares some characteristics with benzodiazepine class depressants. Other reports tell of zolpidem dependence developing in individuals who had a history of drug abuse. Two clinical studies giving the drug to persons for four weeks also produced dependence. Normally dependence is light enough to cause only mild discomfort upon stopping the drug, but withdrawal seizures are known among persons who have taken huge doses of zolpidem for months. However, zolpidem's abuse liability is low enough that the substance is believed to have special potential for treating ailments in persons prone to drug abuse.

Drug interactions. The antifungus drug ketoconazole lengthens and increases zolpidem effects. The tuberculosis drug rifampin shortens and decreases zolpidem effects.

Cancer. Standard laboratory tests have not indicated that zolpidem causes cancer. In studies using many times the recommended human dose, no evidence emerged of the drug causing cancer in mice. Rats receiving such high doses developed tumors with no more frequency than rats receiving no dose at all.

Pregnancy. Offspring from pregnant rats and rabbits receiving several times the maximum human therapeutic dosage showed no obvious birth defects, although there were indications of delayed fetal bone development. Standard advice for women is to be cautious about using zolpidem during pregnancy. Although tests have shown only minute quantities of zolpidem to pass into a mother's milk (less than 0.02% of a dose taken by a mother), the effect on infants is unknown.

Additional scientific information may be found in:

Boyle, J.A. "Look Again at Information on Zolpidem Tartrate." *American Journal of Hospital Pharmacy* 51 (1994): 1354, 1356–57.

Fleming, J., et al. "Comparison of the Residual Effects and Efficacy of Short Term Zolpidem, Flurazepam and Placebo in Patients with Chronic Insomnia." *Clinical Drug Investigation* 9 (1995): 303–13.

Hoehns, J.D., and P.J. Perry. "Zolpidem: Nonbenzodiazepine Hypnotic for Treatment of Insomnia." *Clinical Pharmacy* 12 (1993): 814–28.

Lobo, B.L., and W.L. Greene. "Zolpidem: Distinct from Triazolam?" *Annals of Pharmacotherapy* 31 (1997): 625–32.

Rush, C.R. "Behavioral Pharmacology of Zolpidem Relative to Benzodiazepines: A Review." *Pharmacology, Biochemistry, and Behavior* 61 (1998): 253–69.

Toner, L.C., et al. "Central Nervous System Side Effects Associated with Zolpidem Treatment." *Clinical Neuropharmacology* 23 (2000): 54–58.

"Zolpidem for Insomnia." *Medical Letter on Drugs and Therapeutics* 35 (1993): 35–36.

Sources for More Information

Many sources of drug information are available. Some of the more reliable ones are listed here. A good strategy is to consult sources that take differing stands on the subject. In addition to objective scientific authorities noted below, authorities approaching drug use from different slants are noted. Each advocacy group noted below offers scientific information, but each tends to emphasize findings supporting the group's stance. By consulting groups taking different stances a more complete picture of a specific topic can emerge.

Unlike books, the content of Internet Web sites may change, as may the addresses of those sites. Such transformations are inherent to the Internet and part of its strength, and users of the World Wide Web must deal with those changes. Many of these print and electronic sources refer users to additional sources for more information about covered topics, so the references below are excellent guides that can direct persons to paths of information going as deeply as anyone would want to go into a particular aspect of a particular drug.

Internet Web sites listed here can be accessed free of charge. Some sites are particularly valuable for tracking information published in scientific journals. Summaries of these articles are often available directly on a site, and if a person looks up the original article in a library, that article will likely provide references to still more sources of scientific information about a substance. Many discoveries are detailed in these journal articles. They are a primary source of scientific information.

PRINT SOURCES

AHFS Drug Information. Bethesda, MD: American Society of Health-System Pharmacists, various years. This frequently updated manual of the American Hospital

Formulary Service is a standard source of information used by heath care professionals seeking information about therapeutic drugs.

Brecher, E.M., and the Editors of Consumer Reports. *Licit and Illicit Drugs: The Consumers Union Report on Narcotics, Stimulants, Depressants, Inhalants, Hallucinogens, and Marijuana—Including Caffeine, Nicotine, and Alcohol.* Boston: Little, Brown, 1972. This classic volume remains unsurpassed for frank and accurate information about drugs of abuse.

Dollery, C., ed. *Therapeutic Drugs.* 2d ed. New York: Churchill Livingstone, 1999. The alphabetical format of listings make this source easy to use, and it also contains references to scientific studies.

Goodman, L.S., and A. Gilman. *The Pharmacological Basis of Therapeutics.* 10th ed. New York: McGraw-Hill, 2001. Often referred to as "Goodman & Gilman," this reference work has gone through many editions as decades have passed, demonstrating its continued usefulness for key information about therapeutic drugs. Earlier editions remain well worth consulting.

Lewis, W.H., and M.P.F. Elvin-Lewis. *Medical Botany: Plants Affecting Man's Health.* New York: John Wiley and Sons, 1977. This is a reputable source of information about natural products having drug actions.

Martindale: The Extra Pharmacopoeia. 31st ed. London: Pharmaceutical Press, 1996. Health care givers around the world rely on this standard reference book containing information about therapeutic drugs. As with many multi-edition reference works, earlier editions can be useful.

McGuffin, M., ed. *American Herbal Products Association's Botanical Safety Handbook.* Boca Raton, FL: CRC Press, 1997. This book provides cautions about natural products.

Millspaugh, C.F. *American Medicinal Plants.* Philadelphia: John C. Yorston & Company, 1892. Reprint, New York: Dover Publications, 1974. This classic guide is of historical interest, showing how natural products were once used.

Morton, J.F. *Major Medicinal Plants: Botany, Culture and Uses.* Springfield, IL: Charles C. Thomas, 1977. This volume is a reliable source of information.

Mosby's GenRx: A Comprehensive Reference for Generic and Brand Prescription Drugs. St. Louis, MO: Mosby, various years. This reference book is frequently updated. Its alphabetical format makes it easy to use. The title has slightly changed from earlier editions.

PDR for Herbal Medicines. 2d ed. Montvale, NJ: Medical Economics Company, 2000. This authoritative book does for herbal products what the *Physicians' Desk Reference* does for prescription drugs. Hundreds of herbal preparations are described.

Physicians' Desk Reference. Montvale, NJ: Medical Economics Company. Often called simply *PDR*, this reference source describes thousands of legal drugs, with the descriptions containing information approved by the U.S. Food and Drug Administration, making this volume one of the most authoritative and widely used books on the topic. The printed version is updated annually, and a CD-ROM version is updated more often.

Weiner, Michael A. *Weiner's Herbal.* New York: Stein and Day, 1980. This is a reliable source of information about natural products that contain drugs.

INTERNET SOURCES

Building Better Health
http://www.buildingbetterhealth.com/drugindex/a

This excellent source of therapeutic drug information is sponsored by a health services and products company.

Bureau of Justice Statistics
810 Seventh Street, NW
Washington, DC 20531
(202) 307-0765
http://www.ojp.usdoj.gov/bjs/drugs.htm
This agency of the U.S. Department of Justice provides a wide variety of current and historical statistics about illegal usage of drugs and about many other crime-related issues. The Internet Web site includes links to statistical information at other sites.

Centers for Disease Control and Prevention
1600 Clifton Road
Atlanta, GA 30333
(404) 639-3534
(800) 311-3435
http://www.cdc.gov/tobacco/issue.htm
Although this federal agency's site has relatively little about drugs in general, this Internet address is useful for data about tobacco.

ChemIDplus
http://chem.sis.nlm.nih.gov/chemidplus
This service of the National Library of Medicine allows persons to obtain brief descriptions of drugs, including Chemical Abstracts Service Registry Numbers, molecular formulas, and alternate names for substances. The CAS numbers can be particularly valuable, not only for confirming identity of a drug but for getting more information from other databases.

Code of Federal Regulations
http://www.access.gpo.gov/nara/
At this address a person can access the Code of Federal Regulations (CFR), among other items. The official federal schedules of controlled substances can be found in the CFR under Title 21, part 1308. A drug's schedule status can change, and the CFR can be used to confirm a drug's current status. Another official source is the United States Code (see below).

Drug Abuse Warning Network (DAWN)
http://www.samhsa.gov/oas/dawn.htm
DAWN is an important information system supervised by the Office of Applied Studies in a federal agency called the Substance Abuse and Mental Health Services Administration (see below). DAWN produces reports concerning statistics it gathers about drug-related injuries and deaths. Those numbers do not necessarily reveal whether drug-*related* incidents are drug *caused* but are useful for tracking trends in popularity of various drugs.

Drug Enforcement Administration
Information Services Section (CPI)
2401 Jefferson Davis Highway
Alexandria, VA 22301
http://www.usdoj.gov/dea/
In addition to information about law enforcement efforts, in links to "Drugs of Concern" and "Drugs of Abuse" the DEA's Web site provides official information about individual substances. Another link leads to assorted statistics.

Drug Enforcement Administration Diversion Control Program
http://www.deadiversion.usdoj.gov/schedules/
This web site has lists of schedules and also statistics on amounts of various drugs legally manufactured in various years. The home page of Diversion Control Program has links to the Code of Federal Regulations. The schedules index page has a link to a list of controlled substances scheduling actions, giving a brief chronology showing when various drugs were put into various schedules.

Drug Policy Alliance
925 9th Avenue
New York, NY 10019
(212) 548-0695
925 15th Street NW
Washington, DC 20005
(202) 216-0035
http://www.drugpolicy.org
This organization encourages drug control through means other than harsh criminal sanctions, and the organization questions many standard government policies. Through this Web site a person can obtain information about specific drugs, submit questions, and link to other drug information sources. The organization has offices in more than one city.

Drugs.com
http://www.drugs.com/
This Web site is run by Drugsite Trust, described on the site as "a not for profit trust dedicated to providing free, unbiased information on over the counter (OTC) and prescription medicines." Information includes technical monographs.

E-Doc
http://www.edoc.co.za/medilink/actives/
This index of therapeutic drugs originates in South Africa and includes information about drug varieties having no medical use in the United States.

Erowid
http://www.erowid.org/index.shtml
This site contains a vast amount of information about drugs of abuse, along with links to still more sources. Site visitors can submit questions. The sponsoring organization believes that current government drug control policy is misguided. Although the site contains comments from persons who advocate recreational drug use, the site also contains stories from persons who suffered catastrophic consequences from such use. Used judiciously, the site can produce substantial quantities of solid data.

Food and Drug Administration
5600 Fishers Lane
Rockville, MD 20857-0001
(888) 463-6332
http://www.fda.gov/
The home page of this prestigious and respected source of scientific drug information gives a visitor various choices for obtaining information, including a search function that scans enormous numbers of government documents, and offers selections relevant to a person's inquiry.

Gateway
http://gateway.nlm.nih.gov/gw/Cmd

This is one of several Web sites from the National Library of Medicine. Through Gateway visitors can search various scientific databases for information about drugs.

Google
http://www.google.com/
If any Web site deserves the adjective "awesome," Google is it. In a few seconds Google can search hundreds of millions of Web sites to find information about a topic. The quality of information may vary greatly, as Google will locate not only sites of great scientific institutions but personal Web sites of persons who are long on ranting and short on knowledge. If, however, an Internet user is at a loss on where to find information about a topic or is merely curious about the variety of data available, Google may well provide a jumpstart.

HerbMed
http://herbmed.org
Many natural product descriptions can be found at this site. The organization is friendly to using herbs for medical purposes.

Lycaeum
http://leda.lycaeum.org/quickindex.shtml
This address leads a person to an index of information about many drugs of abuse. The sponsoring organization favors fewer legal restrictions on drug use, but for that very reason a person can find information about nonmedical substances that are ignored in sources devoted strictly to describing therapeutic pharmaceuticals.

Multidisciplinary Association for Psychedelic Studies (MAPS)
http://www.maps.org/
This advocacy organization seeks data that will allow various prohibited drugs to become accepted. Links on the page provide access to such information.

National Institute on Drug Abuse
6001 Executive Boulevard, Room 5213
Bethesda, MD 20892-9651
(301) 443-1124
http://www.drugabuse.gov/
NIDA is a U.S. government agency that sponsors many scientific studies. Much of that information is accessible through this Web site. Statistics may be found here.

National Library of Medicine
http://www.nlm.nih.gov/
This site can be used to obtain vast amounts of scientific information about drugs.

Novartis
http://www.healthandage.com/Home/gm=3
The drug database page of Novartis Foundation for Gerontology is at this address.

Office of National Drug Control Policy
Drug Policy Information Clearinghouse
P.O. Box 6000
Rockville, MD 20849-6000
(800) 666-3332
http://www.whitehousedrugpolicy.gov/
The so-called Drug Czar heads this agency. Its Web site can lead users to information about drugs and about many facets of drug control policy.

Partnership for Responsible Drug Information
14 West 68th Street
New York, NY 10023
(212) 362-1964
http://www.prdi.org/
Partnership for Responsible Drug Information (PRDI) is an organization that strives to present drug information from experts who disagree with some government drug control policies. Many links to still more sources can be found at: http://www.prdi.org/drugindx.html

PubMed
http://www.ncbi.nlm.nih.gov/entrez/query.fcgi
PubMed is another service from the National Library of Medicine. PubMed includes Medline, one of medicine's first electronic databases, which can direct a person to science journal articles about many drugs. Typically PubMed allows users to see summaries of those articles.

RxList
http://www.rxlist.com/
This index of information about therapeutic drugs is sponsored by a company selling various health-related products.

Schaffer Library of Drug Policy
http://www.druglibrary.org/schaffer/
This information resource includes electronic versions of classic reports about drugs, along with large quantities of recent information. The home page of DRCNet Online Library of Drug Policy at http:/www.druglibrary.org/ contains links to still more sources. "DRC" is the Drug Reform Coordination Network, which is an activist group opposing government drug policies.

Substance Abuse and Mental Health Services Administration (SAMHSA)
5600 Fishers Lane
Rockville, MD 20857
Office of Communications (OC)
(301) 443-8956
http://www.drugabusestatistics.samhsa.gov/
SAMHSA is a federal government agency. Many statistics and other types of drug information are available at this site. An important part of this site is the Office of Applied Studies, which offers many reports. The Drug Abuse Warning Network (see above) is part of the Office of Applied Studies.

Tobacco BBS (Electronic Bulletin Board System)
P.O. Box 359
Village Station
New York, NY 10014-0359
(212) 982-4645
http://www.tobacco.org/
This massive collection of information specializes in tobacco and is sponsored by an organization concerned about health problems caused by smoking.

Toxnet
http://toxnet.nlm.nih.gov/
This database is another service of the National Library of Medicine, providing information from science journals. From this page a person can access Toxline, ChemIDPlus, PubMed, and other information services.

United States Code
http://www4.law.cornell.edu/uscode/
The U.S. Code (USC) is an official collection of all federal laws currently in effect. These include the schedule status of controlled substances found in Title 21, chapter 13, section 812. Like the Code of Federal Regulations (see above), USC is an authoritative source for substances' schedule status.

Drug Name Index

Pages in **bold** indicate the location of the main entry

Subject Index

About the Author

RICHARD LAWRENCE MILLER is an independent scholar. He has written many books including *The Case for Legalizing Drugs* (1991) and *Drug Warriors and Their Prey: From Police Power to Police State* (1996).

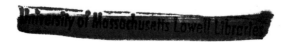